Handbook of Drug Design, Delivery and Therapy

Handbook of Drug Design, Delivery and Therapy

Edited by **Abby Calvin**

SYRAWOOD
PUBLISHING HOUSE

New York

Published by Syrawood Publishing House,
750 Third Avenue, 9th Floor,
New York, NY 10017, USA
www.syrawoodpublishinghouse.com

Handbook of Drug Design, Delivery and Therapy
Edited by Abby Calvin

International Standard Book Number: 978-1-68286-193-6 (Hardback)

The publisher's policy is to use permanent paper from mills that operate a sustainable forestry policy. Furthermore, the publisher ensures that the text paper and cover boards used have met acceptable environmental accreditation standards.

Trademark Notice: Registered trademark of products or corporate names are used only for explanation and identification without intent to infringe.

Printed in the United States of America.

Contents

Preface

Medical science is constantly progressing. Curing diseases is a primary focus of current research in this field. Thus, the field of drug design and delivery is also rapidly advancing. This book includes some of the vital pieces of work being conducted across the world, on various topics related to drug design, delivery and therapy, such as drug targets, antipsychotic drugs, pharmacogenetics, pharmacokinetics, etc. Different approaches, evaluations, methodologies and advanced studies on drug design and delivery as well as drug therapy have been included in this book. It aims to serve as a resource guide for students and experts alike and contribute to the growth of pharmaceutical sciences.

The information shared in this book is based on empirical researches made by veterans in this field of study. The elaborative information provided in this book will help the readers further their scope of knowledge leading to advancements in this field.

Finally, I would like to thank my fellow researchers who gave constructive feedback and my family members who supported me at every step of my research.

Editor

Use, tolerability and compliance of spironolactone in the treatment of heart failure

Jean Lachaine[1*], Catherine Beauchemin[1] and Elodie Ramos[2]

Abstract

Background: Risk of morbidity and mortality in patients with severe heart failure (HF) is reduced by blockade of aldosterone receptors with spironolactone. However, benefits of spironolactone are potentially limited by treatment compliance and adverse events profile. The aim of this study was to estimate use of spironolactone by patients with HF, incidence of key adverse events, and patient compliance.

Methods: This study was performed using data from the Quebec provincial medical and drug plans (*Régie de l'Assurance Maladie du Québec*, RAMQ) for patients who had a diagnosis of HF. Relative incidence of gynecomastia and hyperkalemia was estimated for users and non-users of spironolactone. Treatment adherence was estimated for users of spironolactone and compared to adherence with angiotensin converting enzyme (ACE) inhibitors, beta-blockers (β-blockers), and angiotensin receptor blockers (ARBs).

Results: RAMQ data were obtained for a total of 82,018 patients with a diagnosis of HF. Of these patients, 59.9% used an ACE inhibitor, 59.5% used a beta-blocker, 28.4% used an ARB, and 15.1% (n = 12,344) used spironolactone. Despite underestimation due to limitation of the database, the documented incidence of hyperkalemia (3.3% versus 1.4%) and gynecomastia (1.8% versus 0.7%) was significantly higher in spironolactone users than non-users (p < 0.001). Treatment compliance was significantly lower with spironolactone compared to ACE inhibitors, β-blockers, and ARBs (45.6% versus 56.1%, 59.7%, and 57.0%, respectively; p < 0.001). Persistence to treatment over a one-year period was also lower with spironolactone compared to ACE inhibitors, β-blockers, and ARBs (50.7% versus 64.5%, 70.4%, and 66.3%, respectively; p < 0.001).

Conclusion: Use of spironolactone is associated with an incidence of adverse events, which may have an impact on treatment compliance.

Background

Heart failure (HF) is a chronic condition defined as the inability of the heart to maintain a sufficient pumping activity to meet the body's metabolic demands under normal filling pressure [1]. It is usually characterized by breathlessness (including orthopnea and dyspnea), effort intolerance, swelling of the legs, and fluid retention [2]. In Canada, HF affects over 500,000 individuals, with approximately 50,000 incident cases diagnosed yearly [3]. A retrospective Canadian study comprising 72 patients who had two or more visits to a heart failure clinic revealed that 71% and 21% of subjects were having a severe HF (NYHA class III and IV respectively, with a mean ejection fraction of 31%) [4]. HF is associated with a substantial clinical and

economical burden. In Canada, more than 54,330 patients were hospitalized for HF between 2005 and 2006. Moreover, 4,430 Canadians with HF died in 2004, representing 2% of all deaths [5]. The average cost incurred by HF patients during their last six months of life was $27,983 in Canadian dollars in 2006 [6].

Aldosterone, a steroid hormone known to enhance sodium retention and potassium secretion, plays a major role in the pathophysiology of heart failure (HF). According to the results of the Randomized Aldactone Evaluation Study (RALES), the use of spironolactone, a competitive aldosterone antagonist, an angiotensin converting enzyme (ACE) inhibitor, a loop diuretic, and in most cases digoxin, significantly reduces the risk of mortality and morbidity in patients with severe HF (NYHA class III-IV, LVEF ≤35%) [7]. Results of this randomized trial suggested that adding spironolactone to standard treatment for severe HF

* Correspondence: jean.lachaine@umontreal.ca
[1]Faculty of Pharmacy, University of Montreal, Montreal, Quebec, Canada
Full list of author information is available at the end of the article

reduces death rates (all causes and cardiac causes) and hospitalization rates due to cardiac conditions. In fact, plasma aldosterone concentrations in HF patients may reach 20 times the normal level, because of both increased aldosterone production and decreased rate of hepatic clearance [8]. Thus, ACE inhibitors are not sufficient to suppress the production of aldosterone in HF patients, hence the importance of adding an aldosterone antagonist, such as spironolactone, to severe HF therapy [9].

However, spironolactone is associated with serious adverse events, including hyperkalemia and gynecomastia [10,11]. Consequently, clinical benefits related to the use of spironolactone are potentially limited by the adverse events profile, which may lead to premature treatment cessation and poor treatment adherence.

The purpose of this study was to estimate, in real clinical practice, the utilization rate of spironolactone in patients with HF, the incidence of key adverse events (hyperkalemia and gynecomastia), and patient adherence to spironolactone in terms of compliance and persistence.

Methods

This study was performed using data from the database of the Quebec provincial health plans (*Régie de l'Assurance Maladie du Québec*, RAMQ). Like other Canadian provinces, Quebec has a universal health care program that covers physician services and hospitalization for the entire population. This universal health program is complemented, for a large proportion of the population, by a public drug plan. The provincial drug reimbursement program covers all people aged 65 and over, beneficiaries of the social assistance program, and individuals who do not have access to a private medication insurance plan. As opposed to the health care plan, for which all costs are covered, the drug plan involves limited financial participation on the part of the beneficiaries. More than 40% of Quebec's population is covered by the drug program [12].

The RAMQ medical services database contains information from physicians' claims for services provided within and outside the hospital. The RAMQ pharmaceutical services database includes information from pharmacists' claims for dispensed medications reimbursed by the program, but not for medications received in a hospital. In addition, data obtained from the RAMQ include an encrypted patient identifier, which enables linkage of individual patient information while preserving anonymity. Because patient data used in this study were anonymous, ethical approval was not required for data analyses.

Data on medical and pharmaceutical services from January 2000 to September 2008 were obtained from the RAMQ for patients who had a diagnosis of HF (*The International Classification of Diseases, Ninth Revision*: ICD-9 codes: 4280 - 4289) [13] during that period.

Patient characteristics were described in terms of gender, age, and comorbidities. Comorbidity level was estimated by calculating a chronic disease score, based on the Von Korff score, and updated to account for the medications introduced since its initial development [14]. Occurrences of selected medications use during the study period were used to calculate the chronic disease score. Use of spironolactone, ACE inhibitors, beta-blockers (β-blockers), and angiotensin receptor blockers (ARBs) was also estimated. In addition, use of spironolactone with an ACE inhibitor, an ARB, or a β-blocker was defined as concomitant when the usage overlap period for the two medications was at least 60 days.

Relative incidence of adverse events associated with the use of spironolactone, such as gynecomastia or mastopathy (ICD-9 codes: 6110 - 6119) and hyperkalemia (ICD-9 code: 2767) [13], was estimated by the occurrence of the corresponding ICD-9 codes found in the medical services data for users and non-users of spironolactone.

Treatment adherence was estimated for initial users of standard therapy (ACE inhibitors, ARBs, or β-blockers) or spironolactone. Patients were considered new users if the first script for one of these treatments had not been preceded by any other script for the same treatment in the 12 previous months. In this analysis, treatment adherence comprises two specific dimensions: compliance to treatment and persistence to treatment. Compliance refers to the consistency and accuracy with which the patient follows the recommended treatment regimen, while persistence represents the long-term continuation of treatment.

For each study subject, treatment compliance was estimated by calculating the ratio of effective treatment duration over expected treatment duration. Effective treatment duration was estimated by the quantity of medication received and the corresponding number of days of treatment. Treatment compliance was estimated over a one-year period. Patients were considered compliant if their compliance ratio was equal to or greater than 80%. In a complementary analysis, patients were considered compliant if their compliance ratio was equal to or greater than 50%.

Treatment persistence was estimated over a 3-, 6-, and 12-month period. Patients were considered persistent for as long as the treatment (spironolactone, ACE inhibitors, ARBs, or β-blockers) had not definitively ceased. Treatment cessation was determined when the patients had not received treatment for at least six months.

Differences in incidence of adverse events in spironolactone users and non users were tested for significance using Pearson's chi square test. This statistical test was also performed to compare treatment compliance and persistence with spironolactone and standard therapy (ACE inhibitors, ARBs, β-blockers).

Results

During the period from January 1, 2000 to September 30, 2008, a total of 238,721 patients had received at least one diagnosis of HF. In accordance with the RAMQ's restrictions on the number of subjects available for analysis by external parties, data were obtained on a random sample of 82,018 of these patients. Of this sample, 15.1% (n = 12,344) used spironolactone. There was a higher proportion of men among spironolactone users, as opposed to the overall HF group, where the proportion of women was higher. In addition, comorbidity level, estimated by the modified Von Korff score, was higher for patients using spironolactone. A large proportion of spironolactone users received concomitant treatment with ACE inhibitors and β-blockers, and to a lesser extent with ARBs (Table 1).

Incidence of hyperkalemia, breast complications in men, and more specifically gynecomastia, was significantly higher in spironolactone users than in non-users (Table 2).

Over a one-year period, treatment compliance was significantly lower with spironolactone compared to ACE inhibitors, β-blockers, and ARBs, according to both 80%

Table 1 Patient characteristics

	CHF n = 82 018	CHF using spironolactone n = 12,344
Age group		
<20	518 (0.6%)	11 (0.1%)
20-39	1,366 (1.7%)	62 (0.5%)
40-59	6,114 (7.5%)	716 (5.8%)
60-79	31,499 (38.4%)	5,093 (41.3%)
80+	42,521 (51.8%)	6,462 (52.3%)
Average age (SD)	77.2 (14.1)	78.5 (11.4)
Gender		
- male	39,132 (47.7%)	6,368 (51.6%)
- Female	42,886 (52.3%)	5,976 (48.4%)
Average Von Korff score (SD)	7.6 (3.4)	8.8 (2.9)
Selected drug use		
- ACE	49,140 (59.9%)	9,493 (76.9%)
- ARB	23,326 (28.4%)	4,455 (36.1%)
- β-blocker	48,772 (59.5%)	9,260 (75.0%)
Concomitant use with		
- ACE		6,702 (54.3%)
- ARB		2,654 (21.5%)
- β-blocker		7,217 (58.5%)

Table 2 Incidence of adverse events

	Spironolactone users	Spironolactone non-users
Hyperkalemia	408/12,344 (3.3%)	955/69,674 (1.4%)*
Breast complications in men	158/6,368 (2.5%)	380/32,764 (1.2%)*
Breast hypertrophy in men (gynecomastia)	117/6,368 (1.8%)	233/32,764 (0.7%)*

* $p < 0.001$ (Pearson's chi square test).

and 50% thresholds (Table 3). Moreover, persistence to treatment after 3-, 6-, and 12-month periods was also lower with spironolactone compared to ACE inhibitors, β-blockers, and ARBs (Table 4).

Diagnosis of HF was received after a diagnosis of acute myocardial infarction (AMI) for 9,288 (11.3%) of the HF patients. Of these HF post-AMI patients, 1,016 (10.9%) used spironolactone after the diagnosis was received, while only 686 (7.4%) patients used spironolactone in the first year following the diagnosis. Of the HF post-AMI patients, 45.4% were compliant over a one-year period, based on the 80% threshold, and 47.6% showed persistence to treatment after a 12-month period.

Discussion

Although spironolactone has proven beneficial for patients with HF, only a small proportion of HF patients in this study (15.1%) used this medication. As previously reported [7], this study found that spironolactone use was associated with higher incidence of adverse events, including hyperkalemia and gynecomastia. Treatment adherence was less than optimal for all medications considered in this analysis, particularly for spironolactone. In fact, both compliance and persistence with spironolactone were significantly lower compared to standard therapies (ACE inhibitors, β-blockers, or ARBs). Similarly, treatment persistence related to spironolactone was found to be a major issue in the study by Bouvy and al., where 40.8% and 58.8% of patients discontinued treatment after 6 months and 7 years, respectively [10].

Table 3 Treatment compliance

	Compliance	
	50%	80%
ACE	66.4%	56.1%
ARB	68.1%	57.0%
β-blockers	71.1%	59.7%
Spironolactone	58.4%*	45.6%*

* Spironolactone versus ACE, ARB and β-blockers: $p < 0.001$ (Pearson's chi square test)

Table 4 Treatment persistence

	Persistence		
	3 months	6 months	12 months
ACE	83.6%	75.3%	64.5%
ARB	84.8%	77.5%	66.3%
β-blockers	86.3%	80.0%	70.4%
Spironolactone	76.3%*	65.3%*	50.7%*

* Spironolactone versus ACE, ARB and β-blockers: p < 0.001 (Pearson's chi square test)

As this study used data from an administrative database, it enabled the inclusion of a very large number of subjects who are assumed to accurately represent a real-world clinical setting, contrary to a clinical trial with a small sample size and controlled clinical environment. However, as in other studies based on administrative databases, there are some inherent limitations. It is assumed that the reimbursed medications retrieved from the databases were taken by the patient, although this may not always be the case. This could result in overestimation of treatment adherence. Moreover, medications received while hospitalized and medications that were not reimbursed by the drug plan were not taken into account.

Another limitation of this study is related to the use of ICD-9 codes to identify patients with HF as well as occurrence of hyperkalemia and breast complications. In Quebec, physicians are not required to record an ICD-9 code when meeting their patients, although the vast majority of them do. In addition, because only a single ICD-9 code can be recorded on the form for each claim submitted to the RAMQ for reimbursement of a medical service, the prevalence of a specific diagnosis can be underestimated when patients present more than one medical condition. For example, the diagnosis of gynecomastia in HF patients may not be captured when a diagnosis of HF was first reported. In fact, the incidence of gynecomastia in spironolactone users in the present study (1.8%) was much lower than that reported in the RALES study (9.0%) [7]. As opposed to data from clinical studies, the severity of adverse events is unknown in studies based on claims data. For example, cases of serious hyperkalemia (>6 mmol/L) were reported in the RALES study, whereas only the overall incidence of hyperkalemia could be estimated in the present study [7]. Moreover, studies conducted by the RALES investigators found that hyperkalemia was a dose-dependent effect of spironolactone, as well as gynecomastia, and required monitoring of the patient [7,15]. This monitoring, which includes serum creatinine and potassium measurements, must have been reinforced in the present study population, as most patients were older than 60 and were susceptible to take concomitant medications and therefore, to require a spironolactone dose adjustment. For example, non-steroidal anti-inflammatory drugs (NSAIDs) prescribed in rheumatoid arthritis and in other immune diseases may exacerbate hyperkalemia when used with potassium sparing diuretics such as spironolactone [16,17]. However, these monitoring measurements are not available in RAMQ data. As the purpose of the present study was to assess the global incidence of gynecomastia and hyperkalemia, treatment regimen has not been considered. Further studies are needed to evaluate the impact of the treatment regimen on the incidence of these side effects in Canadian real-life setting. Furthermore, although digitalis, diuretics and nitrates are also used in severe HF, they have not been considered in the present study. However, as there is ample evidence supporting the use of β-blockers, ACE-I and/or ARB in patients with heart failure, which include current guidelines [18-20], results of this analysis could give a good estimate of spironolactone use in a real-life context despite study limitations.

Conclusion
The analysis results suggest that the use of spironolactone is associated with an incidence of adverse events, which may have an impact on treatment compliance.

Acknowledgements
This study was financially supported by Pfizer Canada Inc.

Author details
[1]Faculty of Pharmacy, University of Montreal, Montreal, Quebec, Canada. [2]Health Economics and Outcomes Research, Pfizer Canada Inc., Kirkland, Quebec, Canada.

Authors' contributions
JL and CB designed the study, acquired, analyzed and interpreted the data, and drafted the article. ER revised the manuscript for important intellectual content. All authors read and approved the final manuscript.

Competing interests
At the time of the manuscript was prepared, Elodie Ramos was an employee of Pfizer Canada Inc. Jean Lachaine and Catherine Beauchemin had no competing interests.

References
1. McKelvie R: Heart Failure. Clinical Evidence. *Electronic source* 2009 [http://www.clinicalevidence.bmj.com], Access date: 2011-04-21.
2. Arnold JM, Liu P, Demers C, Dorian P, Giannetti N, Haddad H, Heckman GA, Howlett JG, Ignaszewski A, Johnstone DE, Jong P, McKelvie RS, Moe GW, Parker JD, Rao V, Ross HJ, Sequeira EJ, Svendsen AM, Teo K, Tsuyuki RT, White M: Canadian Cardiovascular Society consensus conference recommendations on heart failure 2006: diagnosis and management. *Can J Cardiol* 2006, **22(1)**:23-45.
3. Ross H, Howlett J, Arnold JM, Liu P, O'Neill BJ, Brophy JM, Simpson CS, Sholdice MM, Knudtson M, Ross DB, Rottger J, Glasgow K: Treating the right patient at the right time: access to heart failure care. *Can J Cardiol* 2006, **22(9)**:749-754.
4. Martineau P, Frenette M, Blais L, Sauve C: Multidisciplinary outpatient congestive heart failure clinic: impact on hospital admissions and emergency room visits. *Can J Cardiol* 2004, **20(12)**:1205-1211.

5. Public Health Agency of Canada: **Tracking Heart Disease and Stroke in Canada.** Ottawa; 2009.
6. Kaul P, McAlister FA, Ezekowitz JA, Bakal JA, Curtis LH, Quan H, Knudtson ML, Armstrong PW: **Resource use in the last 6 months of life among patients with heart failure in Canada.** *Arch Intern Med* 2011, **171(3)**:211-217.
7. Pitt B, Zannad F, Remme WJ, Cody R, Castaigne A, Perez A, Palensky J, Wittes J: **The effect of spironolactone on morbidity and mortality in patients with severe heart failure. Randomized Aldactone Evaluation Study Investigators.** *N Engl J Med* 1999, **341(10)**:709-717.
8. Struthers AD: **Impact of aldosterone on vascular pathophysiology.** *Congest Heart Fail* 2002, **8(1)**:18-22.
9. Weber KT: **Aldosterone and spironolactone in heart failure.** *N Engl J Med* 1999, **341(10)**:753-755.
10. Bouvy ML, Heerdink ER, Herings RM: **Long-term therapy with spironolactone.** *Pharm World Sci* 2001, **23(4)**:132-134.
11. Wrenger E, Muller R, Moesenthin M, Welte T, Frolich JC, Neumann KH: **Interaction of spironolactone with ACE inhibitors or angiotensin receptor blockers: analysis of 44 cases.** *BMJ* 2003, **327(7407)**:147-149.
12. Gearry RB, Richardson AK, Frampton CM, Dodgshun AJ, Barclay ML: **Population-based cases control study of inflammatory bowel disease risk factors.** *J Gastroenterol Hepatol* 2010, **25(2)**:325-333.
13. Nikolaus S, Schreiber S: **Diagnostics of inflammatory bowel disease.** *Gastroenterology* 2007, **133(5)**:1670-1689.
14. Von Korff M, Wagner EH, Saunders K: **A chronic disease score from automated pharmacy data.** *J Clin Epidemiol* 1992, **45(2)**:197-203.
15. **Effectiveness of spironolactone added to an angiotensin-converting enzyme inhibitor and a loop diuretic for severe chronic congestive heart failure (the Randomized Aldactone Evaluation Study [RALES]).** *Am J Cardiol* 1996, **78(8)**:902-907.
16. Hay E, Derazon H, Bukish N, Katz L, Kruglyakov I, Armoni M: **Fatal hyperkalemia related to combined therapy with a COX-2 inhibitor, ACE inhibitor and potassium rich diet.** *J Emerg Med* 2002, **22(4)**:349-352.
17. Webster J: **Interactions of NSAIDs with diuretics and beta-blockers mechanisms and clinical implications.** *Drugs* 1985, **30(1)**:32-41.
18. Krum H, Jelinek MV, Stewart S, Sindone A, Atherton JJ, Hawkes AL: **Guidelines for the prevention, detection and management of people with chronic heart failure in Australia 2006.** *Med J Aust* 2006, **185(10)**:549-557.
19. Poole-Wilson PA: **The Cardiac Insufficiency Bisoprolol Study II.** *Lancet* 1999, **353(9161)**:1360-1361.
20. **Effect of enalapril on survival in patients with reduced left ventricular ejection fractions and congestive heart failure. The SOLVD Investigators.** *N Engl J Med* 1991, **325(5)**:293-302.

3-D DNA methylation phenotypes correlate with cytotoxicity levels in prostate and liver cancer cell models

Arkadiusz Gertych[1,3], Jin Ho Oh[1,2], Kolja A Wawrowsky[1,4], Daniel J Weisenberger[5] and Jian Tajbakhsh[1,2]*

Abstract

Background: The spatial organization of the genome is being evaluated as a novel indicator of toxicity in conjunction with drug-induced global DNA hypomethylation and concurrent chromatin reorganization. 3D quantitative DNA methylation imaging (3D-qDMI) was applied as a cell-by-cell high-throughput approach to investigate this matter by assessing genome topology through represented immunofluorescent nuclear distribution patterns of 5-methylcytosine (MeC) and global DNA (4,6-diamidino-2-phenylindole = DAPI) in labeled nuclei.

Methods: Differential progression of global DNA hypomethylation was studied by comparatively dosing zebularine (ZEB) and 5-azacytidine (AZA). Treated and untreated (control) human prostate and liver cancer cells were subjected to confocal scanning microscopy and dedicated 3D image analysis for the following features: differential nuclear MeC/DAPI load and codistribution patterns, cell similarity based on these patterns, and corresponding differences in the topology of low-intensity MeC (LIM) and low in intensity DAPI (LID) sites.

Results: Both agents generated a high fraction of similar MeC phenotypes across applied concentrations. ZEB exerted similar effects at 10–100-fold higher drug concentrations than its AZA analogue: concentration-dependent progression of global cytosine demethylation, validated by measuring differential MeC levels in repeat sequences using MethyLight, and the concurrent increase in nuclear LIM densities correlated with cellular growth reduction and cytotoxicity.

Conclusions: 3D-qDMI demonstrated the capability of quantitating dose-dependent drug-induced spatial progression of DNA demethylation in cell nuclei, independent from interphase cell-cycle stages and in conjunction with cytotoxicity. The results support the notion of DNA methylation topology being considered as a potential indicator of causal impacts on chromatin distribution with a conceivable application in epigenetic drug toxicology.

Keywords: DNA methylation phenotype, Chromatin distribution, High-throughput cell assay, 3D image analysis, MethyLight, Repetitive element, Epigenetic drug

Background

DNA methylation is a crucial epigenetic modification of the human genome beyond the DNA sequence level that is involved in regulating many cellular processes [1]. Cancer cells frequently exhibit abnormally high levels of DNA methylation in gene-specific CpG-rich promoter regions [2-5]. Furthermore, DNA methylation also occurs at non-CpG islands within the major part of the genome known as heterochromatin [6,7], which plays a key role in nuclear architecture and genome stability [8-10]. It is now clear that DNA hypomethylation in human cancer is also very frequent and affects more cytosine residues than does DNA hypermethylation, accounting for a net loss of 5-methylcytosine (global DNA hypomethylation), as observed in many cancers [11-14]. The reversible nature of epigenetic imbalances in various types of cancers constitutes an attractive therapeutic target. The goal of epigenetic therapy in cancer is the reprogramming of aberrant cells towards normal phenotypes. In this regard,

* Correspondence: tajbakhshj@cshs.org
[1]Translational Cytomics Group, Department of Surgery, Cedars-Sinai Medical Center, Los Angeles, CA 90048, USA
[2]Chromatin Biology Laboratory, Department of Surgery, Cedars-Sinai Medical Center, Los Angeles, CA 90048, USA
Full list of author information is available at the end of the article

the drug discovery field has so far been mostly focusing on screening the effect of candidate agents on the levels of molecular cell signaling and metabolism. However, in recent years of the post-genomic era, chromatin conformation and the higher–order genome organization, which set the framework for the global orchestration as well the locus-specific regulation of gene expression in the human cell nucleus [15-18], are gaining more attention in therapy; the reason being that these functional structures can become affected as a consequence of epigenetic interference by chromatin-modifying agents such as inhibitors of DNA methylation [19].

Catalytic DNA methyltransferase (DNMT) inhibitors have been so far categorized into two classes: nucleoside analogues and non-nucleoside analogues [20]. The two nucleoside analogues, 5-azacytidine (AZA, Vidaza™) and 5-aza-2′-deoxycytidine (decitabine, Dacogen™) are the most advanced in their category, having received US Federal Drug Agency (FDA) approval for their use in treating myelodysplastic syndrome (MDS) and hematopoietic malignancies [21,22]. Zebularine (ZEB) or 1-β-D-ribofuranosyl-2(1H)-pyrimidone has recently emerged as a new DNMT inhibitor (DNMTi), with properties that makes it a potential drug candidate for oral administration: (i) stability at pH ranges between 1.0 and 7.0 in aqueous solutions, (ii) far less toxicity than AZA and decitabine to cultured cells, and (iii) no detectable toxicity in a T-cell lymphoma mouse model [23-27].

The specific mechanism of DNA methylation alterations induced by azacytidine nucleoside analogues is complex and not fully understood. Azacytidine is thought to form a stable covalent bond with DNMTs after its incorporation into genomic DNA, thereby trapping the enzyme and sequestering it from transferring methyl groups to other regions of the genome [28-30]. Such a passive mechanism of DNA demethylation as a result of exposure to DNMTi has been proposed and is thought to progress with several cell divisions, after which DNMT levels increase and specific gene regions show re-methylation. Azacytidine treatment of cells also was shown to induce degradation of DNMT1 via the ubiquitin-activating proteosomal pathway [31], as well as p53-mediated cell cycle arrest and DNA repair [32]. Chromatin packaging and organization are altered in cells treated with azacytidine. Nucleosome depletion of symmetrically demethylated gene loci have been demonstrated after drug treatment [33]. However, it should be noted that there are additional reports indicating that genomic regions with AZA DNA-DNMT adducts are improperly packaged and transcriptional activation can only occur with DNA repair and recruitment of other protein factors [34,35].

To date, differential DNA methylation analysis has been quantitatively performed mostly by means of molecular approaches including electrophoretic, chromatographic, PCR-based, array-based, and sequencing technologies [36,37]. Furthermore, evidences indicate that DNMTi also influence repressive histone marks leading to changes in nucleosome positioning [33,34]. Hence, a novel nucleosome footprinting assay was developed, which takes advantage of improvements in these technologies and focuses on the characterization of locus-specific as well as genome-wide chromatin conformation with respect to DNA methylation on a single molecule level [38,39]. Such an analytical tool can be used to characterize the differential chromatin states and changes thereof that can occur under drug influence and would benefit therapeutic design: as demethylating drugs may, in addition to their physiologic role, also affect chromatin architecture and related gene expression programs in cells [40-47]. The structure and function of the human genome are so intricately intertwined that understanding its regulation requires viewing the genome as a dynamic three-dimensional entity that emerges from iterations of dynamic folding of the primary chromatin structure, the so-called nucleosomal array: also considering the mass of heterochromatin that is largely repressed and condensed through DNA methylation and histone-tail modifications, which are perturbed in complex diseases [17,18]. The immunodeficiency, centromere instability and facial anomalies (ICF) syndrome is a classic example, in which normally highly compacted juxtacentromeric satellite DNA is found hypomethylated and decondensed in chromosomes 1 and 16 [48]. Therefore, the higher genome organization of DNA provides an additional layer of cell-specific information that could render itself valuable in the evaluation of drug action, as it has potential to be translated into high-throughput and cost-efficient pre-clinical genotoxicity assays [19]. In this sense, little is known about the spatial progression of DNA hypomethylation in cell nuclei in response to DNMTi. The analysis of global nuclear DNA methylation patterns could provide a useful means in assessing said epigenetic effect of this class and possibly other classes of drugs in a large number of single cells, as the underlying molecular processes may involve large-scale chromatin reorganization visible by light microscopy [40-44,49-51]. Recently introduced, 3D-qDMI, can measure DNA methylation changes *in situ*, through the differential analysis of relevant nuclear structures that are represented by methylated CpG-dinucleotides (MeC) and global DNA [40-42] (Figure 1). Our analyses revealed significant differences in image patterns of MeC and heterochromatin-derived signals between untreated AtT20 mouse pituitary tumor cells and a subpopulation of these cells treated with AZA, which has been reported to change DNA methylation patterns on a genomic scale [52]. Furthermore, the recently upgraded methodology was able to monitor the dual effect of demethylating agents in

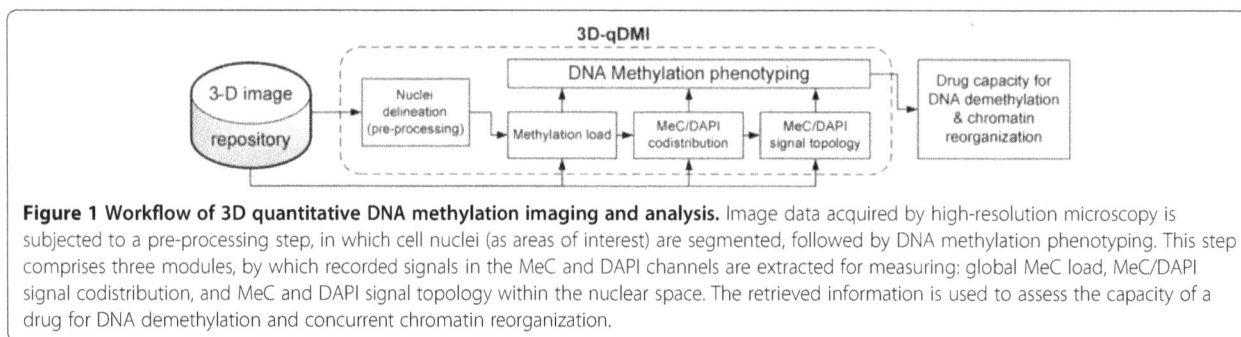

Figure 1 Workflow of 3D quantitative DNA methylation imaging and analysis. Image data acquired by high-resolution microscopy is subjected to a pre-processing step, in which cell nuclei (as areas of interest) are segmented, followed by DNA methylation phenotyping. This step comprises three modules, by which recorded signals in the MeC and DAPI channels are extracted for measuring: global MeC load, MeC/DAPI signal codistribution, and MeC and DAPI signal topology within the nuclear space. The retrieved information is used to assess the capacity of a drug for DNA demethylation and concurrent chromatin reorganization.

human cancer cells: (a) a global decrease in MeC content, and (b) the subsequent reorganization of highly compact heterochromatic regions of the genome as reflected by a significant decrease of DAPI intensity in the relevant nuclear areas. The effects resulted in LIM and LID sites, whose distributions can be mapped within cell nuclei [44]. This approach supports profiling at single-cell level, and provides a rapid display of cell-specific DNA methylation (MeC) phenotypes that is related to drug response in targeted cells. Initial results obtained with 3D-qDMI indicated towards the relatively gentle effect of zebularine on the genome, an observation that is concordant with reported studies based on molecular profiling. Initial proof-of-principle analyses focusing more on technology development were restricted to the application of one concentration per epigenetic drug. Here we report on the first-time probing of the 3D-qDMI system's utility in a dose-dependent manner: by administration of a larger concentration range of the relatively more gentle nucleoside zebularine in comparison to its extensively characterized more aggressive analogue 5-azacytidine [23-27,53,54]. The notion was to follow a more gradual DNA demethylation effect of the agents on 5-methylcytosine topology, along with cytotoxicity evaluations, in the two *in vitro* models, DU145 prostate cancer cells and Huh-7 hepatocarcinoma cells, which have known sensitivity to both drugs [55-59].

Methods
Cell culture and drug treatment
DU145 human prostate cancer cells were obtained from American Tissue Culture Collection (catalog number HTB-81, ATCC). The vendor certifies authentication of cells using a variety of techniques such as short tandem repeat (STR) analysis and cytogenetic analyses (G-banding, fluorescence *in situ* hybridization). Huh-7 cells were a gift from Dr. Vaithilingaraja Arumugaswami (Cedars-Sinai Medical Center, Los Angeles, CA). The cells were propagated for less than six months after receipt and resuscitation. Cells were grown in Dulbecco's modified Eagle's medium (DMEM, Cellgro) supplemented with 10% newborn calf serum, and 1% antibiotic/antimycotic (1000 units/ml penicillin G sodium, 10 mg/ml streptomycin

sulfate) (Gemini Bio-Products), in 5% CO_2, 37°C. Cells were plated at 1×10^5 cells onto coverslips in multi-well plates in replicates, and allowed to attach for 24 hours. For dose dependency assay, wells were divided into two groups: (i) control populations that were not treated for 72 hours, and (ii) populations of cells treated with two different drugs at different concentrations for 72 hours: 0.5 μM, 1 μM, 2.5 μM, 5 μM, 10 μM and 20 μM of 5-azacytidine (Sigma-Aldrich), and 8 μM, 40 μM, 200 μM, 500 μM and 1000 μM of zebularine (Sigma-Aldrich), all in DMEM. For all cells, drug concentrations were freshly prepared prior to administration, and the drug-medium mixture was changed every 24 hours. Subsequently, cells were partially fixed for immunofluorescence and partially harvested for cytotoxicity testing by flow cytometry.

Cell synchronization
DU145 prostate cancer cells were arrested in G0/G1 and G2-phases following previously established protocols [60,61]. Briefly, cells were seeded onto glass coverslips at a concentration of 10^5 cells/ml for immunofluorescence staining and subsequent imaging via confocal microscopy. A parallel set of cultures (at the same concentration) was maintained in culture flasks, for flow cytometry. All cells were first allowed to attach and grow for 24 hours in regular proliferative medium (DMEM/10% FBS/1% penicillin/ 1% streptomycin), which was then replaced by serum-deprived DMEM for 72 hours, followed by a recovery period of 4 hours, in which cells were maintained again in regular proliferative medium. G0/G1 populations were partially fixed at this point for use in either immunocytochemistry or FACS. The remainder cultures were processed for a double-thymidine block to enrich cells in G2-phase: (i) first blocking with deoxythymidine (Sigma) at 2 mM for 18 hours, (ii) recovery in regular proliferative medium for 12 hours to escape S-phase, (iii) second blocking with 2 mM deoxythymidine for another 18 hours, and (iv) second recovery in regular proliferative medium for 8 hours, to release cells into G2. At this point G2-cells were fixed for further experimentation. Enrichment efficiency was checked by propidium iodide (PI) staining of cells and nuclear DNA content analysis, following standard

protocols as previously described in Wong et al. [62]: cells were fixed in 70% ethanol/PBS and maintained for at least 4 hours at 4°C; then incubated in 5 μg/ml PI (Sigma) for 30 minutes at 37°C immediately prior to flow cytometry with a FACScan (Becton Dickinson). FACS data were analyzed using the ModFit LT program (Verity Software House, Topsham, ME, USA).

Cytotoxicity assay

Induction of apoptosis and cell viability was analyzed in cells that were treated as replicates in parallel to cells that were subsequently analyzed by immunofluorescence. For that purpose, 2×10^5 cells/ml were stained with Annexin V (7-AAD) and PI, respectively [63]. In essence, trypsinated cells from parallel wells were processed with the Annexin V-FITC Apoptosis Detection Kit I (BD Biosciences). Cells (1×10^5) were incubated for 15 minutes at room temperature with 7-AAD and PI in a total volume of 510 μl comprised of 5 μl of each of the fluorescent dyes, each and 500 μl of 1X binding buffer. Controls with unstained cells and cells stained with either dye alone were used for FACS setup. Samples were analyzed at emission wavelengths of 530 nm (for Annexin V-FITC) and 650 nm (for PI) using FACScan. The fluorescence of 10^4 cells was acquired and analyzed with CellQuest software (Becton Dickinson).

Immunofluorescence and image acquisition

In order to preserve the three-dimensional structure, cells cultured on glass coverslips in 12-well microplates (Costar, Corning) were fixed with 4% paraformaldehyde/phosphate buffered saline (PBS) (Sigma-Aldrich) and processed for immunofluorescence as previously described [64]. The following antibody sets were used: a monoclonal mouse anti-5-MeC antibody (Clone 33D3, Aviva Systems Biology, San Diego, CA) together with an Alexa488-conjugated polyclonal donkey anti-mouse IgG (H + L) (Invitrogen), and a polyclonal rabbit anti-H3K9me3 antibody (Active Motif) together with an Alexa647-conjugated chicken anti-rabbit IgG (H + L) (Invitrogen). All specimens were counterstained with DAPI. Specimens were imaged by a confocal laser-scanning microscope (TCS SP5 X Supercontinuum, Leica Microsystems Inc.) that allows for any excitation line within the continuous range of 470 to 670 nm, in 1 nm increments. The system was additionally equipped with a 405 nm diode laser line for excitation of DAPI fluorescence. Serial optical sections were collected at increments of 200–300 nm with a Plan-Apo 63X 1.3 glycerol immersion lens (pinhole size was 1.0 Airy unit). To avoid bleed-through, the imaging of each channel was performed sequentially. The typical image size was 2048 × 2048, with a respective voxel size of 116 nm × 116 nm × 230.5 nm (x, y, and z axes), and resolution was 12 bits per pixel in all channels. Fluorescence intensity of MeC-signals and DAPI-signals from optical two-dimensional sections were recorded into separate 3D channels. Raw images were obtained as Leica Image Format (lif) and offline-converted to a series of TIFFs for downstream image analysis.

3D image analysis

Image analysis was performed in three main steps, as comprehensively described in [43,44]: 1) image segmentation resulting in the delineation of a 3D shell for each individual nucleus; 2) extraction of MeC and DAPI signal intensity distributions within each 3D shell; 3) assessment of cell population heterogeneity through 2D histograms of MeC versus DAPI distribution patterns, utilizing K-L divergence, and 4) the mapping of LIMs and LIDs within individual nuclei. A newly added analytical component for this study was the calculation of mean intensity of MeC signals. Images in each two-channel 3D stack were acquired under nearly identical conditions and modality settings, and so the drift of the settings during acquisition is considered minimal and can be neglected. For codistribution analysis, the MeC and DAPI signals were mapped as respective 2D scatter plots, and following [43] the Kullback–Leibler (KL) divergences were calculated between individual 2D plots (nuclei) and the reference 2D plot (cumulative plot from all nuclei in one drug/concentration experiment). Based on the KL value, cells were categorized as: *similar* $KL_G \in [0, 0.5)$, *likely similar* $KL_G \in [0.5, 2)$, *unlikely similar* $KL_G \in [2, 4.5)$, and *dissimilar* $KL_G \in [4.5, \infty)$ in order to evaluate a ratio of similar and dissimilar cells. For localization of resulting LIM and LID sites, the nuclei were analyzed by an algorithm introduced in [44]. Briefly, segmented nuclei were eroded at a constant voxel rate of 1.32 μm × 1.3 μm × 0.25 μm, and MeC and DAPI signals were recorded as integrated intensity values within each nuclear shell. Then, local densities of LIM and LID sites as well as LIM and LID profiles were determined for each nuclear shell as the subset of voxels within a defined intensity range between two thresholds measured separately for each channel (MeC and DAPI): t_{bcg} is the threshold value for the background, and t_Q, which separates high-amplitude from low-amplitude intensities, as explicitly described in [44]. All analytical findings related to image processing including numerical results, MeC/DAPI codistribution patterns, individual and combined MeC/DAPI images, LIM/LID outputs of cells were exported by means of a graphical user interface to text or graphics files respectively for further statistical analyzes. A built-in pseudo-coloring of KL divergence, and LIM and LID site shading was superimposed onto original images to facilitate visual reading and evaluation of experimental data.

Antibody specificity and sensitivity test

The specificity and sensitivity of the applied anti-5-methyl-cytosine antibody used in this study was assessed with a test-microarray as shown in Figure 2. Antibody testing was performed by an immunofluorescence assay utilizing a custom made spotted microarray (Full Moon Biosystems) comprising multiple copies of two synthesized 24-mer oligonucleotide probes that were immobilized onto glass microscopic slides: 5′-TCGTTTTTTTTTTTTTTTTTTTT CGT-3′ (C-oligo) (MWG Biotech), and its counterpart 5′-T ^{me}CGTTTTTTTTTTTTTTTTTT^{me}CGT-3′ (MeC-oligo) (Biopolymers-Thermo Scientific), in which the two cytosine molecules were replaced by methylcytosine. Immuno-fluorescence was performed with the primary anti-methylcytosine antibody and the Alexa488 conjugated secondary antibody, and alternatively a Cy3-conjugated goat anti-mouse IgG1, using a denaturing step with hydrochloric acid, a blocking step with 3% BSA in PBS, and stringency washes as described for the *in situ* immunofluorescence

assay above. Fluorescence detection was performed comparatively at 5 microns resolution with a micro-array scanner (G2565BA, Agilent Technologies) equipped with a helium-neon laser (633 nm) to excite Cy3, and the above-mentioned confocal microscope with a Plan-Apo 10X 0.7 lens.

MethyLight assay for repetitive elements

MethyLight assays for measuring DNA methylation content of Alu, Satα and Sat2 repeat sequences were performed as previously described by Weisenberger et al. [65]. Briefly, genomic DNA was extracted from harvested Huh-7 cells and 1 µg of genomic DNA was converted with bisulfite and recovered using the Zymo EZ DNA methylation kit (Zymo Research, Irvine, CA), as recommended by the manufacturer. Aliquots of the bisulfite-converted DNAs were used in separate MethyLight assays as previously described [65]. MethyLight data specific for the three types of

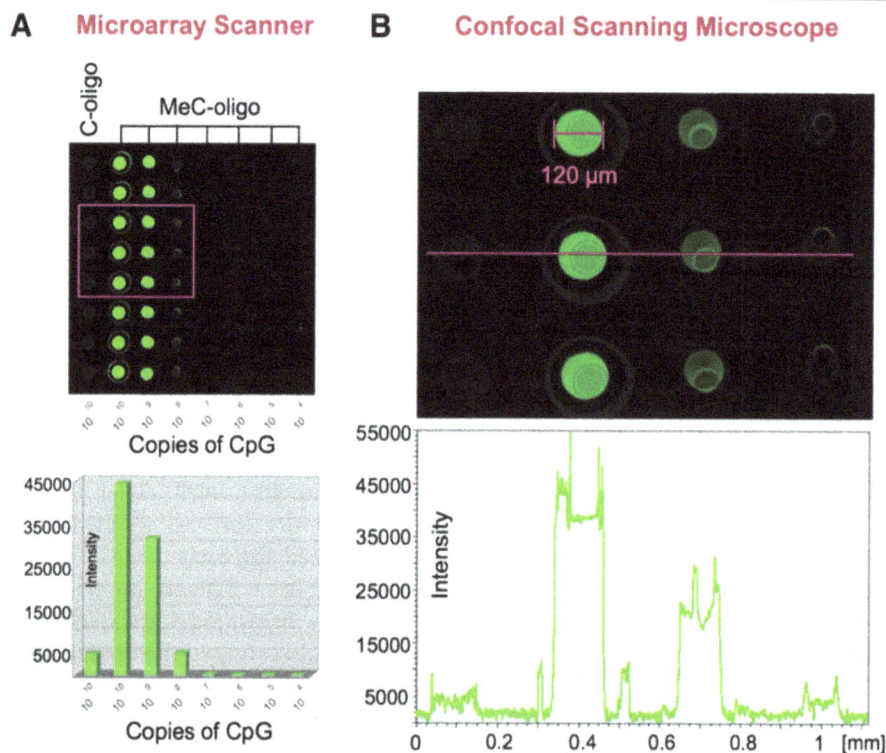

Figure 2 Specificity and sensitivity of used anti-methylcytosine antibody. (**A**) The antibody properties were assessed by an indirect immunofluorescence assay, in which the monoclonal anti-MeC antibody for this study — used at the concentration of 1 µg/ml in combination with a secondary antibody (Cy3-conjugated anti-mouse IgG1 at 5 µg/ml), i.e. at the same concentrations as in the cellular assay — was hybridized to a spotted array with two types of short 24-mer oligonucleotides immobilized onto a glass slide: C-oligo that included two CG dinucleotides and its methylated counterpart, the MeC-oligo printed at various dilutions that correlate with different approximate CpG copy numbers (10^{10}–10^4). Each DNA probe was spotted as octuple. The specific antibody, detected with a microarray scanner at 5 microns resolution, shows best signal-to-noise (background and non-specific binding to unmethylated C-oligo) ratio at a copy number of 10^{10}. The signal (false-colored in green) decreases in a CpG copy number-dependent manner. (**B**) Similar average intensities were obtained, when a sub-area (magenta box in Figure 2A) of the same array was subjected to confocal scanning microscopy at 200 nm horizontal resolution. The line scan (magenta) shows the more detailed intensity profile across the four different types of spots and the intermediate gaps (coated glass slide/background).

repetitive elements were expressed as percent of methylated reference (PMR).

Results

Zebularine exerts a comparably lower degree of cytotoxicity than 5-azacytidine

We evaluated cultured DU145 prostate cancer cells and Huh-7 hepatocellular carcinoma cell lines for imaging-based DNA methylation analysis using the 3D-qDMI system to determine DNA methylation phenotypes of cells after 5-zacytidine and zebularine administration. These drugs have been used with a variety of cancer cell lines, including DU145 and Huh-7 cells, and described as being compatible to a large extent with cell viability and cell division [25,40,53-59]. The azanucleoside drug concentrations applied here were in the range as previously reported by investigations utilizing molecular nucleic acids-based assays.

For cytotoxicity analysis, we tested cells that were cultured in parallel to those used for imaging-based DNA methylation analysis. Cytotoxicity analysis was divided into an initial cell counting with an aliquot of trypsinized cells, followed by staining of the remainder of the cells with Annexin V and propidium iodide, and subsequent flow cytometry. Zebularine was administered at molar concentrations (8–1000 μM) that were one to two orders of magnitude higher than AZA (0.5–20 μM) with comparable cytotoxic effects (Figure 3A, 3B). Therefore, ZEB can be categorized as an agent with a much lower cytotoxic potential. This has also been described in previous reports [23,27]. In more detail, flow cytometry revealed a higher sensitivity of DU145 for ZEB compared to Huh-7 cells: IC_{10} and IC_{50} of ZEB were 8 μM and 500 μM, respectively for DU145 versus 200 μM and 1000 μM for Huh-7. In the case of AZA we experienced fewer discrepancies: IC_{10} was 0.5 μM for both cell types and IC_{50} was measured at 10 μM for DU145 and 5 μM for Huh-7. A greater than two-fold increase of the apoptotic fraction (Annexin V-positive) for AZA-treated cells of both types was detected at 2.5 μM, and for ZEB-treated DU145 cells at 200 μM, whereas same effects were registered in Huh-7 cells at 1000 μM (Figures 3C and 3D). For the comparative analysis of the two drugs at different concentrations, 2.5×10^5 cells were initially seeded onto coverslips. After 72 hours we recorded a tripling of naïve cells and only a doubling for both cell types at the drugs' IC_{10} levels. Analogously, at IC_{50} ZEB-treated cells did not show any population growth, whereas AZA-treated cells showed significant reduction of their populations: Huh-7 cells were reduced to 50% and DU145 cells even to 10% of their original confluency. The results underline the ability of ZEB to reduce proliferation at higher doses without acting discernibly cytotoxic as demonstrated by AZA.

High variation in DNA demethylation and differential drug sensitivity revealed by cell-by-cell imaging

Untreated cells as well as cells treated separately with AZA and ZEB were automatically imaged from different areas of each coverslip. Imaged sub-populations were batch-processed off-line using 3D-qDMI software. We evaluated drug action by measuring two parameters on a per-cell basis: (i) the 5-methylcytosine load of nuclei, which we refer to as the mean intensity of the MeC signal (I_{MeC}), and (ii) the nuclear topology of the MeC versus DAPI signals. The number of cells that we could extract the MeC-specific signals from depended on the cytotoxicity level of the drugs: resulting in a certain density of intact cells for each drug type, and subsequently the number of analyzable nuclei per image frame. We determined I_{MeC} across all resulting nuclei for each drug type. Figure 4 illustrates relevant statistics in naïve cells and each of the treated populations. The mean intensity was evaluated by a two-sample Kolmogorov-Smirnov test run for the experiments with each combination of drug and cell line. In DU145 (ZEB) cells, a significant difference was observed between all distributions of I_{MeC}, except for the 200 μM dose that was not significantly different from 40 μM and 500 μM. In DU145, cells treated with AZA the distributions of I_{MeC} for untreated and 0.5 μM were not significantly different. Also, no significant difference was observed between 10 μM and 20 μM in Huh-7 (AZA) cells, as well as between untreated and 8 μM dose, and the three highest concentrations in Huh-7 (ZEB) cells. The significance level in each test (β) was determined by Bonferroni correction (β = α/n) for α = 0.05, n = 6 or 7 for ZEB and AZA treatments, respectively.

The experimental results confirm the hypomethylating effect of both drugs; the increase of drug concentration causes a progressive loss of globally measured MeC-specific signal in nuclei (I_{MeC}) and a decrease of I_{MeC} spread (Figure 4). Interestingly, AZA, at the highest concentration applied (20 μM), reduced the I_{MeC} stronger in Huh-7 cells (88%) than in DU145 cells (75%), whereas ZEB at the highest concentration (1000 μM) reduced I_{MeC} in DU145 cells at 72% versus 50% in Huh-7 cells, on average. However, when comparing global DNA methylation of cell nuclei at the equitoxic levels, ZEB showed a much stronger DNA hypomethylation effect than its nucleoside analogue at IC_{10} — 15% versus 5% for DU145 and 43% versus 18% for Huh-7 — then a milder effect at IC_{50}: 54% versus 69% for DU145 and 50% versus 80% for Huh-7 cells. These results are in agreement with previous studies [24,26,54], and underline the less toxic effect of zebularine on cells and the milder nature of the drug when compared to AZA. In other words, AZA-treatment in both cell lines showed an approximate reduction of I_{MeC} at 63% between IC_{10}

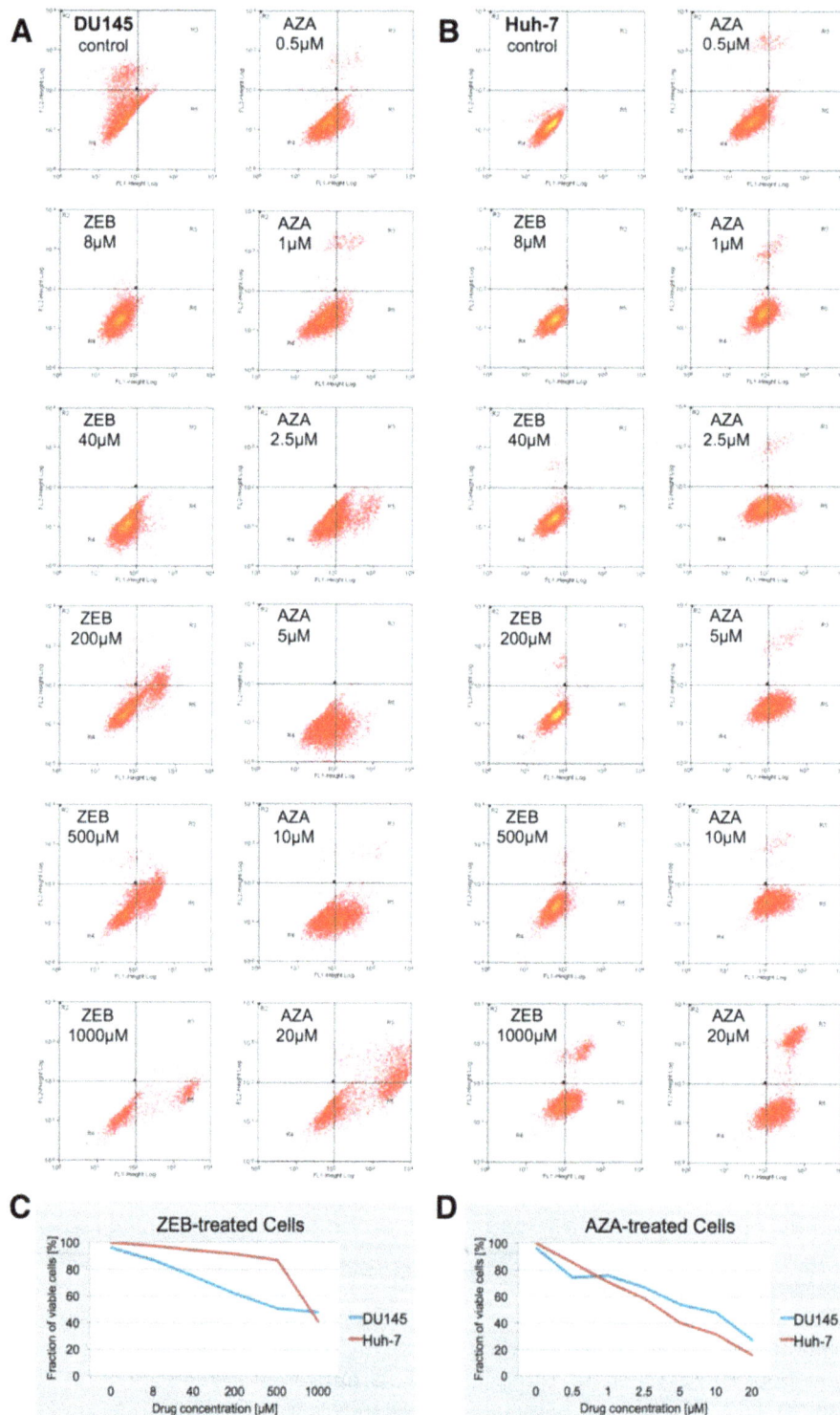

Figure 3 Cytotoxicity of agents analyzed by FACS. Results for the comparative analysis of the effects of zebularine (**A**) and 5-azacytidine (**B**). FL1-Height and FL2-Height represent Annexin V-staining and PI staining, respectively. Untreated control cell populations of DU145 and Huh-7 cells consist of a major portion of viable cells (> 90%). This reference profile changes with treatment of cells with different drug concentrations applied for 72 hrs. The viability of cells was normalized against the viability in the control population (considered as 100%) and displayed as a chart for zebularine (**C**) and 5-azacytidine (**D**).

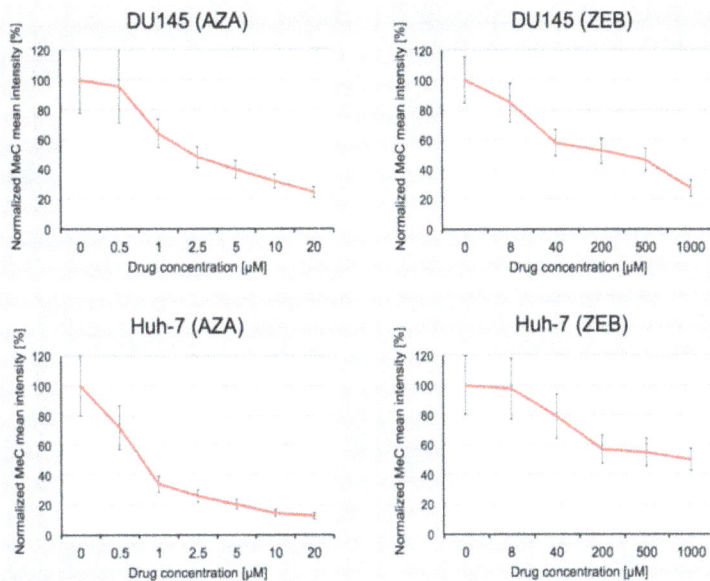

Figure 4 Normalized MeC mean intensity in untreated and drug-treated cells. Decline of signal intensity is plotted as a function of drug concentration. Standard deviation of I_{MeC} for untreated cells and cells treated with lower drug concentration is significantly greater than for cells treated with higher drug concentration. Comparative reduction in overall DNA methylation (as percentage drop compared to untreated controls) can be inferred for both drugs in DU145 cells, although at concentrations of one to two magnitudes lower for AZA than for ZEB. Huh-7 cells show comparatively less loss of I_{MeC} at highest zebularine concentration (1000 µM).

and IC_{50} concentrations, whereas the I_{MeC} reduction leap was significantly different between ZEB-treated cells: $I_{MeC} \approx 39\%$ for DU145 and only 7% for Huh-7 cells. The data indicate that if DNA hypomethylation effects would be influencing cytotoxicity, dose–response may vary for different drugs in different cells.

Dose-dependent topological progression of DNA hypomethylation correlates with cytotoxicity

The analysis of the MeC/DAPI codistribution showed a high fraction of cells with pooled all *similar* categories in response to both drugs for all concentrations (Figure 4). ZEB-treated populations contained ≥ 90% similar cells, compared with AZA-treated populations with an average ≥ 85% and a slight tendency to drop for DU145 cells at 0.5 µM and 10 µM (82% and 79%, respectively). The cell population heterogeneity analysis was performed with an average total cell number of n = 300. Figure 5 displays normalized proportions of the two resultant categories of cells, and example MeC/DAPI codistributions are presented in Figure 6.

The effect of the drugs can be perceived as a reduction in the MeC signal, with a similar effect in both cell systems, when compared to nuclei of untreated cells. In case of each drug, we observed a dose-dependent reduction of the MeC-specific signal. At lower drug concentrations (ZEB: 8 µM and 40 µM; AZA: 0.5 µM and 1 µM) the nucleus still shows significant DNA methylation in its periphery, which becomes hypomethylated at

medium to higher drug doses (ZEB: 200–1000 µM, AZA: 5–20 µM). This is accompanied by a decrease of DNA methylation at interior nuclear regions, gradually affecting also DAPI-dense areas that are attributed to heterochromatin. Zebularine at the 1000 µM dose shows extremely strong hypomethylation in the entire nuclear space, including a large portion of heterochromatin in the nuclear interior (Figure 5). In comparison, AZA shows similar effects already at 5 µM (data not shown). These observations support our findings presented in Figure 3. The visual impressions of DNA hypomethylation in response to drug type and concentration were confirmed by quantitation of MeC and DAPI signal codistributions in the respective nuclei and displayed as accompanying scatter plots (Figure 6).

In addition to AZA-treatments, a subset of Huh-7 cells was separately stained for covisualizing differential spatial distribution of histone H3 lysine 9 trimethylation (H3K9me3) and global DNA. H3K9me3 is associated with heterochromatin and is involved in the recruitment and binding of heterochromatin protein 1 (HP1), with subsequent chromatin condensation and compaction [66,67]. Therefore, we monitored this marker in sample cells to specifically record changes in higher-order heterochromatin organization in conjunction with AZA drug application (Figure 7). Our findings show a high degree of colocalization between the H3K9me3 and DAPI signals in untreated cells and cells treated with the entire spectrum of applied AZA concentrations.

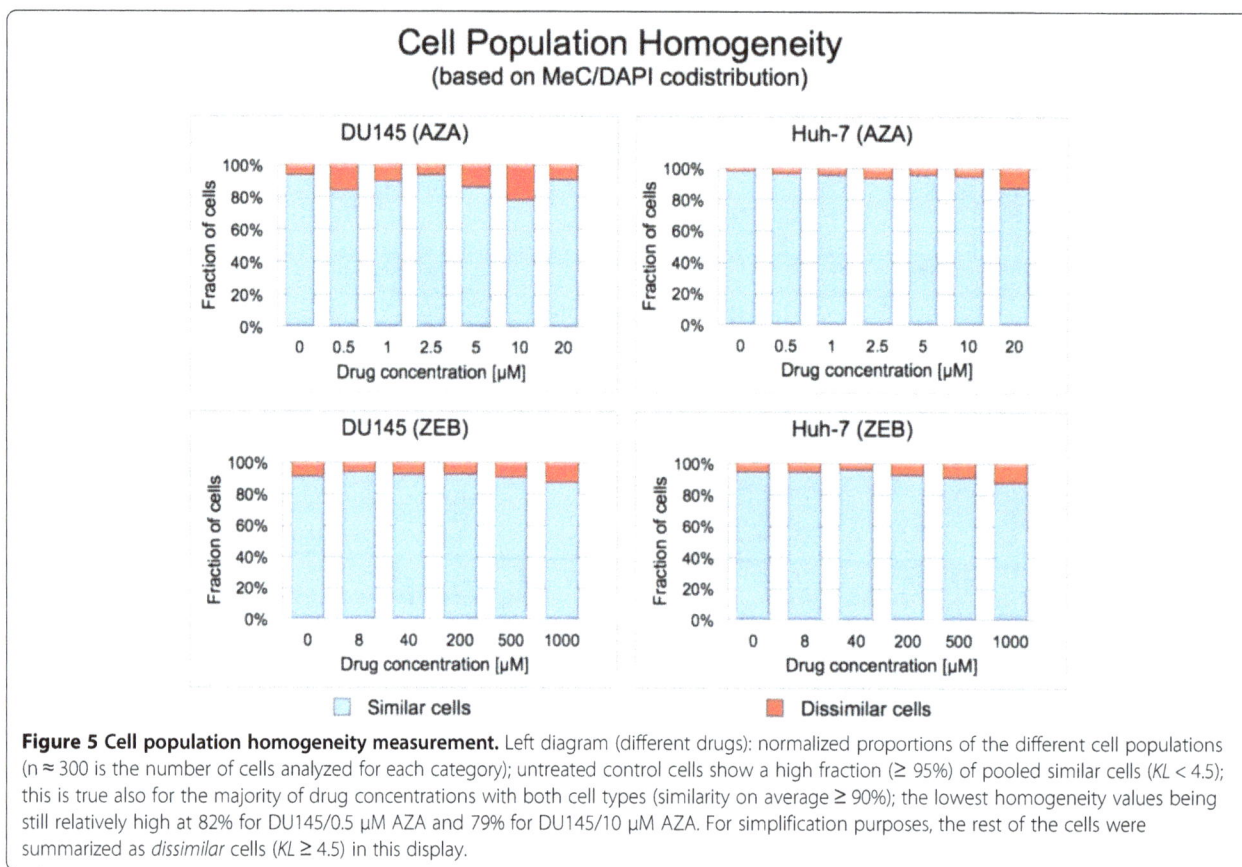

Figure 5 Cell population homogeneity measurement. Left diagram (different drugs): normalized proportions of the different cell populations (n ≈ 300 is the number of cells analyzed for each category); untreated control cells show a high fraction (≥ 95%) of pooled similar cells (*KL* < 4.5); this is true also for the majority of drug concentrations with both cell types (similarity on average ≥ 90%); the lowest homogeneity values being still relatively high at 82% for DU145/0.5 μM AZA and 79% for DU145/10 μM AZA. For simplification purposes, the rest of the cells were summarized as *dissimilar* cells (*KL* ≥ 4.5) in this display.

Therefore, one can assume that DAPI signals could be utilized as a surrogate marker for visualizing changes of global heterochromatin organization. Furthermore, it is conceivable that a reduction in H3K9me3 could lead to local DNA decondensation as extensively reported elsewhere [10,68]. These findings support our topologic approach in using DAPI signals as a convenient way of reporting changes in heterochromatin organization and distribution, extensively discussed in previous works [43,44]: as we found that DAPI staining is compatible with the hydrochloric acid-treatment conditions of fixed cells we applied for MeC-signal retrieval without any detectable obscuring of both signals [64].

To further emboss the differential spatial distribution of global DNA and its methylated portion, we focused on the changes in the localization of LIMs and LIDs, as subsets of nuclear signals that represent hypomethylated sites and areas of lower DNA density in naïve and treated cells. As illustrated in Figure 8, both LIM and LID sites in the untreated cells have a rim-like localization at or close to the nuclear border ($LIM_{0.5}$ = 0.80–0.85, and $LID_{0.5}$ = 0.85) for both cell types after zebularine treatment, while only 15–20% of LIMs were located in nuclei. In cells comparatively treated with ZEB and AZA, the nuclei showed an increased portion of interior LIM

and LID sites after treatment with each drug. The increase in LIM sites is correlated with the increase in ZEB concentration: on average the LIM-portion in DU145/Huh-7 is raised to ~30%/~40% at 8 μM, ~40%/~40% at 40 μM, ~45%/~50% at 200 μM, 50%/60% at 500 μM, and ~55%/~65% at 1000 μM, respectively. In comparison, the LID-portion in the nuclear interior significantly expanded at lower ZEB concentrations: up to 50% at 8 μM for DU145 and 40% at 40 μM for Huh-7, but did not significantly change beyond this concentration in either cell type. In AZA-treated cells the change for LIDs was very similar, however, LIM sites increased up to 60% on average as can be inferred from the subset of data displayed for the equitoxic drug concentrations in Figure 9. For the two drugs, the responding distributions of LIM and LID sites are quite similar between equitoxic concentrations with a slight difference of IC_{50} for DU145 cells. Interestingly in this context, LID distributions did not vary substantially compared to LIM distributions between IC_{10} and IC_{50} concentrations. From these results we glean that an increase of global DNA hypomethylation can be traced in a dose-dependent manner. However, a significant concurrent reorganization of the genome based on changes in DAPI densities occurs already at the lower applied drug concentrations, and does not seem to become stronger at

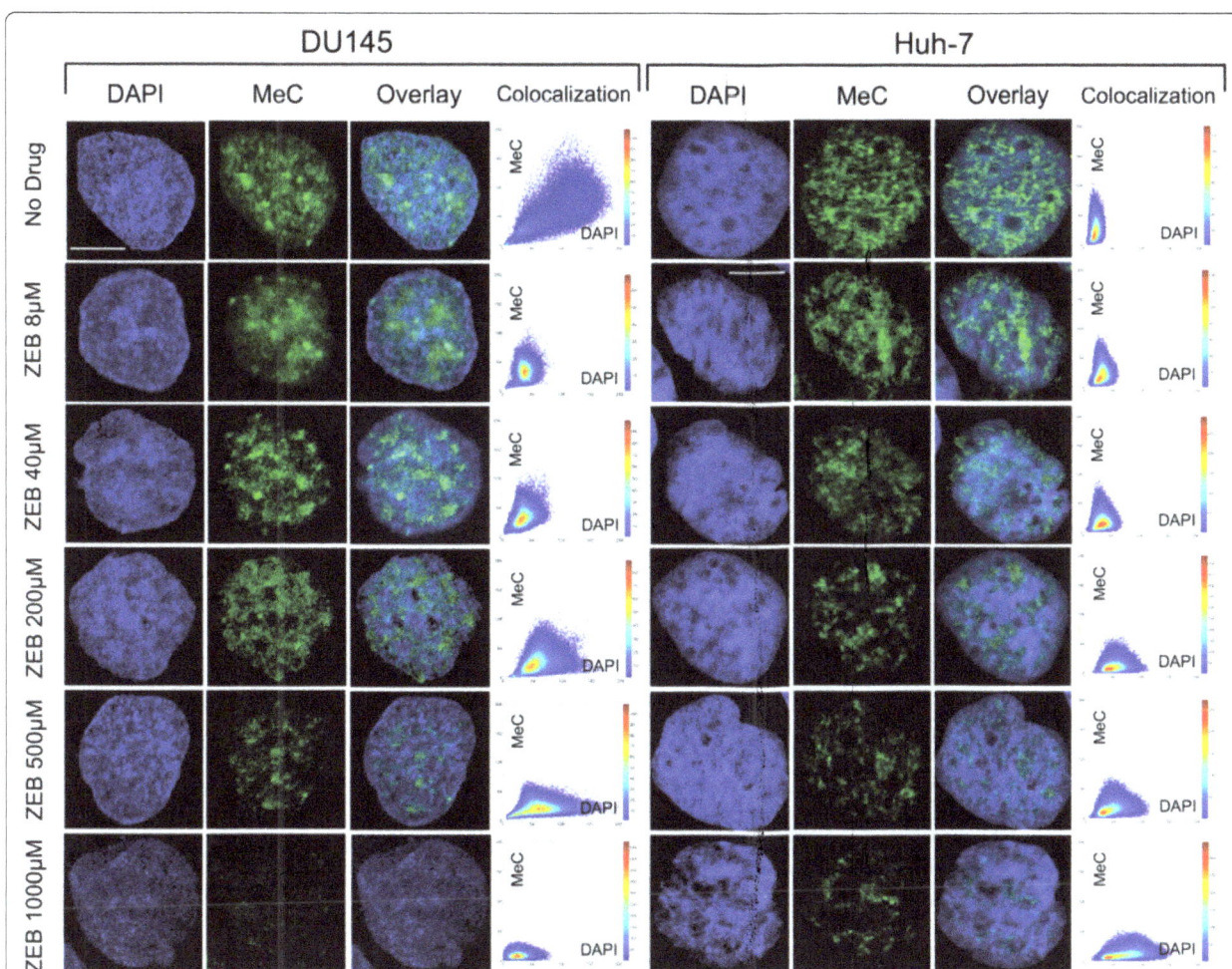

Figure 6 Global differential DNA methylation phenotypes in response to zebularine concentration. Maximum intensity projections (MIP) of 3D-imaged nuclei of DU145 cells with high similarity values within their population category are selected for display (bars are 5 μm). Gradual increase in reduction of MeC sites (false-colored green) was observed in correlation with an increase in zebularine concentration, similarly in both cell types. At lower concentrations (8 and 40 μM) global demethylation seems to be preferentially stronger at the nuclear periphery (delineated by DAPI, false-colored blue) and less DAPI-dense areas (supposedly euchromatin), and gradually affects more interior regions with increased drug concentrations. At higher drug doses (200 μM and especially 500–1000 μM), also more DAPI-dense areas (heterochromatin) have been demethylated. This latter effect is even more pronounced in the AZA-treated cell nuclei (data not shown in here). However, the majority of heterochromatic regions seem to retain their compact conformation. The respective scatter plots of the nuclei provide more quantitative information regarding changes in the MeC/DAPI codistribution as a consequence of drug application, especially for the lower drug doses: a demethylation of non-heterochromatic sites (MeC-positive, low-DAPI signals) is indicated for 40 μM compared to 8 μM, as judged by the decline of the graph slope. This trend correlates with increasing drug concentration. At 200–1000 μM the leveling of the slope towards the x-axis becomes obvious; additionally also strong DAPI-positive sites (heterochromatin) have started to become hypomethylated.

concentrations that are 25–100-fold higher. Therefore, the differential LIM and LID topology supplements the MeC/DAPI codistribution findings described in Figure 6. The respective diagrams of the cells show a flattening of MeC/DAPI codistribution and the increase of LIM sites concurrent with increasing dosage. Stronger hypomethylating effects at higher concentrations of AZA or ZEB were not accompanied by an additional increase of LID sites. Also, the increase in LIM distribution towards higher LIM densities reflects the spatial progression of DNA hypomethylation, which seems to positively correlate with drug-based cytotoxicity.

MeC/DAPI codistribution patterns are independent from cell cycle interphases

Interphase cells are largely divided into two prominent groups based on their cell cycle stage: G0/G1-phase and G2-phase, differing in DNA content. Compared to haploid G1-cells diploid G2-cells normally contain two copies of the genome after having undergone the intermediate S-phase, in which DNA is replicated. Therefore, we investigated the possibility of existing differences in MeC/DAPI distribution patterns between these two cell cycle phases. DU145 cells were synchronized in culture and arrested in G0/G1 and G2-phases. Cell stage-enriched

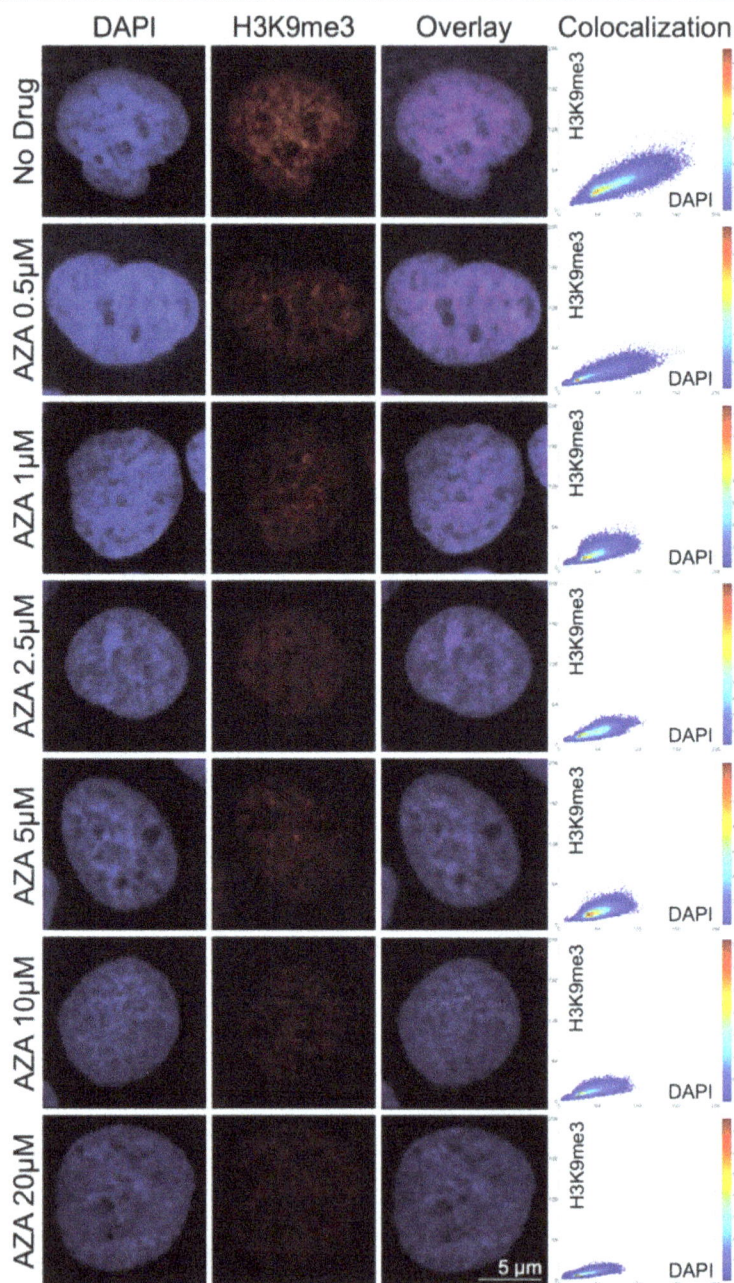

Figure 7 Nuclear codistribution of H3K9me3 and global DNA. Heterchromatin-associated H3K9me3 (red) significantly colocalizes with DAPI-intense areas (blue) in untreated and AZA-treated Huh-7 cells. The scatter plots show that the signal in both channels gradually decreases with increasing drug concentration. The relatively stable inclination of the colocalization graph indicates that both signals regress proportionally, which could be interpreted as a tight correlation between heterochromatin and DAPI-intense regions.

populations were processed for immunofluorescence and 3-D imaging. We found that synchronized cell populations were comprised of an absolute majority of cells in interphase, as most of the barely attached and round metaphase cells are usually lost during the early synchronization steps (Figures 10A and 10B). Utilizing 3D-qDMI, we did not detect any significant differences for MeC/DAPI codistribution patterns between the two major cell cycle phases. Sample signatures of selected (*similar*) G1 and G2-cells with a low KL-value that represent typical global nuclear MeC phenotypes are shown in Figure 10 (C–F), and demonstrate similar codistribution patterns seen for untreated DU145 cells (Figure 5). Based on these results, we conclude that significant changes in MeC/DAPI patterns detected by 3D-qDMI are a result of drug action and not influenced by eventual cell cycle phase variability.

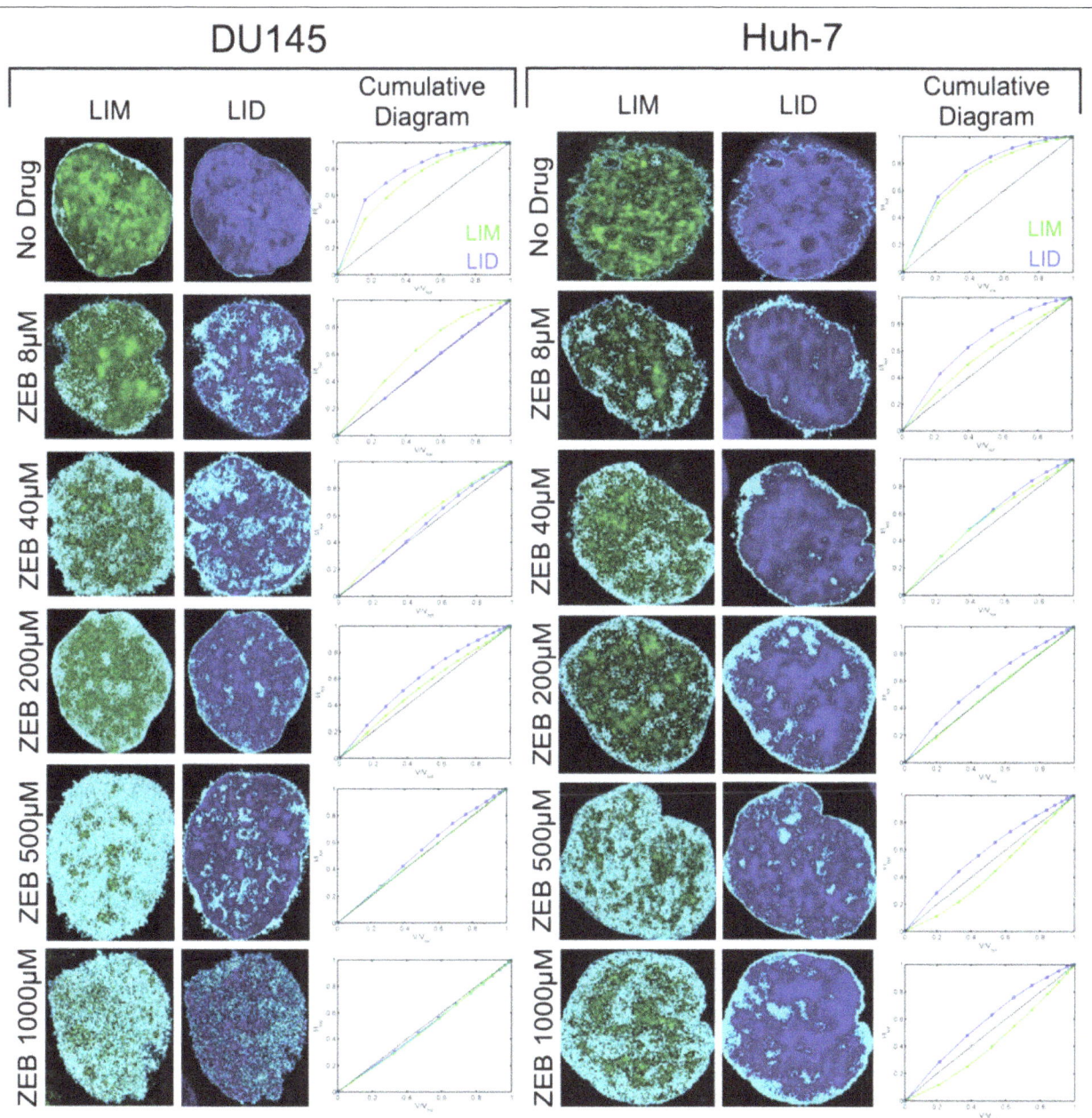

Figure 8 Differential LIM and LID topology in zebularine-treated cells. LIM and LID sites detected in the range of (t_{pcg}, t_Q) in individual cells from Figure 6 (marked in cyan color) are superimposed onto an intermediate optical section in the respective MeC (green) and DAPI (blue) channels (left and middle columns). LIM/LID density curves obtained through morphological erosion of nuclei are shown as cumulative diagrams (right column). These sites correspond with codistribution patterns in Figure 4 for the respective nuclei. The number of graph points in the third column is associated with the number of detected shells; the value of each point refers to the fraction of all sites found in the nucleus up to the next shell. V is the shell volume and V_{tot} is the total volume of a nucleus. The argument $V/V_{tot} = 0.5$ distinguishes all LIM sites that are localized in the peripheral half of the nucleus from LIMs of the interior half ($V/V_{tot} > 0.5$). The diagonal line across each plot in represents hypothetically equal density of LIM or LID sites across the nuclear volume. Similar degrees of high rim-like LIM and LID densities are apparent in untreated prostate and hepatic cancer cell nuclei. LIM sites quasi-linearly expand towards the nuclear interior upon the increase of zebularine concentration, with ZEB at 500–1000 μM show large coverage in Huh-7 nuclei and nearly full coverage throughout DU145 nuclei. Also LIDs show an increased distribution in treated cells versus naïve cells, but the changes are more similar across all the applied ZEB and AZA concentrations in both cell types, with most increases occurring in the exterior shells of the nuclei.

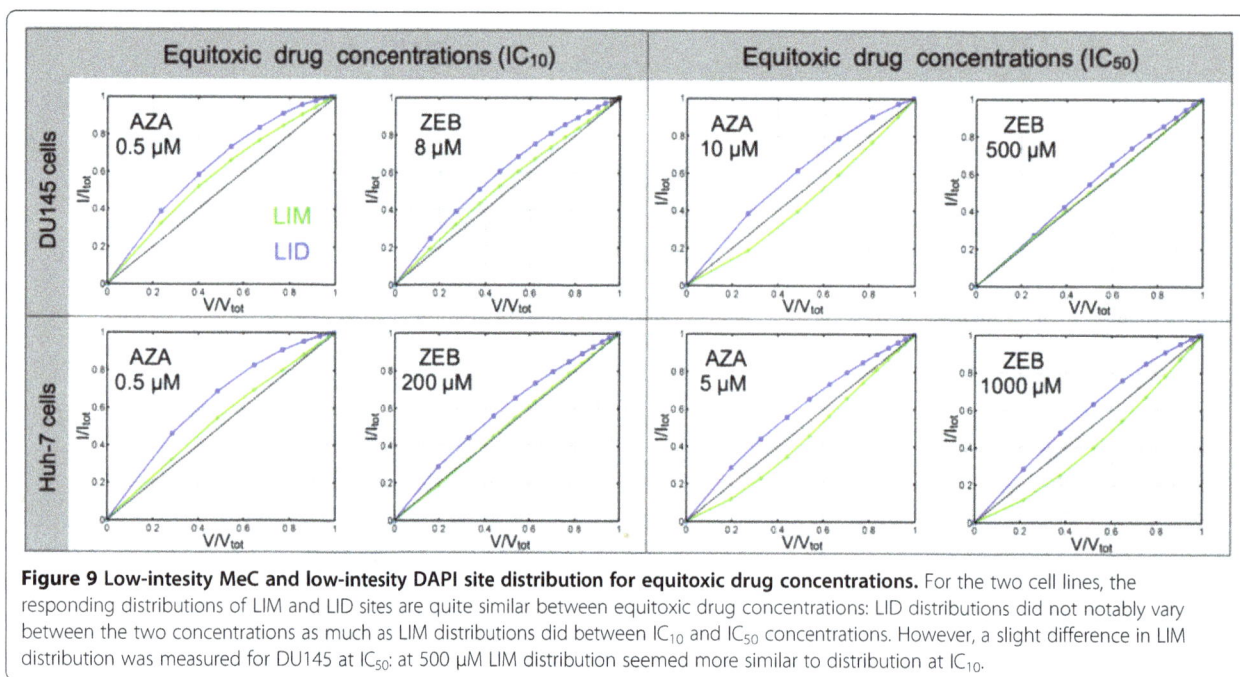

Figure 9 Low-intesity MeC and low-intesity DAPI site distribution for equitoxic drug concentrations. For the two cell lines, the responding distributions of LIM and LID sites are quite similar between equitoxic drug concentrations: LID distributions did not notably vary between the two concentrations as much as LIM distributions did between IC$_{10}$ and IC$_{50}$ concentrations. However, a slight difference in LIM distribution was measured for DU145 at IC$_{50}$: at 500 μM LIM distribution seemed more similar to distribution at IC$_{10}$.

In comparison, when analyzing DNA methylation and DAPI loads of nuclei in synchronized cell populations, we found that the amplitude of the respective mean intensities I_{MeC} and I_{DAPI} has nearly doubled in G2 versus G0/G1 phase. However, the distribution of these two values shows a large spread in both phases (Figure 11). This fact demonstrates that although we could measure general load trends that most probably correlate with the doubling of the genome between G1 and G2 phases, overall mean intensities of global DNA and total MeC content can drastically vary, even between synchronized cells; therefore making it difficult to distinguish between their natural variation and strictly drug-induced changes. On the contrary, when MeC/DAPI codistribution data of the same G1 and G2 arrested cells were combined, the computationally merged population presented a high degree of homogeneity, as calculated by KL-divergence measurement. This confirms the high similarity between the MeC phenotypes of cells from the two different populations, and emphasizes on the robustness of MeC/DAPI patterns in evaluating drug-induced effects on nuclear DNA methylation topology.

Analysis of DNA methylation levels in repeat sequences correlates with imaging results

For comparative analysis of differential DNA methylation loads and to verify the quantitative accuracy of 3D-qDMI, Huh-7 cells were subjected to AZA treatment under the same conditions (concentrations and exposure times) as for cells interrogated by image and flow cytometry, and analyzed using MethyLight technology, a

real-time PCR based DNA methylation assay [65]. MethyLight assays measuring DNA methylation of repetitive element sequences have been previously described as accurate surrogates for quantitating global DNA methylation levels. Using this technique, we measured DNA methylation levels in the three of the most prevalent and highly methylated human repeat sequences: the short interspersed nuclear element (SINE) Alu sequences that are highly abundant in the human genome, as well as the pericentromeric Sat2 and the centromeric Satα, which both belong to constitutive heterochromatin. The choice of said targets was based on the facts that DNA hypomethylation of these sequences can lead to local chromatin decondensation and genomic instability, which have been well characterized in diverse cancers and other types of complex traits such as ICF syndrome [8,13,48]. Also, these repetitive elements have been shown to become hypomethylated after exposure to DNMTi [12-14,69]. The molecular assay revealed that DNA methylation levels in all three classes of repetitive elements showed similar trends and were in strong agreement with results observed for global DNA methylation with 3D-qDMI: the untreated cells record the highest level of MeC content with a gradual decline as the drug concentration increases, and a re-increase of DNA methylation for the 20 μM AZA dose. We believe that because of the purportedly extensive damage to cell integrity at the 20 μM AZA concentration, the more methylated (possibly drug-resistant) cells may have selectively survived (Figure 12). This was observed with microscopic imaging, in which the cell populations were significantly reduced

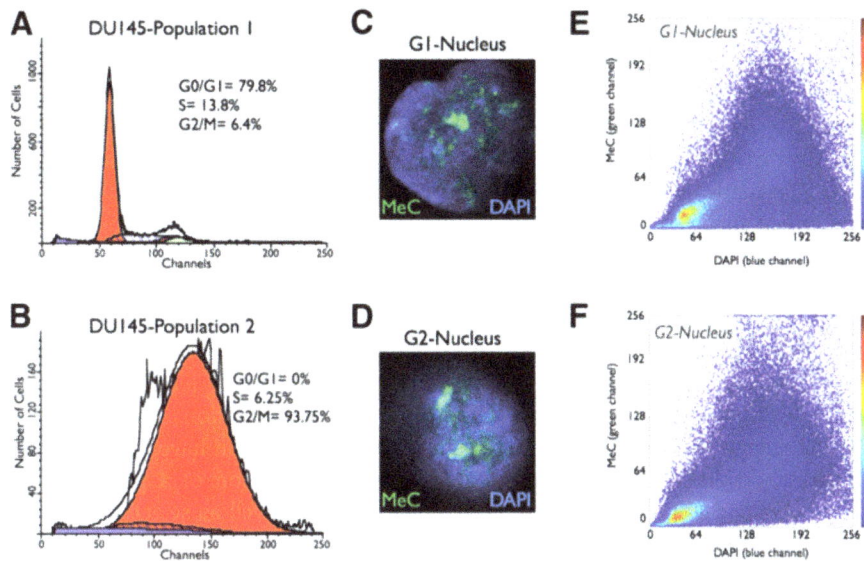

Figure 10 Cell cycle-specific MeC/DAPI codistribution patterns. Flow cytometry results show DU145 cell populations were efficiently arrested in G0/G1-phase (**A**) and enriched in G2-phase (**B**). The culture conditions were chosen to skip an enrichment of the cells in S-Phase. G1-cells and G2-cells from parallel populations were subjected to immunofluorescence and confocal imaging. The prototypic nuclei (**C** and **D**) of the two cell cycle phases (with a low KL-value) show very similar MeC (green) and DAPI/gDNA (blue) codistribution patterns, also confirmed by their respective scatter plots (**E** and **F**).

compared to lower drug doses and contained larger numbers of highly methylated cells, which were excluded as outliers in 3D-qDMI analysis.

In order to draw direct comparisons between image-derived data and molecular sequenced-based results a correlation coefficient was calculated between *in situ* global DNA methylation levels, i.e. normalized MeC mean intensities of analyzed Huh-7 cells (obtained by 3D-qDMI, Figure 4) and DNA methylation levels measured (normalized PMR values) for each class of repeat sequence across AZA concentrations up to the 10 μM dose, as shown in Table 1. The comparison

resulted in high correlations between the outcome of the two platforms, the highest being for the interspersed Alu sequences (R = 0.96), followed by pericentromeric Sat2 and centromeric Satα (R = 0.89 and 0.86, respectively).

Discussion

Epigenetic drugs including DNA methyltransferase inhibitors, which are meant to correct for DNA methylation imbalances in cells, constitute promising therapeutic approaches in the battle against cancer. The FDA-approved azanucleotides 5-azacytidine and decitabine are already administered to patients with hematologic neoplasias.

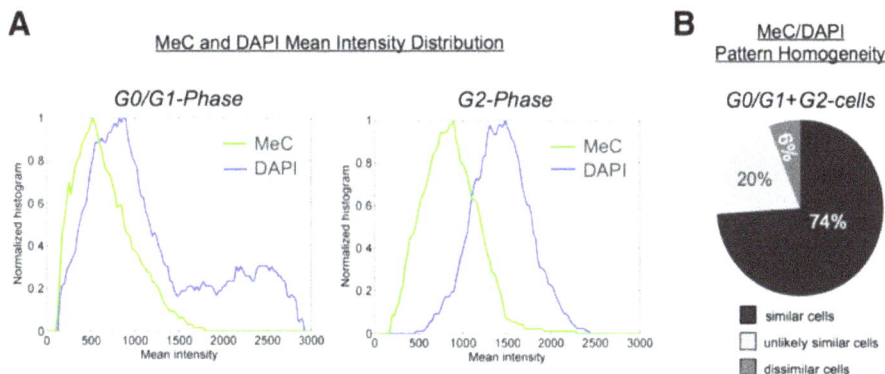

Figure 11 Variability of MeC and DAPI intensities in synchronized cells. (**A**) Mean intensities (normalized for n = ~200 cells for each) of global methylcytosine (MeC) and overall DNA (DAPI) nearly doubled between G0/G1-phase and G2-phase, with a large spread in MeC and DAPI signal distributions indicating high signal variabilities in synchronized cells. (**B**) In comparison MeC/DAPI codistribution patterns in the combined data of the same cells from the two phases exposed a high degree of homogeneity, which is a sign for high similarity in MeC phenotypes between cells of the two phases.

Zebularine has emerged as a new member of this type of agents that has shown potentials for long-term oral applications, as a result of systematic comparative analyses [23-27,70,71]. However, most of the assessments have been performed utilizing molecular methods that reveal precise information regarding CpG methylation profiles of non-repetitive sequences, but are currently costly and time-consuming, if not challenged, when applied in a cell-by-cell mode. Nevertheless, we believe that analysis of cultured cell models *at single-cell resolution* is necessary to obtain a more global and cell systemic picture of drug action and efficacy in the search for new drugs as well as the epigenetic evaluation of existing drugs. Thus, high-content and high-throughput analyses, which have been supported by recent advancements in imaging technology and computational capacities, offer valuable means for rapid and cost-effective cellular phenotyping in drug screening [72]. Furthermore, the vast majority of studies so far have been focusing on assessing the hypomethylating potential of drugs on selected gene promoters in combination with cell viability testing for drug cytotoxicity and genotoxicity. However, hypomethylating agents can also perturb the epigenetic regulation of chromatin conformation, thus having an impact on the higher-order genome organization and nuclear architecture that regulate genome integrity and gene expression [19]. We were interested in tracking the progression and extent of such global structural changes, also in correlation with drug cytotoxicity to additionally elaborate on the verification of the 3D-qDMI system's utility for the therapeutic field. Towards this end, we have conducted a comparative cell-by-cell evaluation of zebularine and its extensively characterized isoform 5-azacytidine based on their effects on global nuclear DNA and its higher-order organization in the cell nucleus. For the purpose of generating comparable topological data, we chose human cell culture models that have rendered themselves as sensitive to both agents, as well as cell culture conditions and drug doses that have been used previously in comprehensive studies to explore differential changes on the level of DNA methylation for targeted single-copy CpG sites. Our study includes standard viability testing for measuring cytotoxicity and upgraded 3D-qDMI for evaluating the demethylation effects on two levels: (i) changes in the load of nuclear MeC (I_{MeC}), and (ii) alterations in the spatial codistribution of MeC and global DNA, including condensed heterochromatin regions that are represented by bright DAPI areas in the nuclei of cells. Our cytotoxicity data as well as the results of our topologic approach are strongly concordant with data presented by other investigators [23,25,26,73-75]. Drug response efficacy, as judged by the degree of spatial nuclear MeC/DAPI patterns, was comparably high for the two drugs across all concentrations.

In terms of cytotoxicity, we found that the Huh-7 hepatocarcinoma cells reacted more sensitively to zebularine than the prostate cancer cells. Nevertheless, for both cell types, zebularine elicited similar cytotoxicity levels at doses that were one to two orders of magnitude higher than for 5-azacytidine, thus can be considered as much less cytotoxic at near-equimolar concentrations. The results are in accordance with data from other investigations that have probed the two agents in various other cancer cell models such as bladder (T24), colon (HCT-116), ovarian (A2780 and HEY) and breast (MBA-MD-231 and MCF-7) cancer cell lines, as well as in acute myeloid leukemia cells (AML 193) [23,25,73-75]. Investigations addressing the chemistry behind this phenomenon have led to cumulative evidence indicating the formation of a permanent covalent bond between human as well as selected bacterial DNMTs and 5-azacytidine that can trap the enzyme in a suicide complex (triggering apoptosis). In comparison, only a stable but no permanent covalent bond has been proven between zebularine and the same DNMTs, which would allow the enzymes' release after binding *in vitro* as well as *in vivo*. This may explain why higher concentrations of zebularine are necessary for similar levels of global DNA hypomethylation in cell nuclei and its lower cytotoxicity (at equimolar concentrations), compared with AZA [76,77].

Furthermore, we observed that the increase in cytotoxicity correlates with global 5-methylcytosine levels, especially the extent of DNA hypomethylation at DAPI-positive heterochromatic sites as revealed by 3D-qDMI through scatter plotting of MeC/DAPI codistribution. This was also true for AZA-treated cells (data not shown). Along the same lines, when localizing low-intensity MeC and DAPI sites in the same nuclei, we could map the gradual increase in LIMs from the nuclear periphery into the more interior parts of the nuclei. However, we experienced that a strong level of LID increase within the nuclei interior was already seen at the lower zebularine concentration (8–40 µM), compared to naïve cells, which did not significantly change up to the highest concentration applied (1000 µM). These LID-patterns were very similar to the one in AZA-treated cells (Figure 8), in which the majority of LIDs were found to be located in the nuclear periphery. These conclusions are drawn from images of cells with seemingly intact nuclear envelope. In fact, for drug concentrations ≥5 µM for 5-azacytidine and ≥500 µM for zebularine, a large number of cells were found to present DAPI and MeC signals outside of their nuclei, leading to the assumption that the drugs had also affected the nuclear envelope and caused DNA leakage. In these cells the respective LID curves were located below the diagonal of the graphs (not

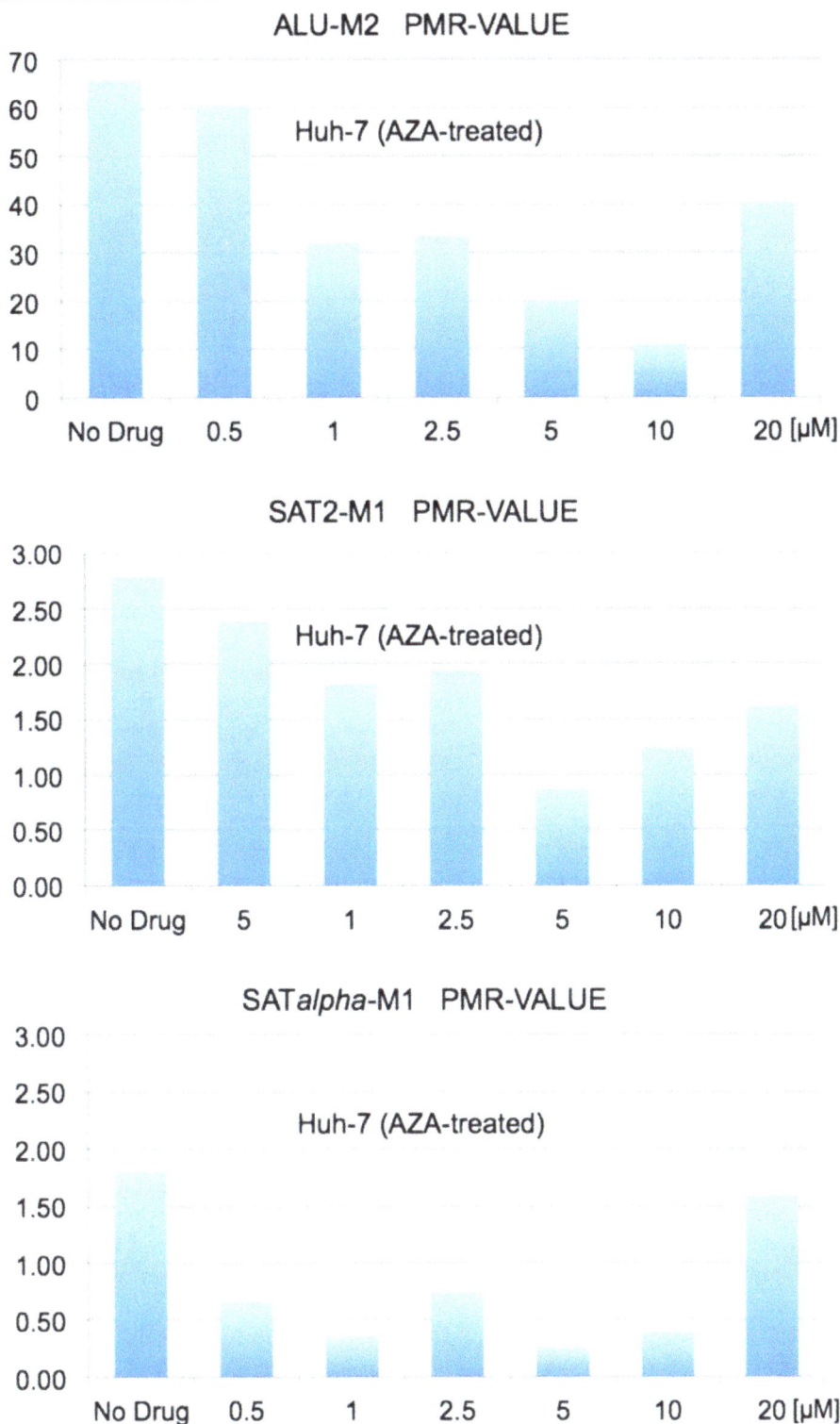

Figure 12 Drug-induced changes in DNA methylation levels of repetitive elements. DNA methylation levels of the three classes of repeat sequences Alu, Satα, and Sat2, assessed by specific MethyLight assays, significantly decreased in Huh-7 cells upon treatment with AZA. The degree of hypomethylation correlated with drug concentration, with the exception of an increase in DNA methylation seen for all three repetitive elements at the 20 μM AZA concentration.

Table 1 Correlation between imaging and sequence-based methylcytosine levels

AZA concentration	3D-qDMI Normalized MeC intensity	MethyLight		
		Normalized Alu PMR value	Normalized Sat2 PMR value	Normalized Satα PMR value
No Drug	1.00	1.00	1.00	1.00
0.5 μM	0.72	0.92	0.86	0.37
1 μM	0.34	0.49	0.65	0.20
2.5 μM	0.26	0.51	0.69	0.42
5 μM	0.20	0.31	0.31	0.15
10 μM	0.14	0.17	0.45	0.22
20 μM	0.13	0.61	0.58	0.88
Correlation coefficient R*		0.96	0.89	0.86

* Correlation coefficient R was calculated between the normalized MeC intensities measured by 3D-qDMI and normalized PMR values of the three classes of repetitive elements obtained by MethyLight, excluding the values for 20 μM of AZA.

shown). Due to the cytotoxic effect induced by high drug concentrations, such cells were not included in our further analyses.

Therefore we cannot exclude any contribution of topological changes of gDNA/heterochromatin to cytotoxicity. On the contrary, we assume that global DNA demethylation may lead to both DNA hypomethylation as well as gDNA reorganization, which are bilateral and together could lead to cellular decline. Although, our data here suggest that cytotoxicity is more fine-correlated with DNA hypomethylation than with bulk DNA reorganization. However, it may also be possible that only local gDNA rearrangements occurred under the conditions applied in our study. The latter effect is conceivable from the increase of LIMs in nuclear areas that harbor heterochromatin: as a significant LIM increase was detected for cells already at low zebularine doses, a compounding of both DNA demethylation effects may have triggered cellular disruption. Figure 6 underlines the fact that 5-azacytidine has equivalent effects at concentrations that are much lower than of zebularine.

The mode of action of azanucleosides is quite complex [78]. Cytosine hypomethylation by azanucleosides, including zebularine, has been extensively reported to reactivate tumor suppressor genes and apoptosis-related genes [79-81] but also the relaxation of highly compacted chromatin that can be seen as a loss of gDNA (DAPI) signal per voxel [43,44], as chromatin conformation is linked to DNA methylation and its bilateral relationship to histone tail modifications [82]. Therefore, we believe that cell-by-cell topological analysis as used in our approach, i.e. the topology of LIMs and LIDs in combination with the display of differential MeC/DAPI colocalization patterns shows a potential to serve as a valuable indicator for the observed phenomena: cytotoxicity-correlated global DNA hypomethylation and DNA reorganization, as consequences of drug effects. For the selected combinations of cell types and agents, the measurement of mean MeC signal (I_{MeC}) — a

derivative of DNA methylation load, across all imaged cells — corresponded well with the level of cytotoxicity (Figure 4). However, for the majority of cases I_{MeC} presented a relatively high standard deviation, whereas for the same cell populations we observed a low fraction of dissimilar cells in terms of MeC/gDNA distribution (Figure 5). The discrepancy between the two signatures becomes more plausible with the analysis of synchronized DU145 cells: high similarity was measured between G0/G1-cells and G2-cells in MeC/DAPI codistribution (Figure 10). On the contrary, individual intensity values for global 5-methylcytosine (MeC) and overall DNA (DAPI) nearly doubled between G0/G1-phase and G2-phase as expected, although with a large spread in both signal distributions indicating high signal variability even in synchronized cells (Figure 11). Based on these findings, we believe that signatures based on spatial MeC/DAPI codistribution are more robust in MeC-phenotyping of cells than simply measuring DNA methylation loads, as they can better distinguish between drug-induced demethylation effects and the variation of methylation among individual cells. In combination with K-L divergence measurement, such a cell-by-cell cross-examination as performed with 3D-qDMI can provide structure-based quantities for studying epigenetic drug response.

Finally, in order to test the quantitative accuracy of 3D-qDMI a comparative analysis was performed utilizing MethyLight assays that have been specifically designed for and proven to measure differential levels of DNA methylation in repeat sequences such as Alu, Sat2, and Satα with high confidence [65]. These sequences are highly methylated in human cells and also represent a significant portion of their genomes. Therefore, they have been proven to serve as surrogates for measuring the global content of 5-methylcytosine in cells. Our comparative analyses revealed a significantly high degree of correlation between the outcomes of the two methods. We chose MethyLight as a validated technique over high-pressure liquid chromatography (HPLC), used as a standard method for measuring global DNA methylation: as the latter method requires significantly more input DNA (5–10 μg).

We conclude that the results of our work strongly support the idea of utilizing the spatial higher-order genome organization as a sentinel for drug-induced toxicity effects in liaison with global DNA hypomethylation. In particular, nuclear DNA methylation distribution patterns have proven to serve as an indicator of topological changes of the genome that could perturb spatial interactions of genomic loci and subsequent expression programs leading to cytotoxicity in treated cells. This is quite conceivable as it has been observed that DNA hypomethylation after treatment with DNMTi can be accompanied by additional changes in histone-tail modifications and nucleosome depletion that decrease DNA-repressive mechanisms and support a more open chromatin conformation [83-86], an effect that we could reconcile with 3D image analysis for H3K9me3. A decrease in this repressive and compacting chromatin landmark with increasing doses of 5-azacytidine correlates well with a decrease in gDNA signal, and could be interpreted as chromatin decondensation (Figure 7). These downstream effects remain to be evaluated by determining the underlying molecular effects of possible cellular reprogramming, including the degree of heterochromatin demethylation [87]. Especially, the loss of global DNA methylation at heterochromatic areas of the genome that harbor highly repetitive DNA sequences such as highly abundant Alu repeats, transposable long interspersed nuclear elements (LINEs) and satellite DNAs can be associated with multiple risks towards genome instability [8,88]; through an adverse reorganization of the genome with side effects, such as transcriptional activation of oncogenes, activation of latent retrotransposons, chromosomal instability, and telomere elongation of chromosomes [11,89-92]. More specifically, Satα and Sat2 DNA hypomethylation may favor centromeric and pericentromeric instability, respectively. Alu retroelements, if left unchecked, would insert throughout the genome into noncoding and coding regions. The result would be mutations, and activation of oncogenes: spontaneous insertion of an Alu element causes nearby promoters to be hypomethylated, increasing gene expression [93,94]. Diseases directly associated with Alu insertion into coding regions include neurofibromatosis, haemophilia, agammaglobulinaemia, leukemia, breast cancer and ovarian cancer [95]. Any malignancy caused by Alu insertion is both heritable along somatic cell lines as well as in the germline. This concern has been recently strengthened by observations, in which specific genomic areas were found to become re-methylated during a following DNA replication step after initial drug-induced demethylation; as a possible mechanism to protect these sequences from permanent hypomethylation [96]. The study showed that exposure of cancer cells to agents such as 5-azacytidine and decitabine preferentially led to demethylation of CpGs not located in CpG-islands, whereas island-associated CpGs became preferentially re-methylated, suggesting that CG-dinucleotides in repetitive elements could become more persistently hypomethylated than gene-associated CGs.

Conclusions

In light of these observations, it appears reasonable to point out the necessity of new assays and complementary bioinformatics for detecting unwanted genomic-scale adverse effects such as heterochromatin reorganization, that could be used as endpoints in the cytotoxic and genotoxic risk assessment of already existing demethylating drugs and next-generation chromatin-targeting agents under development. Recent advancements in cellular imaging and computational image analysis have made it feasible for large volumes of images from thousands of cells to be analyzed in relatively short amount of time at substantially lower costs. Imaging-based cytomics also enables the quantification of spatial and temporal distribution of molecules and cellular components within their native environment [97], which can boost understanding drug activity at the cell systemic level. Within this context, MeC phenotyping appears to provide a valuable technology, and further investigations will be crucial to evaluate its performance for a broader spectrum of epigenetic drugs in cytotoxicity and eventually genotoxicity testing. Hence, the combination of 3D-qDMI with comparative techniques that provide genome-wide sequence-specific MeC-profiles and detail concurrent changes in chromatin conformation could lead to validation of MeC phenotypes in assessment of drug-induced chromatin states. A variety of impressive high-resolution sequencing-based techniques have recently become available such as NOMe-Seq [39], which provides nucleosome positioning landscapes; chromosome conformation capture (3C) methodology and its whole-genomic version Hi-C, which map the 3D architecture of the genome by proximity-based ligation and subsequent next-generation sequencing [98,99]; a related method called chromatin interaction analysis using paired-end tag sequencing (ChIA–PET) [100], and newer attempts that focus on increasing the sensitivity of chromatin immunoprecipitation-based assays towards single-cell analysis [101]. For example: the correlation of chromatin textures derived from MeC patterns with matching nucleosome depleted regions and proximity-ligation profiles can lead to the identification of MeC phenotypes indicative of risky and genotoxic drug effects.

Abbreviations

CSMC: Cedars-Sinai Medical Center; Cy3: Cyanine 3; FBS: Fetal bovine serum; IC_{10}: Inhibitory concentration at which 10% of cells are nonviable.

Competing interest

The authors declare that they have no competing interests.

Authors' contributions

JT designed and conducted the study, and performed all drug experiments. JHO contributed with cell synchronization assays. KAW performed imaging. AG and JT conceptualized image analyses. AG contributed analytical software tools. AG and JT performed image and statistical data analysis. JT wrote the manuscript together with AG. DJW was in charge of the comparative MethyLight assays and helped with manuscript revision. All authors read and approved the final manuscript.

Acknowledgements

We thank Patricia Lin (CSMC Research Flow Cytometry Core) for helping us with flow cytometry and Vaithilingaraja Arumugaswami (CSMC) for Huh-7 cells. This work was supported by the DOD-CDMRP Award W81XWH-10-1-0939 (to JT), the NIH grant 1R21CA143618-01A1 (to AG), and institutional grants from the Department of Surgery at CSMC.

Author details

[1]Translational Cytomics Group, Department of Surgery, Cedars-Sinai Medical Center, Los Angeles, CA 90048, USA. [2]Chromatin Biology Laboratory, Department of Surgery, Cedars-Sinai Medical Center, Los Angeles, CA 90048, USA. [3]Bioinformatics Laboratory, Department of Surgery, Cedars-Sinai Medical Center, Los Angeles, CA 90048, USA. [4]Department of Biomedical Sciences, Cedars-Sinai Medical Center, Los Angeles, CA 90048, USA. [5]USC Epigenome Center, Keck School of Medicine, University of Southern California, Los Angeles, CA 90089, USA.

References

1. Jaenisch R, Bird A: **Epigenetic regulation of gene expression: how the genome integrates intrinsic and environmental signals.** *Nat Genet* 2003, **33**:245–254.
2. Jones PA, Baylin SB: **The epigenomics of cancer.** *Cell* 2007, **128**:683–692.
3. Herman JG, Baylin SB: **Gene silencing in cancer is associated with promoter hypermethylation.** *N Engl J Med* 2003, **349**:2042–2054.
4. Esteller M: **Epigenetics in cancer.** *N Engl J Med* 2008, **358**:1148–1159.
5. Costello JF, Frühwald MC, Smiraglia DJ, Rush LJ, Robertson GP, Gao X, Wright FA, Feramisco JD, Peltomäki P, Lang JC, Schuller DE, Yu L, Bloomfield CD, Caligiuri MA, Yates A, Nishikawa R, Su Huang H, Petrelli NJ, Zhang X, O'Dorisio MS, Held WA, Cavenee WK, Plass C: **Aberrant CpG-island methylation has non-random and tumour-type-specific patterns.** *Nat Genet* 2000, **24**:132–138.
6. Ehrlich M, Gama-Sosa MA, Huang LH, Midgett RM, Kuo KC, McCune RA, Gehrke C: **Amount and distribution of 5-methylcytosine in human DNA from different types of tissues of cells.** *Nucleic Acids Res* 1982, **10**:2709–2721.
7. Gardiner-Garden M, Frommer M: **CpG islands in vertebrate genomes.** *J Mol Biol* 1987, **196**:261–282.
8. Ehrlich M: **DNA Hypomethylation in cancer cells.** *Epigenomics* 2009, **1**:239–259.
9. Puitri EL, Robertson KD: **Epigenetic mechanisms and genome stability.** *Clin Epigenetics* 2011, **2**:299–314.
10. Peng JC, Karpen GH: **Epigenetic regulation of heterochromatic stability.** *Curr Opin Genet Dev* 2008, **18**:204–211.
11. Feinberg AP, Vogelstein B: **Hypomethylation distinguishes genes of some human cancers from their normal counterparts.** *Nature* 1983, **301**:89–92.
12. Gama-Sosa MA, Slagel VA, Trewyn RW, Oxenhandler R, Kuo KC, Kuo KC, Gehrke CW, Ehrlich M: **The 5-methylcytosine content of DNA from human tumors.** *Nucleic Acid Res* 1983, **11**:6883–6894.
13. Ehrlich M: **NA hypomethylation and cancer.** In *DNA Alterations in Cancer: Genetic and Epigenetic Changes.* Edited by Ehrlich M. Natick, MA: Eaton Publishing; 2000:273–291.
14. Dunn BK: **Hypomethylation: one side of a larger picture.** *Ann N Y Acad Sci* 2003, **983**:28–42.
15. Fraser P, Bickmore W: **Nuclear organization of the genome and the potential for gene regulation.** *Nature* 2007, **447**:413–417.
16. Deal RB, Henikoff S: **Capturing the dynamic epigenome.** *Genome Biol* 2010, **11**:218.
17. Misteli T: **Higher-order genome organization in human disease.** *Cold Spring Harb Perspect Biol* 2010, **2**:a000794.
18. Li G, Reinberg D: **Chromatin higher-order structures and gene regulation.** *Curr Opin Genet Dev* 2011, **21**:175–186.
19. Tajbakhsh J: **DNA methylation topology: potential of a chromatin landmark for epigenetic drug toxicology.** *Epigenomics* 2011, **3**:761–770.
20. Yoo CB, Jones PA: **Epigenetic therapy of cancer: past, present and future.** *Nat Rev Drug Discov* 2006, **5**:37–50.
21. Gore SD, Jones C, Kirkpatrick P: **Decitabine.** *Nat Rev Drug Discov* 2006, **5**:891–892.
22. Issa JP, Kantarjian H: **5-azacytidine.** *Nat Rev Drug Discov* 2005, (Suppl):S6–S7.
23. Cheng JC, Matsen CB, Gonzales FA, Ye W, Greer S, Marquez VE, Jones PA, Selker EU: **Inhibition of DNA methylation and reactivation of silenced genes by zebularine.** *J Natl Cancer Inst* 2003, **95**:399–409.
24. Yoo CB, Cheng JC, Jones PA: **Zebularine: a new drug for epigenetic therapy.** *Biochem Soc Trans* 2004, **32**:910–912.
25. Marquez VE, Kelley JA, Agbaria R, Ben-Kasus T, Cheng JC, Yoo CB, Jones PA: **Zebularine: a unique molecule for an epigenetically based strategy in cancer chemotherapy.** *Ann N Y Acad Sci* 2005, **1058**:246–254.
26. Herranz M, Martín-Caballero J, Fraga MF, Ruiz-Cabello J, Flores JM, Desco M, Marquez V, Esteller M: **The novel DNA methylation inhibitor zebularine is effective against the development of murine T-cell lymphoma.** *Blood* 2006, **107**:1174–1177.
27. Stresemann C, Bokelmann I, Mahlknecht U, Lyko F: **5-azacytidine causes complex DNA methylation responses in myeloid leukemia.** *Mol Cancer Ther* 2008, **7**:2998–3005.
28. Santi DV, Norment A, Garrett CE: **Covalent bond formation between a DNA-cytosine methyltransferase and DNA containing 5-azacytosine.** *Proc Natl Acad Sci USA* 1984, **81**:6993–6997.
29. Bender CM, Gonzalgo ML, Gonzales FA, Nguyen CT, Robertson KD, Jones PA: **Roles of Cell Division and Gene Transcription in the Methylation of CpG Islands.** *Mol Cell Biol* 1999, **19**:6690–6698.
30. Weisenberger DJ, Velicescu M, Cheng JC, Gonzales FA, Liang G, Jones PA: **Role of the DNA Methyltransferase Variant DNMT3b3 in DNA Methylation.** *Mol Cancer Res* 2004, **2**:62–72.
31. Ghoshal K, Datta J, Majumder S, Bai S, Kutay H, Motiwala T, Jacob ST: **5-Aza-Deoxycytidine Induces Selective Degradation of DNA Methyltransferase 1 by a Proteasomal Pathway That Requires the KEN Box, Bromo-Adjacent Homology Domain, and Nuclear Localization Signal.** *Mol Cell Biol* 2005, **25**:4727–4741.
32. Zhu WG, Hileman T, Ke Y, Wang P, Lu S, Duan W, Dai Z, Tong T, Villalona-Calero MA, Plass C, Otterson GA: **5-aza-2′-deoxycytidine activates the p53/p21Waf1/Cip1 pathway to inhibit cell proliferation.** *J Biol Chem* 2004, **279**:15161–15166.
33. Yang X, Noushmehr H, Han H, Andreu-Vieyra C, Liang G, Jones PA: **Gene reactivation by 5-aza-2′-deoxycytidine-induced demethylation requires SRCAP-mediated H2A.Z insertion to establish nucleosome depleted regions.** *PLoS Genet* 2012, **8**:e1002604.
34. Patra SK, Patra A, Rizzi F, Ghosh TC, Bettuzzi S: **Demethylation of (Cytosine-5-C-methyl) DNA and regulation of transcription in the epigenetic pathways of cancer development.** *Cancer Metastasis Rev* 2008, **27**:315–334.
35. Patra SK, Bettuzzi S: **Epigenetic DNA-(cytosine-5-carbon) modifications: 5-aza-2′-deoxycytidine and DNA-demethylation.** *Biochemistry (Mosc)* 2009, **74**:613–619.
36. Ammerpohl O, Martin-Subero JI, Richter J, Vater I, Siebert R: **Hunting for the 5th base: Techniques for analyzing DNA methylation.** *Biochim Biophys Acta* 2009, **1790**:847–862.
37. Laird PW: **Principles and challenges of genome-wide DNA methylation analysis.** *Nat Rev Genet* 2010, **11**:191–203.
38. Fatemi M, Pao MM, Jeong S, Gal-Yam EN, Egger G, Weisenberger DJ, Jones PA: **Footprinting of mammalian promoters: use of a CpG DNA methyltransferase revealing nucleosome positions at a single molecule level.** *Nucleic Acids Res* 2005, **33**:e176.
39. Kelly TK, Liu Y, Lay FD, Liang G, Berman BP, Jones PA: **Genome-wide mapping of nucleosome positioning and DNA methylation within individual DNA molecules.** *Genome Res* 2012, **22**:2497–2506.
40. Haaf T: **The effects of 5-azacytidine and 5-azadeoxycytidine on chromosome structure and function: implications for methylation-associated cellular processes.** *Pharmacol Ther* 1995, **65**:19–46.

41. De Capoa A, Menendez F, Poggesi I, Giancotti P, Grappelli C, Marotta MR, Di Leandro M, Reynaud C, Niveleau A: Cytological evidence for 5-azacytidine-induced demethylation of the heterochromatic regions of human chromosomes. *Chromosome Res* 1996, **4**:271–276.

42. Tajbakhsh J, Wawrowsky KA, Gertych A, Bar-Nur O, Vishnevsky E, Lindsley EH, Farkas DL: Characterization of tumor cells and stem cells by differential nuclear methylation imaging. In *Imaging, Manipulation, and Analysis of Biomolecules, Cells, and Tissues. Proceedings of the SPIE: 19–24 January 2008*. Edited by Farkas DL DL, Nicolau DV, Robert C, Leif RC. San Jose, CA: SPIE Publications; 2008:6859F1–6859F10.

43. Gertych A, Wawrowsky KA, Lindsley E, Vishnevsky E, Farkas DL, Tajbakhsh J: Automated quantification of DNA demethylation effects in cells via 3D mapping of nuclear signatures and population homogeneity assessment. *Cytometry A* 2009, **75**:569–583.

44. Gertych A, Farkas DL, Tajbakhsh J: Measuring topology of low-intensity DNA methylation sites for high-throughput assessment of epigenetic drug-induced effects in cancer cells. *Exp Cell Res* 2010, **316**:3150–3160.

45. Szyf M: Epigenetics, DNA methylation, and chromatin modifying drugs. *Annu Rev Pharmacol Toxicol* 2009, **49**:243–263.

46. Tajbakhsh J, Gertych A, Farkas DL: Utilizing nuclear DNA methylation patterns in cell-based assays for epigenetic drug screening. *Drug Discovery World* 2010, 27–35. spring edition.

47. Tong WG, Wierda WG, Lin E, Kuang SQ, Bekele BN, Estrov Z, Wei Y, Yang H, Keating MJ, Garcia-Manero G: Genome-wide DNA methylation profiling of chronic lymphocytic leukemia allows identification of epigenetically repressed molecular pathways with clinical impact. *Epigenetics* 2010, **5**:499–508.

48. Ehrlich M: DNA hypomethylation, cancer, the immunodeficiency, centromeric region instability, facial anomalies syndrome and chromosomal rearrangements. *J Nutr* 2002, **132**:2424S–2429S.

49. Espada J, Esteller M: Epigenetic control of nuclear architecture. *Cell Mol Life Sci* 2007, **64**:449–457.

50. Santos AP, Abranches R, Stoger E, Beven A, Viegas W, Shaw PJ: The architecture of interphase chromosomes and gene positioning are altered by changes in DNA methylation and histone acetylation. *J Cell Sci* 2002, **115**:4597–4605.

51. Gilbert N, Thomson I, Boyle S, Allan J, Ramsahoye B, Bickmore WA: DNA methylation affects nuclear organization, histone modifications, and linker histone binding but not chromatin compaction. *J Cell Biol* 2007, **177**:401–411.

52. Christman JK: 5-azacytidine and 5-aza-2'-deoxycytidine as inhibitors of DNA methylation: mechanistic studies and their implications for cancer therapy. *Oncogene* 2002, **21**:5483–5495.

53. Stresemann C, Brueckner B, Musch T, Stopper H, Lyko F: Functional diversity of DNA methyltransferase inhibitors in human cancer cell lines. *Cancer Res* 2006, **66**:2794–2800.

54. Dote H, Cerna D, Burgan WE, Carter DJ, Cerra MA, Hollingshead MG, Camphausen K, Tofilon PJ: Enhancement of in vitro and in vivo tumor cell radiosensitivity by the DNA methylation inhibitor zebularine. *Clin Cancer Res* 2005, **11**:4571–4579.

55. Schwarze SR, Fu VX, Desotelle JA, Kenowski ML, Jarrard DF: The identification of senescence-specific genes during the induction of senescence in prostate cancer cells. *Neoplasia* 2005, **7**:816–823.

56. Ewald J, Desotelle J, Almassi N, Jarrard D: Drug-induced senescence bystander proliferation in prostate cancer cells in vitro and in vivo. *Br J Cancer* 2008, **98**:1244–1249.

57. Patra A, Deb M, Dahiya R, Patra SK: 5-Aza-2'-deoxycytidine stress response and apoptosis in prostate cancer. *Clin Epigenetics* 2011, **2**:339–348.

58. Venturelli S, Armeanu S, Pathil A, Hsieh CJ, Weiss TS, Vonthein R, Wehrmann M, Gregor M, Lauer UM, Bitzer M: Epigenetic combination therapy as a tumor-selective treatment approach for hepatocellular carcinoma. *Cancer* 2007, **109**:2132–2141.

59. Andersen JB, Factor VM, Marquardt JU, Raggi C, Lee YH, Seo D, Conner EA, Thorgeirsson SS: An integrated genomic and epigenomic approach predicts therapeutic response to zebularine in human liver cancer. *Sci Transl Med* 2010, **2**:54ra77.

60. Heinemann L, Simpson GR, Annels NE, Vile R, Melcher A, Prestwich R, Harrington KJ, Pandha HS: The effect of cell cycle synchronization on tumor sensitivity to reovirus oncolysis. *Mol Ther* 2010, **18**:2085–2093.

61. Whitfield ML, Zheng LX, Baldwin A, Ohta T, Hurt MM, Marzluff WF: Stem-loop binding protein, the protein that binds the 3' end of histone mRNA, is cell cycle regulated by both translational and posttranslational mechanisms. *Mol Cell Biol* 2000, **20**:4188–4198.

62. Wong C, Stearns T: Mammalian cells lack checkpoints for tetraploidy, aberrant centrosome number, and cytokinesis failure. *BMC Cell Biol* 2005, **6**:6.

63. van Engeland M, Nieland LJ, Ramaekers FC, Schutte B, Reutelingsperger CP: Annexin V-affinity assay: a review on an apoptosis detection system based on phosphatidylserine exposure. *Cytometry* 1998, **31**:1–9.

64. Tajbakhsh J, Gertych A: Three-dimensional quantitative DNA methylation imaging for chromatin texture analysis in pharmacoepigenomics and toxicoepigenomics. In *Epigenomics: From Chromatin Biology to Therapeutics*. Edited by Appasani K. Cambridge, UK: Cambridge University Press; 2012:273.

65. Weisenberger DJ, Campan M, Long TI, Kim M, Woods C, Fiala E, Ehrlich M, Laird PW: Analysis of repetitive element DNA methylation by MethyLight. *Nucleic Acids Res* 2005, **33**:6823–6836.

66. Cowell IG, Aucott R, Mahadevaiah SK, Burgoyne PS, Huskisson N, Bongiorni S, Prantera G, Fanti L, Pimpinelli S, Wu R, Gilbert DM, Shi W, Fundele R, Morrison H, Jeppesen P, Singh PB: Heterochromatin, HP1 and methylation at lysine 9 of histone H3 in animals. *Chromosoma* 2002, **111**:22–36.

67. Lachner M, O'Carroll D, Rea S, Mechtler K, Jenuwein T: Methylation of histone H3 lysine 9 creates a binding site for HP1 proteins. *Nature* 2001, **410**:116–120.

68. Peng JC, Karpen GH: Heterochromatic genome stability requires regulators of histone H3 K9 methylation. *PLoS Genet* 2009, **5**:e1000435.

69. Shvachko LP: Alterations of constitutive pericentromeric heterochromatin in lymphocytes of cancer patients and lymphocytes exposed to 5-azacytidine is associated with hypomethylation. *Exp Oncol* 2008, **30**:230–234.

70. Chiam K, Centenera MM, Butler LM, Tilley WD, Bianco-Miotto T: GSTP1 DNA methylation and expression status is indicative of 5-aza-2'-deoxycytidine efficacy in human prostate cancer cells. *PLoS One* 2011, **6**:e25634.

71. Chen M, Shabashvili D, Nawab A, Yang SX, Dyer LM, Brown KD, Hollingshead M, Hunter KW, Kaye FJ, Hochwald SN, Marquez VE, Steeg P, Zajac-Kaye M: DNA methyltransferase inhibitor, zebularine, delays tumor growth and induces apoptosis in a genetically engineered mouse model of breast cancer. *Mol Cancer Ther* 2012, **11**:370–382.

72. Lang P, Yeow K, Nichols A, Scheer A: Cellular imaging in drug discovery. *Nat Rev Drug Discov* 2006, **5**:343–356.

73. Cheng JC, Weisenberger DJ, Gonzales FA, Liang G, Xu GL, Hu YG, Marquez VE, Jones PA: Continuous zebularine treatment effectively sustains demethylation in human bladder cancer cells. *Mol Cell Biol* 2004, **24**:1270–1278.

74. Scott SA, Lakshimikuttysamma A, Sheridan DP, Sanche SE, Geyer CR, Hu YG, Marquez VE, Jones PA: Zebularine inhibits human acute myeloid leukemia cell growth in vitro in association with p15INK4B demethylation and reexpression. *Exp Hematol* 2007, **35**:263–273.

75. Billam M, Sobolewski MD, Davidson NE: Effects of a novel DNA methyltransferase inhibitor zebularine on human breast cancer cells. *Breast Cancer Res Treat* 2010, **120**:581–592.

76. van Bemmel DM, Brank AS, Eritja R, Marquez VE, Christman JK: DNA (Cytosine-C5) methyltransferase inhibition by oligodeoxyribonucleotides containing 2-(1H)-pyrimidinone (zebularine aglycon) at the enzymatic target site. *Biochem Pharmacol* 2009, **78**:633–641.

77. Champion C, Guianvarc'h D, Sénamaud-Beaufort C, Jurkowska RZ, Jeltsch A, Ponger L, Arimondo PB, Guieysse-Peugeot AL: Mechanistic insights on the inhibition of c5 DNA methyltransferases by zebularine. *PLoS One* 2010, **5**:e12388.

78. Stresemann C, Lyko F: Modes of action of the DNA methyltransferase inhibitors 5-azacytidine and decitabine. *Int J Cancer* 2008, **123**:8–13.

79. Huang J, Plass C, Gerhauser C: Cancer chemoprevention by targeting the epigenome. *Curr Drug Targets* 2011, **12**:1925–1956.

80. Khan R, Schmidt-Mende J, Karimi M, Gogvadze V, Hassan M, Ekström TJ, Zhivotovsky B, Hellström-Lindberg E: Hypomethylation and apoptosis in 5-azacytidine-treated myeloid cells. *Exp Hematol* 2008, **36**:149–157.

81. Ruiz-Magaña MJ, Rodríguez-Vargas JM, Morales JC, Saldivia MA, Schulze-Osthoff K, Ruiz-Ruiz C: The DNA methyltransferase inhibitors zebularine and decitabine induce mitochondria-mediated apoptosis and DNA damage in p53 mutant leukemic T cells. *Int J Cancer* 2012, **130**:1195–1207.

82. D'Alessio AC, Szyf M: Epigenetic tête-à-tête: the bilateral relationship between chromatin modifications and DNA methylation. *Biochem Cell Biol* 2006, **84**:463–476.

83. Nguyen CT, Weisenberger DJ, Velicescu M, Gonzales FA, Lin JC, Liang G, Jones PA: Histone H3-lysine 9 methylation is associated with aberrant gene silencing in cancer cells and is rapidly reversed by 5-aza-2′-deoxycytidine. *Cancer Res* 2002, **62**:6456–6461.

84. Lin JC, Jeong S, Liang G, Takai D, Fatemi M, Tsai YC, Egger G, Gal-Yam EN, Jones PA: Role of nucleosomal occupancy in the epigenetic silencing of the MLH1 CpG island. *Cancer Cell* 2007, **12**:432–444.

85. Komashko VM, Farnham PJ: 5-azacytidine treatment reorganizes genomic histone modification patterns. *Epigenetics* 2010, **5**:229–240.

86. Si J, Boumber YA, Shu J, Qin T, Ahmed S, He R, Jelinek J, Issa JP: Chromatin remodeling is required for gene reactivation after decitabine-mediated DNA hypomethylation. *Cancer Res* 2010, **70**:6968–6977.

87. Csoka AB, Szyf M: Epigenetic side-effects of common pharmaceuticals: a potential new field in medicine and pharmacology. *Med Hypotheses* 2009, **73**:770–780.

88. Gaudet F, Hodgson JG, Eden A, Jackson-Grusby L, Dausman J, Gray JW, Leonhardt H, Jaenisch R: Induction of tumors in mice by genomic hypomethylation. *Science* 2003, **300**:489–492.

89. Holliday R, Pugh JE: DNA modification mechanisms and gene activity during development. *Science* 1975, **187**:226–232.

90. Bestor TH, Tycko B: Creation of genomic methylation patterns. *Nat Genet* 1996, **12**:363–367.

91. Ehrlich M: DNA methylation in cancer: too much, but also too little. *Oncogene* 2002, **21**:5400–5413.

92. Vera E, Canela A, Fraga MF, Esteller M, Blasco MA: Epigenetic regulation of telomeres in human cancer. *Oncogene* 2008, **27**:6817–6833.

93. Feltus FA, Lee EK, Costello JF, Plass C, Vertino PM: DNA motifs associated with aberrant CpG island methylation. *Genomics* 2006, **87**:5728–5729.

94. Kang MI, Rhyu MG, Kim YH, Jung YC, Hong SJ, Cho CS, Kim HS: The length of CpG islands is associated with the distribution of Alu and L1 retroelements. *Genomics* 2006, **87**:580–590.

95. Deininger PL, Batzer MA: Alu repeats and human disease. *Mol Genet Metab* 1999, **67**:183–193.

96. Hagemann S, Heil O, Lyko F, Brueckner B: 5-azacytidine and decitabine induce gene-specific and non-random DNA demethylation in human cancer cell lines. *PLoS One* 2011, **6**:e17388.

97. Tárnok A: Cytomics for discovering drugs. *Cytometry A* 2010, **77**:1–2.

98. Dostie J, Richmond TA, Arnaout RR, Selzer RA, Lee WL, Honan TA, Rubio ED, Krumm A, Lamb J, Nusbaum C, Green RD, Dekker J: Chromosome conformation capture carbon copy (5C): a massively parallel solution for mapping interactions between genomic elements. *Genome Res* 2006, **16**:1299–1309.

99. Lieberman-Aiden E, van Berkum NL, Williams L, Imakaev M, Ragoczy T, Telling A, Amit I, Lajoie BR, Sabo PJ, Dorschner MO, Sandstrom R, Bernstein B, Bender MA, Groudine M, Gnirke A, Stamatoyannopoulos J, Mirny LA, Lander ES, Dekker J: Comprehensive mapping of long-range interactions reveals folding principles of the human genome. *Science* 2009, **326**:289–293.

100. Fullwood MJ, Fullwood MJ, Liu MH, Pan YF, Liu J, Xu H, Mohamed YB, Orlov YL, Velkov S, Ho A, Mei PH, Chew EG, Huang PY, Welboren WJ, Han Y, Ooi HS, Ariyaratne PN, Vega VB, Luo Y, Tan PY, Choy PY, Wansa KD, Zhao B, Lim KS, Leow SC, Yow JS, Joseph R, Li H, Desai KV, Thomsen JS, *et al*: An oestrogen-receptor-a-bound human chromatin interactome. *Nature* 2009, **462**:58–64.

101. Goren A, Ozsolak F, Shoresh N, Ku M, Adli M, Hart C, Gymrek M, Zuk O, Regev A, Milos PM, Bernstein BE: Chromatin profiling by directly sequencing small quantities of immunoprecipitated DNA. *Nat Methods* 2010, **7**:47–49.

3

Effects of paliperidone extended release on the symptoms and functioning of schizophrenia

Min-Wei Huang[1,2], Tsung-Tsair Yang[3], Po-Ren Ten[4], Po-Wen Su[5], Bo-Jian Wu[6], Chin-Hong Chan[7], Tsuo-Hung Lan[7], I-Chao Liu[3], Wei-Cheh Chiu[8], Chun-Ying Li[1], Kuo-Sheng Cheng[1,9] and Yu-Chi Yeh[8]*

Abstract

Background: We aimed to explore relations between symptomatic remission and functionality evaluation in schizophrenia patients treated with paliperidone extended-release (ER), as seen in a normal day-to-day practice, using flexible dosing regimens of paliperidone ER. We explored symptomatic remission rate in patients treated with flexibly dosed paliperidone ER by 8 items of Positive and Negative Syndrome Scale (PANSS) and change of Personal and Social Performance (PSP) scale.

Method: This was a 12-week multicenter, open-label, prospective clinical study conducted in in-patient and out-patient populations. Flexible dosing in the range 3-12 mg/day was used throughout the study. All subjects attended clinic visits on weeks 0, 4, 8, and 12 as usual clinical practice for the 12-week observation period. Data were summarized with respect to demographic and baseline characteristics, efficacy measurement with PANSS scale, PSP, and social functioning score, and safety observations. Descriptive statistics were performed to identify the retention rate at each visit as well as the symptomatic remission rate. Summary statistics of average doses the subjects received were based on all subjects participating in the study.

Results: A total of 480 patients were enrolled. Among them, 426 patients (88.8%) had evaluation at week 4 and 350 (72.9%) completed the 12-week evaluation. Patients with at least moderate severity of schizophrenia were evaluated as "mild" or better on PANSS scale by all 8 items after 12 weeks of treatment with paliperidone ER. There was significant improvement in patients' functionality as measured by PSP improvement and score changes. Concerning the other efficacy parameters, PANSS total scale, PSP total scale, and social functioning total scale at the end of study all indicated statistically significant improvement by comparison with baseline. The safety profile also demonstrated that paliperidone ER was well-tolerated without clinically significant changes after treatment administration.

Conclusions: Although the short-term nature of this study may limit the potential for assessing improvements in function, it is noteworthy that in the present short-term study significant improvements in patient personal and social functioning with paliperidone ER treatment were observed, as assessed by PSP scale.

Trial Registration: Clinical Trials. PAL-TWN-MA3

Background

Schizophrenia is a severe form of mental illness affecting about 24 million people worldwide (7 per 1000 adult population), mostly in the age group 15-35 years. Although the incidence is low (3/10,000), the prevalence is high due to chronicity [1]. Deficits in social functioning can be observed throughout the course of

schizophrenia: in the early stages, during acute exacerbations, and over long-term maintenance treatment.

The early course of schizophrenia typically includes a prodromal phase characterized by nonspecific symptoms and behaviors, a formal onset/deteriorative stage with active psychosis, cognitive impairment, negative symptoms, and social deficits, and a period of several years following the initial episode that often includes repeated episodes of psychosis with a progressive increase in residual symptoms and functional decline. There is general

* Correspondence: yeh.yuchi@gmail.com
[8]Department of Psychiatry, Cathay General Hospital, Taipei 10630, Taiwan
Full list of author information is available at the end of the article

agreement that approximately 5 years after the initial psychotic episode patients enter a chronic, but relatively more stable phase with no marked further decline in functioning or increase in residual symptoms [1-5].

With the advancement of new medications, treatment goals of patients with schizophrenia were raised. On the one hand, remission, instead of response was recognized as the optimal treatment goal for patients with schizophrenia. Research on treatments for schizophrenia focused predominantly on symptom improvement; however, outcomes such as cognition, health-related quality of life, and social functioning are now being recognized as important indices of treatment success. The Remission in Schizophrenia Working Group (RSWG) chose 8 items of PANSS (delusions, unusual thought content, hallucinatory behavior, conceptual disorganization, mannerisms/posturing, blunted affect, social withdrawal, and lack of spontaneity) as determinants for the definition of remission [6]. Several studies have already implemented this concept and found that patients achieving remission status had better performance in neuropsychological tests and greater social and occupational functions [7-9]. On the other hand, functionality became an important focus of treatment in psychotic patients. Patients who returned to normal life were considered as undergoing "truly recovery" [5]. The Personal and Social Performance (PSP) scale, developed to measure patients' personal and social functionality, is a convenient tool in clinical practice. Several clinical trials measured patients' functioning as study endpoints with this scale [10].

Typically with antipsychotic drugs, dose titration to the maintenance dose is recommended. Paliperidone is available in a formulation using extended-release (ER) osmotic release technology (OROS®), hereinafter referred to as paliperidone ER. This formulation was designed to deliver paliperidone at a controlled rate over a 24-hour period, resulting in a gradual increase in plasma concentration after the first intake and low peak-to-trough fluctuation at steady state [11]. Paliperidone is the major metabolite of risperidone. It is a prolonged release oral atypical antipsychotic for the treatment of schizophrenia. Based on preclinical experiments and clinical investigations, paliperidone is an effective and safe antipsychotic medication for the treatment of schizophrenia. Some studies showed that paliperidone ER significantly improved symptoms and functioning in schizophrenia patients regardless of time since diagnosis [4,12-15]. The phase III well-controlled pivotal efficacy and safety studies were performed using randomly applied fixed dosages (3, 6, 9, 12, or 15 mg/day) of paliperidone ER. In daily clinical practice, however, flexible dosing is applied based on the individual needs of patients. The pivotal studies were also performed in well-defined homogenous groups of subjects

with schizophrenia. In daily clinical practice, however, a more diverse population is treated, e.g. having higher rates of comorbidities and/or comedications. Pivotal studies also used an initial washout period. Therefore, no data for direct transition from a variety of oral antipsychotics to flexibly dosed paliperidone ER are available today.

In most treatment-related clinical trials, response, measured with certain percent improvement of rating scales, is used as outcome determinant. However, approaches focusing on psychotic patients' real life functioning are the main interest of clinical practice. Achieving symptom-free and normal life ought to be the key measure in clinical studies. Moreover, understanding symptom-free function is of great value for treatment goals in clinical practice. Therefore, we designed this study to explore symptomatic remission and functionality evaluation in patients treated with paliperidone ER, as seen in normal day-to-day practice, using flexible dosing regimens.

Methods
2.1 Study Design
This was a 12-week, multicenter, open-label, prospective clinical study conducted in inpatients and outpatients. Throughout the study flexible dosing in the range 3-12 mg/day was used so as to allow investigators to adjust the dosage of each subject based on individual needs. In general, the recommended paliperidone ER dose was 6 mg once daily, although some subjects benefited from lower or higher doses in the recommended dose range.

After obtaining informed consent, baseline characteristics, PANSS scale, PSP, and social functioning scale were assessed and recorded. Treatment of these subjects was decided by clinicians' opinion. As for patients with pharmacotherapy, dosing was flexible throughout the study period according to investigators' discretion based on individual subjects' clinical response to and tolerability of study drug. During the study observation period, subjects attended clinic visits on weeks 0, 4, 8, and 12 as usual clinical practice. At the preplanned clinic visits, PANSS and PSP scale, reports of adverse events, and treatment information were recorded. Subjects could withdraw from this study at any time; reasons of withdrawal or loss of follow-up were recorded. The study was approved by the Institutional Review Board of Cathay General Hospital (protocol no. PAL-TWN-MA3).

2.2 Patient Population
Participants were male or female and met DSM-IV diagnostic criteria above aged 18 years. They were drug naïve; their previous treatment was considered unsuccessful due to one or more of the following reasons:

lack of efficacy, lack of tolerability or safety, lack of compliance, and/or other reasons. Subjects or their legally acceptable representatives had signed an informed consent document indicating that they understood the purpose of and procedures required for the study and were willing to participate in the study. Female subjects were postmenopausal for ≥ 1 year, surgically sterile, abstinent, or, if sexually active, agreed to practice an effective method of birth control before entry and throughout the study. Effective methods of birth control included prescription hormonal contraceptives, contraceptive injections, intrauterine devices, double-barrier method, contraceptive patch, and male partner sterilization. Female subjects also had a negative urine pregnancy test at screening.

Individuals were excluded from the study if the patients were on clozapine, paliperidone ER, any conventional depot neuroleptic or Risperdal® Consta® during the last 3 months. Subjects experienced serious unstable medical condition including known clinically relevant laboratory abnormalities, history of neuroleptic malignant syndrome, hypersensitivity to paliperidone ER or risperidone or inability to swallow the study medication whole with the aid of water (subjects may not chew, divide, dissolve, or crush the study medication because this may affect the release profile) were excluded. Pregnant or breast-feeding woman and participation in another investigational drug trial in the 30 days prior to selection were also excluded from the study. Of course, employees of the investigator or study center, persons with direct involvement in the proposed study or other studies under the direction of that investigator or study center, or family members of the employees or the investigator were not allowable.

At each visit subjects received the amount of medication required until the next visit. Subjects from any oral antipsychotic medication could be switched to an effective dose of paliperidone ER without the need for titration. Subjects could be cross-tapered in different ways from their previous antipsychotic medication, e.g. a decrease of the previous antipsychotic drug may occur at the time of or after initiation of paliperidone ER. The period of cross-tapering also varied among subjects, since both dosing and timing of transition depended on relevant individual subject characteristics such as kind and severity of current symptoms or adverse events, course of previous relapses and rehospitalizations, or type and dose of previous antipsychotic medication (e.g. with or without anticholinergic and/or sedating properties).

The neuropsychiatric symptoms of schizophrenia were assessed by 30-item PANSS scale, which provides a total score (sum of the scores of all 30 items). Each scale is rated 1 (absent) to 7 (extreme). The PANSS assessment was performed by a qualified rater defined as a trained clinician. If possible, for a given subject, the same rater assessed this scale at all visits. Subjects were interviewed at each visit to assess the psychiatric symptoms of schizophrenia.

The following 8 items were used as determinants for remission:
-P1 Delusions
-P2 Conceptual disorganization
-P3 Hallucinatory behavior
-G9 Unusual thought content
-G5 Mannerisms and posturing
-N1 Blunted affect
-N4 Social withdrawal
-N6 Lack of spontaneity/flow of conversation

Subjects were rated for their personal and social performance at each visit by PSP scale. This scale assessed the degree of difficulty a subject exhibited over a 1-month period within 4 domains of behavior: socially useful activities, personal and social relations, self-care, and disturbing and aggressive behavior. The score ranged from 1 to 100, divided into 10 equal intervals to rate the degree of difficulty (absent to very severe) in each of the 4 domains. Subjects with scores 71-100 had a mild degree of difficulty, 31-70 varying degrees of disability, and ≤ 30 functioning so poorly as to require intensive supervision.

2.3 Statistical Analysis

Data were analyzed on intent-to-treat (ITT) principle. All statistical tests were performed with an alpha level of 0.05. Descriptive analysis of the demographic variables and other baseline line variables was conducted using measures of central tendency and variation for quantitative variables and frequency distributions for categorical variables. Assessment of safety included computation of the incidence of AEs and of discontinuation due to AEs, and presented in a frequency distribution table.

Two cohorts were introduced into the study:
- All enrolled subjects (overall);
- An ITT population comprising all enrolled subjects who received paliperidone ER at least once and provided ≥ 1 post-baseline efficacy measurement.

The efficacy analysis was mainly performed on the ITT population, but also performed on all enrolled subjects. The safety profile was assessed for the ITT population.

Data were summarized with respect to demographic and baseline characteristics, efficacy measurement with PANSS scale, PSP, and social functioning score, and safety observations. Descriptive statistics were performed to identify the retention rate at each visit as well as the symptomatic remission rate. Summary statistics of average doses that subjects received were based on all subjects participating in the study. Descriptive analysis was performed including frequency and percentage for categorical parameters, and mean, standard deviation, minimum, and maximum for continuous parameters. Descriptive analyses comprised summary statistics and 95% confidence intervals (95%CI). The paired t test was also performed to compare changes in scores of continuous variables.

The assessment of safety was based mainly on the frequency of AEs. The Medical Dictionary for Regulatory Activities (MedDRA, Version 12.1) AE dictionary was used to map AEs to preferred terms and system organ class. Patients reporting an individual preferred term AE and the total number of patients reporting at least one adverse event per system organ class were tabulated. Each AE based on preferred terminology was counted only once for a given subject for each group. The frequency and percent AEs (preferred terms and system organ class) are presented. Descriptive statistics were provided to evaluate the changes of vital signs at each scheduled time-point.

Results

A total of 480 patients were enrolled. Among them, a total of 426 subjects (88.8%) had evaluation at week 4 and 350 (72.9%) completed the 12-week evaluation. The details of patient disposition are summarized in Figure 1.

Reasons of patient withdrawal before week 4 were AEs (n = 6), insufficient response (n = 2), ineligible to continue (n = 15), lost to follow-up (n = 12), consent withdrawn (n = 16), and noncompliance (n = 3). Therefore these 54 patients did not have any safety and efficacy evaluation, resulting in 426 subjects included in the ITT population.

The initial dose disposition at baseline for these 426 patients was 3 mg/day for 154 patients, 6 mg/day for 232 patients, 9 mg/day for 29 patients, and 12 mg/day for 11 patients. The average dosage was 5.5 mg/day. The end doses for 350 subjects who completed the study were distributed as 45 patients with 3 mg/day, 183 patients with 6 mg/day, 64 patients with 9 mg/day, and 58 patients with 12 mg/day.

The withdrawal reasons are summarized in Table 1. Overall, 130 subjects (27.1%) discontinued the study prematurely. The details are as follows: 1 subject (0.2%) died, 12 subjects (4.8%) withdrew because of adverse events, 18 (3.8%) subjects withdrew because of insufficient response, 15 subjects (3.1%) were ineligible to continue, 28 subjects (5.8%) were lost to follow-up, 35 subjects (7.3%) withdrew their consent, 8 (1.7%) subjects discontinued because of non-compliance, and 2 subjects (0.4%) because of other reasons.

Summary statistics of demographic characteristics for the overall and ITT populations are listed in Table 2. In the ITT population, there were more men (55.9%) than women (44.1%). The mean age was 40.4 (range, 17-72) years; median age was 40 years. Subjects' schizophrenia subtype distribution was paranoid 61.7%, undifferentiated 18.9%, disorganized 10.8%, residual 7.3%, catatonic 1.2%, and other subtypes 0.2%. Overall, 33.3% of the subjects had symptom onset > 10 years but < 20 years. There were 4.9% of subjects with history of drug abuse. The results of all enrolled subjects were similar to those of the ITT population.

The reasons for subjects switching their treatments are displayed for all enrolled patients and the ITT population in Figures 2 and 3, respectively. For the ITT population, there were 4 subjects who did not receive any antipsychotics at enrollment. For the remaining 422 subjects, 409 received antipsychotics within 30 days prior to enrollment. The treatments included oral risperidone for 188 subjects (45.97%), olanzapine for 40 subjects (9.78%), quetiapine for 29 subjects (7.09%), aripiprazole for 28 subjects (6.85%), and other treatments for 166 subjects (40.59%). The major reason of switching treatment was insufficient efficacy, accounting for a total of 321 subjects. AEs (82 subjects), noncompliance (42 subjects), and other (2 subjects) were the reasons for switching. Thirteen subjects received antipsychotics > 30 days prior to enrollment. The switching reasons were insufficient efficacy (n = 7), noncompliance (n = 6), and other (n = 1).

Table 3 summarizes previous antipsychotic treatment received for consecutive 3 months. The most frequently used antipsychotics were oral risperidone (207 subjects; 48.6%) for the ITT population. The results of all enrolled subjects were similar to those of the ITT population.

Table 4 summarizes the complicating diseases for subjects. For the ITT population, the most commonly complained complications were psychiatric (329 subjects; 77.23%), gastrointestinal (145 subjects; 34.04%), and neurological disorders (104 subjects; 24.41%), respectively.

Dose disposition of study medication paliperidone ER of the ITT population and completed population is presented in Table 5 and Table 6, respectively. In the ITT population, the number of subjects who started paliperidone ER treatment with the initial dose of 3 mg/day and increased to 6, 9, and 12 mg/day at the end of study was 69, 17, and 18, respectively. There were 43 and 30 subjects with the initial dose of 6 mg/day and increased to 9 and 12 mg/day, respectively, at the end of study, whereas 11 subjects with the initial dose of 9 mg/day increased to 12 mg/day at the end of study. All subjects with initial dose of 12 mg/day remained on 12 mg/

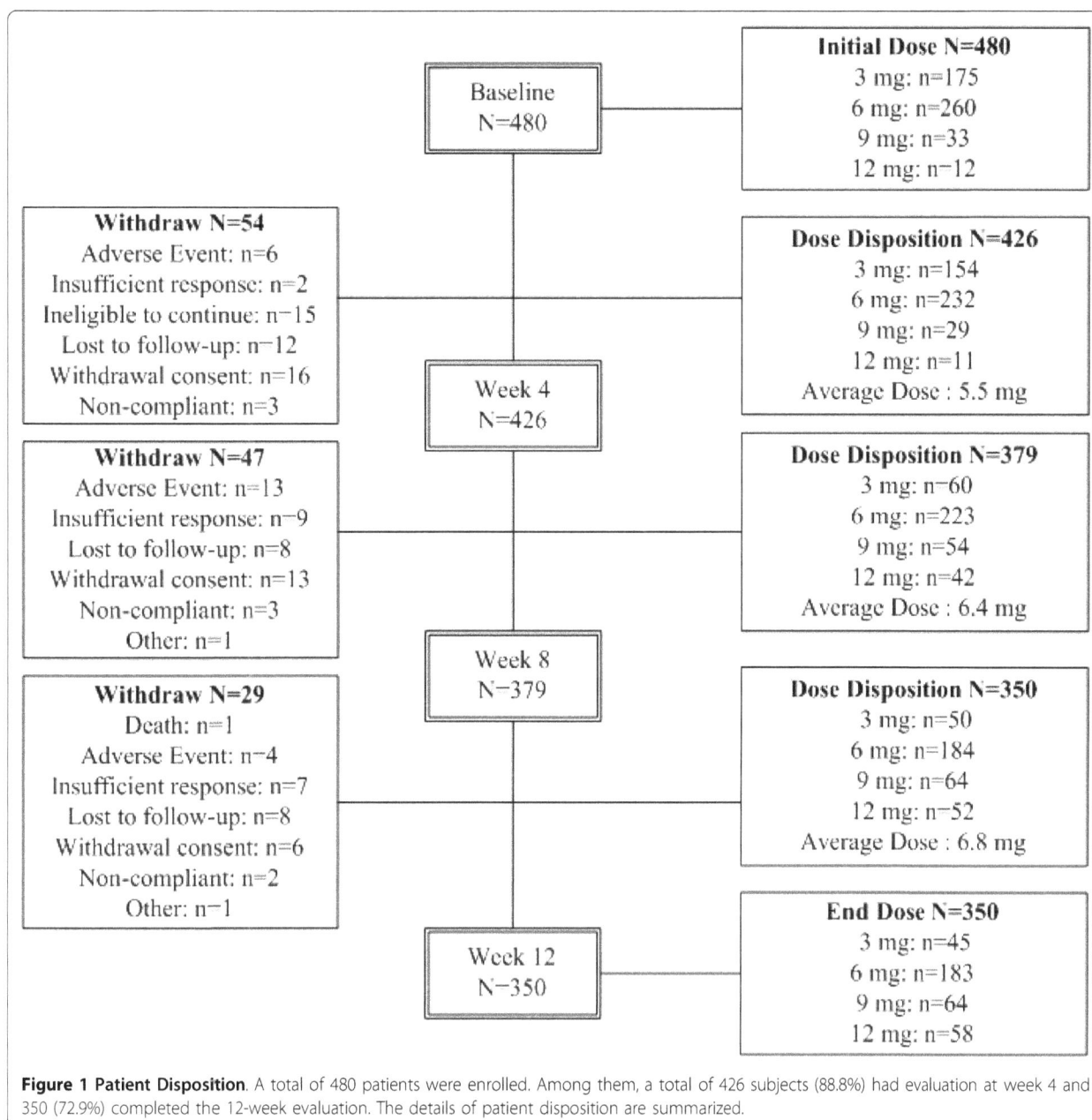

Figure 1 Patient Disposition. A total of 480 patients were enrolled. Among them, a total of 426 subjects (88.8%) had evaluation at week 4 and 350 (72.9%) completed the 12-week evaluation. The details of patient disposition are summarized.

Table 1 Summary of Withdrawal Reason

Time	Overall (N = 480)	ITT (N = 426)
Total	130 (27.1%)	76 (17.8%)
Death	1 (0.2%)	1 (0.2%)
Adverse Event	23 (4.8%)	17 (4.0%)
Insufficient Response	18 (3.8%)	16 (3.8%)
Ineligible to Continue	15 (3.1%)	0 (0.0%)
Lost to Follow-up	28 (5.8%)	16 (3.8%)
Withdrew Consent	35 (7.3%)	19 (4.5%)
Non-Compliant	8 (1.7%)	5 (1.2%)
Other	2 (0.4%)	2 (0.5%)

day till the end of study. The completed population had a similar dose pattern of study dose disposition.

PANSS and PAP total score both showed significant improvements after 12-week treatment (PANSS score, from 89.88 ± 29.20 to 72.72 ± 26.36; PSP score, from 47.07 ± 16.34 to 56.61 ± 14.32; both $p < 0.05$). The results of symptomatic remission are summarized in Figure 4. The symptomatic remission rate was 3.5% (95%CI, 1.98%, 5.74%) at baseline and improved to 11.7% (95%CI, 8.84%, 15.18%) at the end of study ($p < 0.05$). The criteria for PSP improvement was at least one 10-point interval on PSP scale. In the ITT population, subjects showed an increasing PSP improvement after

Table 2 Summary of Demographics

Characteristics		Overall (N = 480)	ITT (N = 426)
Sex	Male	262 (54.6%)	238 (55.87%)
	Female	218 (45.4%)	188 (44.13%)
Age (years)	N	< 480 >	< 426 >
	Mean (SD)	40.3 (10.6)	40.4 (10.6)
	Median	39.5	40.0
	Min. ~ Max.	16.0 ~ 72.0	17.0 ~ 72.0
Diagnosis	Paranoid	300 (62.5%)	263 (61.74%)
	Disorganized	46 (9.6%)	46 (10.80%)
	Catatonic	6 (1.3%)	5 (1.17%)
	Undifferentiated	88 (18.3%)	80 (18.78%)
	Residual	37 (7.7%)	31 (7.28%)
	Other	3 (0.6%)	1 (0.23%)
In/Out Patient	In-patient	218 (45.4%)	207 (48.6%)
	Out-Patient	262 (54.6%)	219 (51.4%)
Symptom onset (years)	Unspecified	46 (9.6%)	41 (9.62%)
	< = 5	95 (19.8%)	78 (18.31%)
	> 5~ < = 10	83 (17.3%)	74 (17.37%)
	> 10~ < = 20	153 (31.9%)	142 (33.33%)
	> 20~ < = 30	78 (16.2%)	67 (15.73%)
	> 30	25 (5.2%)	41 (9.62%)
Drug abuse	No	437 (91.0%)	386 (90.61%)
	Yes	23 (4.8%)	21 (4.93%)
	Unspecified	20 (4.2%)	19 (4.46%)

treatment began. The improvement rate was increased from 28.1% (95%CI, 23.94%, 32.70%) at week 4 to 47.4% (95%CI, 42.59%, 52.28%) at the end of study.

AEs with occurrence ≥ 2% during the study are summarized in Table 7. There were 213 patients (50.0%) with ≥ 1 AE during study. The most commonly experienced AEs were disease progression (33 patients; 7.7%), upper respiratory tract infection (30 patients; 7.0%), extrapyramidal disorder (25 patients; 5.2%), insomnia (17 patients; 4.0%), and constipation (14 patients; 3.3%). Among the 30 schizophrenia events 27 were recorded as serious AEs.

Discussion

The severity of the symptoms and long-lasting, chronic pattern of schizophrenia can impact all areas of daily living including work or school, social contacts, and relationships. Treatment typically involves antipsychotic medications to stabilize the mood and treat the psychotic symptoms for individual patients. Paliperidone ER tablets have been approved in the USA and Europe for the treatment of schizophrenia based on three 6-week, placebo-controlled clinical trials in patients with acute symptoms of schizophrenia [13-15]. These studies indicate that paliperidone ER at dosages 3-15 mg/day was associated with statistically significant improvement (relative to placebo) in schizophrenia symptoms as

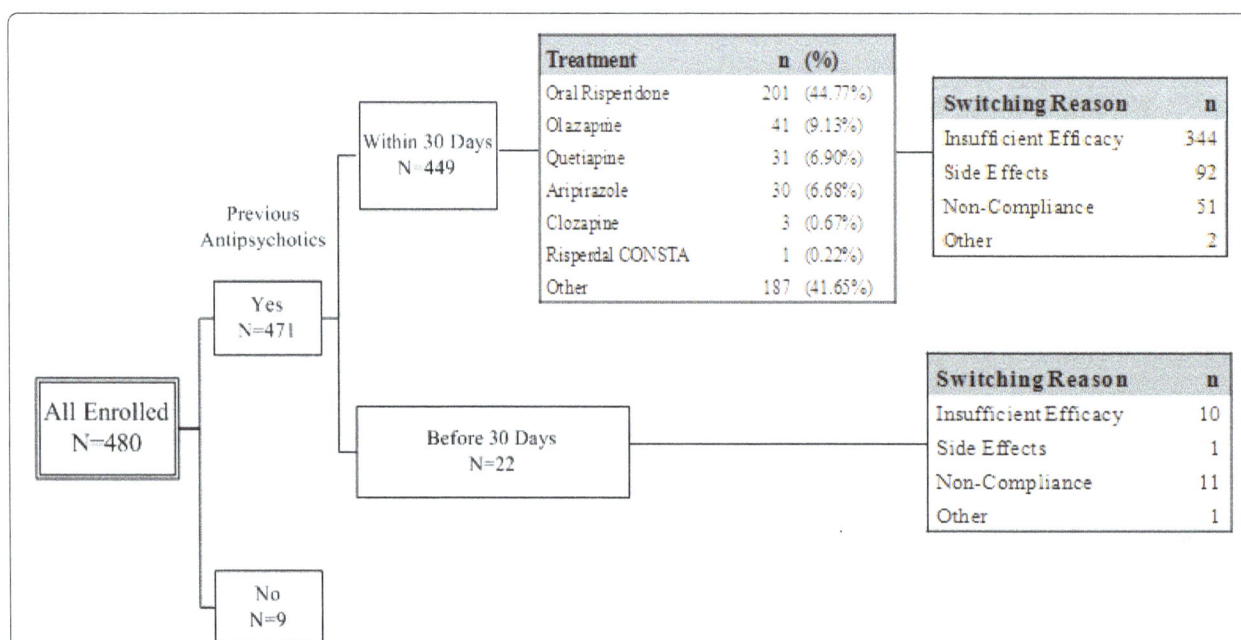

Figure 2 Summary of switching reasons of previous antipsychotic treatment of all enrolled patients. For the enrolled population, there were 9 subjects who did not receive any antipsychotics at enrollment. For the remaining 471 subjects, 449 received antipsychotics within 30 days prior to enrollment. The treatments included oral risperidone for 201 subjects (44.77%), olanzapine for 41 subjects (9.13%), quetiapine for 31 subjects (6.90%), aripiprazole for 30 subjects (6.68%), and other treatments for 187 subjects (41.65%). The major reason of switching treatment was insufficient efficacy, accounting for a total of 344 subjects. AEs (92 subjects), noncompliance (51 subjects), and other (2 subjects) were the reasons for switching. Twenty-two subjects received antipsychotics > 30 days prior to enrollment. The switching reasons were insufficient efficacy (n = 10), side effects (n = 1), noncompliance (n = 11), and other (n = 1).

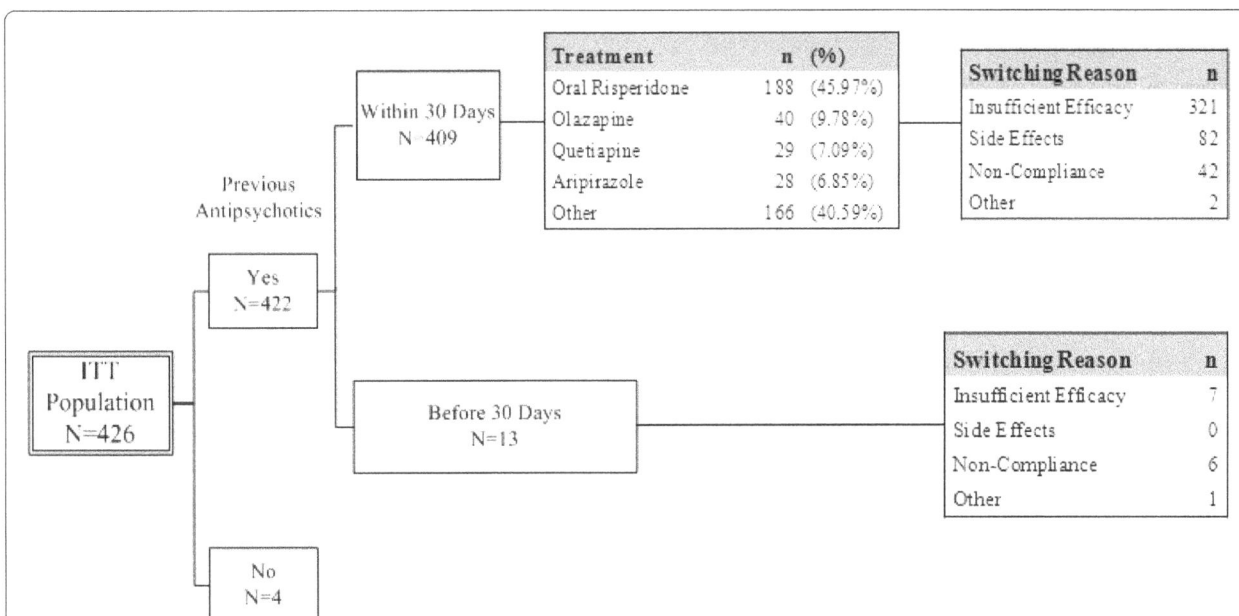

Figure 3 Summary of switching reasons of previous antipsychotic treatment of ITT population. For the ITT population, there were 4 subjects who did not receive any antipsychotics at enrollment. For the remaining 422 subjects, 409 received antipsychotics within 30 days prior to enrollment. The treatments included oral risperidone for 188 subjects (45.97%), olanzapine for 40 subjects (9.78%), quetiapine for 29 subjects (7.09%), aripiprazole for 28 subjects (6.85%), and other treatments for 166 subjects (40.59%). The major reason of switching treatment was insufficient efficacy, accounting for a total of 321 subjects. AEs (82 subjects), noncompliance (42 subjects), and other (2 subjects) were the reasons for switching. Thirteen subjects received antipsychotics > 30 days prior to enrollment. The switching reasons were insufficient efficacy (n = 7), noncompliance (n = 6), and other (n = 1).

measured by PANSS, personal and social functioning as measured by the PSP, and clinician's overall assessment as measured by CGI-S. Paliperidone ER was well tolerated in this patient population during acute treatment, with tolerability measured by low discontinuation rates and low adverse event burden [12,13,16]. The maintenance of social functioning is important treatment objective in the long-term management of schizophrenia. However, the aim of this study is to measure maintenance of social functioning with Personal and Social Performance scale (PSP) to assess treatment benefit in clinical trials. The 10-point PSP decrement is a clinically relevant measure of maintenance of functioning in patients stabilized with antipsychotic therapy.

Paliperidone palmitate demonstrated a statistically significant treatment benefit in terms of maintenance of functioning [17].

The current phase IV, open-label, prospective study was conducted with the main objective of exploring the relationship between achieving symptomatic remission status by means of the 8 items of Positive and Negative Syndrome Scale (PANSS) and personal and social functioning by means of the Personal and Social Performance (PSP) scale in patients treated with flexibly dosed Paliperidone ER. The proportion of patients achieving the definition of symptomatic remission status was 3.52% with 95% C.I. [1.98%, 5.74%] at baseline and

Table 3 Summary of Previous Antipsychotics Treatment Received for Consecutive 3 Months

Antipsychotic Treatments	Overall (N = 480)	ITT (N = 426)
Oral Risperidone	224 (46.67%)	207 (48.59%)
Olanzapine	52 (10.83%)	49 (11.50%)
Quetiapine	35 (7.29%)	32 (7.51%)
Aripiprazole	30 (6.25%)	28 (6.57%)
Clozapine	14 (2.92%)	10 (2.35%)
Risperdal CONSTA	3 (0.63%)	1 (0.23%)
Other	125 (26.04%)	110 (25.82%)

Table 4 Summary of Concurrent Disease with Incidence ≥ 5%

System	Overall (N = 480)	ITT (N = 426)
Psychiatric	364 (75.83%)	329 (77.23%)
Gastrointestinal	156 (32.50%)	145 (34.04%)
Neurological	114 (23.75%)	104 (24.41%)
Cardiovascular	77 (16.04%)	74 (17.37%)
Endocrine	71 (14.79%)	62 (14.55%)
Respiratory	34 (7.08%)	31 (7.28%)
Ears, Nose, Throat	29 (6.04%)	28 (6.57%)
Musculoskeletal	32 (6.67%)	31 (7.28%)

Table 5 Summary of Dose Disposition of ITT Population

ITT Population		Initial Dose			
		3 mg/day	6 mg/day	9 mg/day	12 mg/day
Dose at the End of Study	3 mg/day	50	7	0	0
	6 mg/day	69	152	0	0
	9 mg/day	17	43	18	0
	12 mg/day	18	30	11	11

improved to 11.74% with 95% C.I. [8.84%, 15.18%] at the end of study of the ITT population.(Figure 4) The significant improvements in personal and social functioning that resulted subsequent to paliperidone ER treatment, as measured by the validated and reliable PSP instrument may be an important clinical consideration for patient treatment. Apart from improvement in positive and negative symptoms, medications that improve personal and social function may lead to better social integration and overall functioning [18,19]. The sensitivity demonstrated that the cut point 60 of PSP scale revealed best relationship between PSP scale and symptomatic remission. It would be useful to be able to assess the importance of both PSP scores and changes in PSP scores by relating them to real-life outcomes. Ultimately, a real-life assessment of PSP scores would have to be addressed by long-term observational studies incorporating relatively objective measures of social functioning, possibly drawing on multiple observers (e. g., clinicians, family members, friends, caregivers) as well as patient self-assessment [20-23]. The PSP may be a useful tool to assess social functioning and importantly to predict relapse, enabling management teams to intervene before the deleterious clinical and economic impact of relapse negatively affects the patient's course of illness. The high predictive value of the PSP criteria and relapse is particularly relevant in an illness such as schizophrenia where noncompliance and partial compliance to medication is substantial [24,25]. Patients with schizophrenia may present with negative, cognitive, disorganization and mood symptoms, which persist during periods of acute exacerbation when more overt positive symptoms are evident. The post-hoc analysis showed that acutely ill patients with or without predominant negative symptoms respond similarly to treatment with paliperidone ER [26].

The safety profile also demonstrated that paliperidone ER was well-tolerated without clinically significant changes after treatment administration. The most frequently reported adverse event was disease progression (33 patients, 7.7%), upper respiratory tract infection (30 patients, 7.0%), extrapyramidal disorder (25 patients, 5.2%), insomnia (17 patients, 4.0%) and constipation (14 patients, 3.3%). As well, one patient committed suicide, and another attempted suicide and was comatose in a vegetative state. Vital signs, such as weight, SBP, DBP, and pulse had no clinically significant change. Various clinical studies have demonstrated that paliperidone ER is safe and well-tolerated and have similar adverse event profile. Pooled safety data indicated that paliperidone ER was generally well tolerated. Discontinuations related to treatment-emergent AEs were similarly low for patients receiving paliperidone ER or placebo. Although the incidence of EPS-related AEs was higher in paliperidone ER-treated patients, primarily those receiving higher doses, the severity of EPS was very low throughout the study [27]. Therefore, no safety concerns were raised in this study [28]. In this study, short-term treatment with paliperidone ER significantly improved psychiatric symptoms and functioning, with no unexpected safety or tolerability findings. Paliperidone is the active metabolite of risperidone, and nearly half of the subjects were on risperidone prior to study entry. Oral risperidone may have failed to provide adequate efficacy in patients even though it is metabolized to paliperidone because of the short plasma half-life of paliperidone. This would make the case that paliperidone ER treatment would be more effective since it stays in blood circulation for an extended period of time and hence, the controlled drug release from the osmotic drug delivery system demonstrates clear formulation benefits as highlighted specifically in the title of this study. The

Table 6 Summary of Dose Disposition of Complete Study Subjects

Complete Study Subjects		Initial Dose			
		3 mg/day	6 mg/day	9 mg/day	12 mg/day
Dose at the End of Study	3 mg/day	40	5	0	0
	6 mg/day	61	122	0	0
	9 mg/day	11	42	11	0
	12 mg/day	15	26	8	9

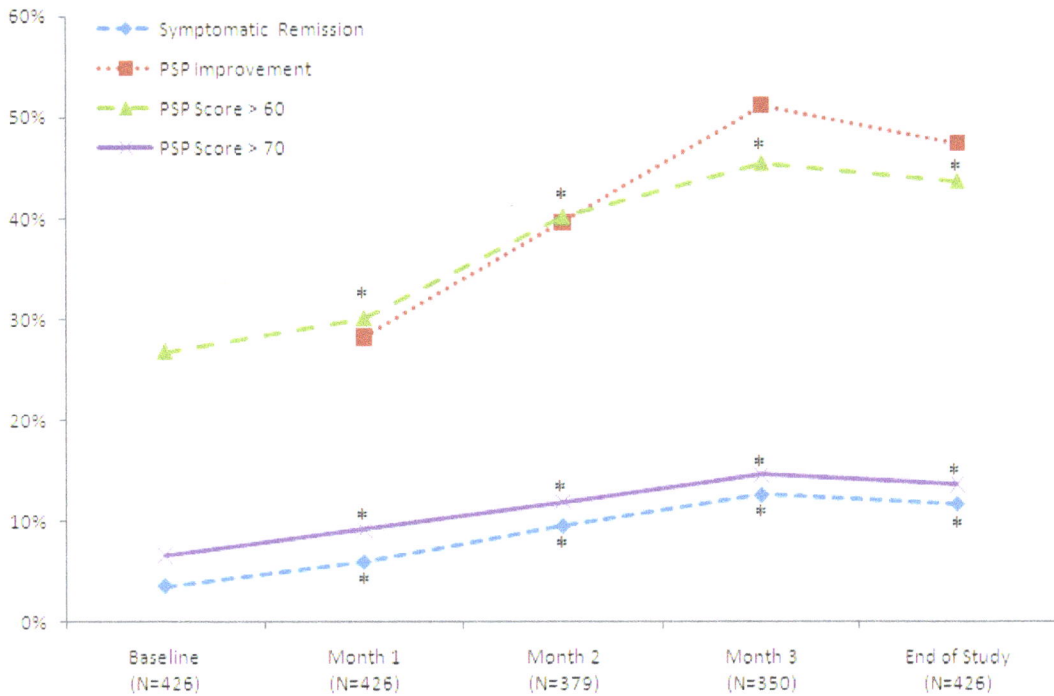

*: p-value of change from baseline <0.05

Figure 4 Summary of Efficacy Result. The symptomatic remission rate was 3.5% (95%CI, 1.98%, 5.74%) at baseline and improved to 11.7% (95%CI, 8.84%, 15.18%) at the end of study (p < 0.05). The criteria for PSP improvement was at least one 10-point interval on PSP scale. In the ITT population, subjects showed an increasing PSP improvement after treatment began. The improvement rate was increased from 28.1% (95% CI, 23.94%, 32.70%) at week 4 to 47.4% (95%CI, 42.59%, 52.28%) at the end of study.

symptomatic remission rate was 3.52% with 95% C.I. [1.98%, 5.74%] at baseline and improved to 11.74% with 95% C.I. [8.84%, 15.18%] at the end of study (p-value < 0.05). The results demonstrated an improvement in

Table 7 Adverse Events with Incidence ≧ 2%

Preferred Term	N = 426 N (%)
Patients with any Adverse Event	213 (50.0%)
Disease progression	33 (7.7%)*
Upper respiratory tract infection	30 (7.0%)
Extrapyramidal disorder	22 (5.2%)
Insomnia	17 (4.0%)
Constipation	14 (3.3%)
Anxiety	11 (2.6%)
Nasopharyngitis	11 (2.6%)
Diarrhoea	9 (2.1%)
Headache	9 (2.1%)
Somnolence	9 (2.1%)
Tachycardia	9 (2.1%)

*27 events were recorded as serious adverse events.

symptomatic remission rate after the 12-week treatment of paliperidone ER. Another study showed that the remission rate was increased from 43.9% at baseline to 51.7% at 12 weeks after aripiprazole treatment [29]. The original RSWG criteria requires 6 month duration, we have not used the criteria for remission as originally defined. There are three key limitations to the study. These are as follows. First, the study is the short study design. The study attempts to explore the relationship between symptomatic remission and function, however, this aspect of the investigation requires additional assessment for validity. A third limitation is the heterogeneous nature of the population, with some patients being remitted at baseline. Prospectively designed and longer-term studies are needed to further assess this finding.

Conclusions

The diminished social functioning in schizophrenia is probably responsible for more burdens in patients, families, and care systems than residual symptoms.

Finding a psychotropic treatment that improves social functioning is critically important. The clinical program of paliperidone ER was designed to incorporate the PSP as a measure of social functioning [30]. The result showed that the 11.74% patients with at least moderate severity of schizophrenia were evaluated as "mild" or better on PANSS scale by all 8 items after 12 weeks of treatment with paliperidone ER. There were also significant improvement in patients' functionality as measured by PSP improvement and score changes. The cut point 60 of PSP scale revealed best relationship between PSP scale and symptomatic remission. Besides, PANSS scale revealed better correlation with PSP scale rather than social functioning scale. Safety profile was also acceptable. This 12-week, multi-center, open-label; prospective study established the efficacy, safety, and tolerability of paliperidone ER and significantly showed that symptom severity and social functioning improve with paliperidone ER treatment. In the future, the correlations between PSP and PANSS to prove the close interplay between social functioning and psychopathology in the chronic course of schizophrenia should be further evaluated. The interaction of psychopathological states and psychosocial functioning determines the long-term course of schizophrenia and its treatment.

Acknowledgements
The statistical analysis will be done by or under the supervision of Janssen-Cilag Taiwan. The study results have not been previously published in a peer review journal. This research was supported by Janssen-Cilag Taiwan, Johnson & Johnson.

Author details
[1]Institute of Biomedical Engineering, National Cheng Kung University, Tainan 70403, Taiwan. [2]Department of Psychiatry, Chiayi Branch, Taichung Veterans General Hospital, Chia-Yi 60090, Taiwan. [3]Department of Psychiatry, Cardinal Tien Ken-Sin Hospital, Taipei 23148, Taiwan. [4]Department of Psychiatry, Show Chwan Memorial Hospital, Changhua 50008, Taiwan. [5]Department of Psychiatry, Chu-Tung Branch, National Taiwan University Hospital, Hsinchu 31064, Taiwan. [6]Department of Psychiatry, Yuli Hospital, Hualien 98147, Taiwan. [7]Department of Psychiatry, Taichung Veterans General Hospital, Taichung 40705, Taiwan. [8]Department of Psychiatry, Cathay General Hospital, Taipei 10630, Taiwan. [9]Medical Devices Innovation Center, National Cheng Kung University, Tainan 70403, Taiwan.

Authors' contributions
YCY and MWH conceived the study, analyzed the data and prepared the manuscript. PPY participated in the study design and provided significant comments on the manuscript. PRT participated in the study design and helped to draft the manuscript. PWS, BJW, CHC, THL, ICL, WCC, CYL and KSC participated in the study design and helped to provide clinical service. All authors have read and approved the final version of the manuscript.

Competing interests
This research was supported by Janssen-Cilag Taiwan, Johnson & Johnson. All the authors are clinical psychiatrists. The authors declare that they have no competing interests.

References
1. World Health Organization: Mental health, Disorder management. 2006 [http://www.who.int/mental_health/management/schizophrenia/en/].
2. Keshavan MS, Schooler NR: First-episode studies in schizophrenia: criteria and characterization. Schizophr Bull 1992, 18:491-513.
3. Jeffrey ALieberman, Diana Perkinsa, Aysenil Belger, Miranda Chakos, Fred Jarskog, Kalina Boteva, John Gilmore: The early stages of schizophrenia: speculations on pathogenesis, pathophysiology, and therapeutic approaches. Biol Psychiatry 2001, 50:884-97.
4. Canuso CM, Bossie CA, Amatniek J, Turkoz I, Pandina G, Cornblatt B: Paliperidone extended-release tablets in patients with recently diagnosed schizophrenia. Early intervention in psychiatry 2010, 4(1):64-78.
5. Rosen K, Garety P: Predicting recovery from schizophrenia: a retrospective comparison of characteristics at onset of people with single and multiple episodes. Schizophr Bull 2005, 31:735-50.
6. Nancy CAndreasen, William TCarpenter, John MKane, Robert ALasser, Stephen RMarder, Daniel RWeinberger: Remission in schizophrenia: proposed criteria and rationale for consensus. Am J Psychiatry 2005, 162:441-449.
7. Emsley R, Oosthuizen P, Koen L, Niehaus DJ, Medori R, Rabinowitz J: Remission in patients with first-episode schizophrenia receiving assured antipsychotic medication: a study with risperidone long-acting injection. Int Clin Psychopharmacol 2008, 23(6):325-31.
8. Emsley R, Chiliza B, Schoeman R: Predictors of long-term outcome in schizophrenia. Current Opinion in Psychiatry 2008, 21(2):173-177.
9. Kane JM, Crandall DT, Marcus RN, Eudicone J, Pikalov A, Carson WH, Swyzen W: Symptomatic remission in schizophrenia patients treated with aripiprazole or haloperidol for up to 52 weeks. Schizophr Res 2007, 95(1-3):143-50.
10. Morosini PL, Magliano L, Brambilla L, Ugolini S, Pioli R: Development, reliability and acceptability of a new version of the DSM-IV Social and Occupational Functioning Assessment Scale (SOFAS) to assess routine social functioning. Acta Psychiatr Scand 2000, 101(4):323-9.
11. Conley R, Gupta SK, Sathyan G: Clinical spectrum of the osmotic-controlled release oral delivery system (OROS), an advanced oral delivery form. Curr Med Res Opin 2006, 22:1879-92.
12. Herbert YMeltzer, William VBobo, Isaac FNuamah, Rosanne Lane, David Hough, Michelle Kramer, Marielle Eerdekens: Efficacy and tolerability of oral paliperidone extended-release tablets in the treatment of acute schizophrenia: pooled data from three 6-week, placebo-controlled studies. J Clin Psychiatry 2008, 69:817-29.
13. Kane J, Canas F, Kramer M, Ford L, Gassmann-Mayer C, Lim P, Eerdekens M: Treatment of schizophrenia with paliperidone extended-release tablets: a 6-week placebo-controlled trial. Schizophr Res 2007, 90(1-3):147-61.
14. Marder SR, Kramer M, Ford L, Eerdekens E, Eerdekens M, Lim P: Efficacy and safety of paliperidone extended-release tablets: results of a 6-week, randomized, placebo-controlled study. Biol Psychiatry 2007, 62:1363-70.
15. Michelle Kramer, George Simpson, Valentinas Maciulis, Stuart Kushner, Ujjwala Vijapurkar, Pilar Lim, Mariëlle Eerdekens: Paliperidone extended-release tablets for prevention of symptom recurrence in patients with schizophrenia: a randomized, doubleblind, placebo-controlled study. J Clin Psychopharmacol 2007, 27:6-14.
16. Priebe S, Watzke S, Hansson L, Burns T: Objective social outcomes index (SIX): A method to summarise objective indicators of social outcomes in mental health care. Acta Psychiatr Scand 2008, 118:57-63.
17. Nicholl D, Nasrallah H, Nuamah I, Akhras K, Gagnon DD, Gopal S: Personal and social functioning in schizophrenia: defining a clinically meaningful measure of maintenance in relapse prevention. Current Medical Research & Opinion 2010, 26(6):1471-84.
18. Michael Davidsona, Robin Emsleyb, Michelle Kramerc, Lisa Fordc, Guohua Pand, Pilar Limd, Mariëlle Eerdekense: Efficacy, safety and early response of paliperidone extended-release tablets (paliperidone ER): results of a 6-week, randomized, placebocontrolled study. Schizophr Res 2007, 93:117-30.
19. Kawata AK, Revicki DA: Psychometric properties of the personal and social performance scale (PSP) among individuals with schizophrenia living in the community. Qual Life Res 2008, 17:1247-1256.
20. Georg Juckela, Daniela Schauba, Nina Fuchsa, Ute Naumanna, Idun Uhla, Henning Witthausa, Ludger Hargarterb, Hans-Werner Bierhoffc, Martin Brünea: Validation of the Personal and Social Performance (PSP)

Scale in a German sample of acutely ill patients with schizophrenia. *Schizophr Res* 2008, **104**:287-293.

21. Kozma CM, Dirani RG, Canuso CM, Mao L: Predicting hospital admission and discharge with symptom or function scores in patients with schizophrenia: pooled analysis of a clinical trial extension. *Ann Gen Psychiatry* 2010, **9**:24.

22. Nasrallah H, Morosini PL, Gagnon D: Reliability validity and ability to detect change of the Personal and Social Performance scale in patients with stable schizophrenia. *Psychiatry Research* 2008, **161**:213-224.

23. Patrick DL, Burns T, Morosini P, Gagnon DD, Rothman M, Adriaenssen I: Measuring social functioning with the personal and social performance scale in patients with acute symptoms of schizophrenia: interpretation of results of a pooled analysis of three Phase III trials of paliperidone extended-release tablets. *Clinical therapeutics* 2010, **32(2)**:275-92.

24. Valenstein M, Ganoczy D, McCarthy JF, Myra Kim H, Lee TA, Blow FCI: Antipsychotic adherence over time among patients receiving treatment for schizophrenia: a retrospective review. *J Clin Psychiatry* 2006, **67**:1542-50.

25. Lacro JP, Dunn LB, Dolder CR, Leckband SG, Jeste DV: Prevalence of and risk factors for medication nonadherence in patients with schizophrenia: a comprehensive review of recent literature. *J Clin Psychiatry* 2002, **63**:892-909.

26. Canuso CM, Bossie CA, Turkoz I, Alphs L: Paliperidone extended-release for schizophrenia: Effects on symptoms and functioning in acutely ill patients with negative symptoms. *Schizophrenia Research* 2009, **13(1)**:56-64.

27. Turkoz I, Bossie CA, Dirks B, Canuso CM: Direct and indirect effects of paliperidone extended-release tablets on negative symptoms of schizophrenia. *Neuropsychiatric disease and treatment* 2008, **4(5)**:949-58.

28. Tzimos A, Samokhvalov V, Kramer M, Ford L, Gassmann-Mayer C, Lim P, Eerdekens M: Safety and tolerability of oral paliperidone extended-release tablets in elderly patients with schizophrenia: a double-blind, placebo-controlled study with six-month open-label extension. *Am J Geriatr Psychiatry* 2008, **16(1)**:31-43.

29. Kim CY, Chung S, Lee JN, Kwon JS, Kim do H, Kim CE, Jeong B, Jeon YW, Lee MS, Jun TY, Jung HY: A 12-week, naturalistic switch study of the efficacy and tolerability of aripiprazole in stable outpatients with schizophrenia or schizoaffective disorder. *Int Clin Psychopharmacol* 2009, **24(4)**:181-8.

30. David Hough, Isaac FNuamah, Pilar Lim, Allan Sampson, Dennis DGagnon, Margaret Rothman: Independent Effect of Paliperidone Extended Release on Social Functioning Beyond Its Effect on Positive and Negative Symptoms of Schizophrenia A Mediation Analysis. *Journal of Clinical Psychopharmacology* 2009, **29(5)**:496-497.

4

R- and S-Equol have equivalent cytoprotective effects in Friedreich's Ataxia

Timothy E Richardson[1,2] and James W Simpkins[1*]

Abstract

Background: Estradiol (E2) is a very potent cytoprotectant against a wide variety of cellular insults in numerous different cell models, including a Friedreich's ataxia (FRDA) model. Previously, we demonstrated that estrogen-like compounds are able to prevent cell death in an FRDA model independent of any known estrogen receptor (ER) by reducing reactive oxygen species (ROS) and the detrimental downstream effects of ROS buildup including oxidative damage to proteins and lipids and impaired mitochondrial function.

Results: We have previously demonstrated by western blot that our cell model lacks ERα and expresses only very low levels of ERβ. Using L-buthionine (S,R)-sulfoximine (BSO) to induce oxidative stress in human FRDA fibroblasts, we determine the potency and efficacy of the soy-derived ERβ agonist S-equol and its ERα-preferring enantiomer, R-equol *in vitro* on cell viability and ROS accumulation. Here we demonstrate that these equol biphenolic compounds, while significantly less potent and efficacious than E2, provide statistically similar attenuation of ROS and cytoprotection against a BSO-induced oxidative insult.

Conclusions: These preliminary data demonstrate that estrogen and soy-derived equols could have a beneficial effect in delaying the onset and decreasing the severity of symptoms in FRDA patients by an antioxidant mechanism. In addition, these data confirm that the protection seen previously with E2 was indeed unrelated to ER binding.

Keywords: Equol, 17β-estradiol, Antioxidants, Friedreich's Ataxia, Fibroblasts, Neuroprotection

Background

First recognized in 1863 [1], Friedreich's Ataxia (FRDA) is the most common hereditary form of ataxia characterized by an autosomal recessive GAA trinucleotide repeat in the *FXN* gene, resulting in the absence of frataxin protein [2,3]. The exact function of frataxin is unclear, however it is necessary for iron metabolism within cells, Fe-S cluster assembly in proteins, and maintenance of cellular redox state. Without sufficient levels of frataxin, reactive oxygen species (ROS) begin to accumulate and cells are unable to maintain function of Fe-S cluster proteins essential for mitochondrial respiration leading to mitochondrial dysfunction, insufficient energy production and ultimately cell death, beginning in organs with greater energy requirements and thus more dependent on aerobic ATP production, such as the heart, brain and spinal cord. Symptoms usually begin in the second decade of life and include ataxia, neural hearing and ocular abnormalities, scoliosis, diabetes and cardiomyopathy, which is the most common cause of premature death in FRDA patients [for review see Ref 4].

First detected in humans in 1982 [5], equol is a biphenolic isoflavone metabolized from the soy product daidzein by intestinal flora [6-8] in 14-59% of the human population [9]. Equol is known to act as an antioxidant [10,11], decreases circulating estrogens and androgens [12], inhibits DHT binding to its receptor [13] and decreases risks of prostate [9,11,14] and breast cancer [15]. Separation of racemic equol mixtures shows that S-equol binds with very high affinity to ERβ ($K_d \sim 0.73$ nM), while its enantiomer, R-equol has a far lower affinity for ERβ, instead showing a preference for ERα ($K_d \sim 15.4$ nM), while E2 has a $K_d \sim 0.05\text{-}0.1$ nM [16,17]. These enantiomers allow for the discrimination

* Correspondence: james.simpkins@unthsc.edu
[1]Institute for Aging and Alzheimer's Disease Research, Department of Pharmacology & Neuroscience, University of North Texas Health Science Center, Fort Worth, TX 76107, USA
Full list of author information is available at the end of the article

between effects due to antioxidant effects and those due to ERβ activation.

We have previously shown that phenolic estrogens are able to prevent BSO-induced FRDA skin fibroblast death, as well as block the formation of ROS [18], prevent lipid peroxidation, protein damage, depletion of ATP and support the mitochondria and oxidative phosphorylation [19]. In the present study, we provide further evidence that E2 acts by an ERα- and ERβ-independent mechanism. In addition, we demonstrated a lack of ERα and a very low level of ERβ in FRDA fibroblasts by western blot [19]. Here, we show pharmacologically that ERβ is not contributing to this process, as R- and S-equol have statistically equivalent efficacies and potencies, represented here as EC_{50} values. These data indicate that it is the phenolic ring present in the compound structure of equol and E2 and not intrinsic receptor binding ability that is responsible for cytoprotective effects in this FRDA cell model. Although these compounds are substantially less efficacious and potent than compounds previously used [18], this pharmacologic model lends support to the non-receptor mediated, non-genomic antioxidant mechanism of E2.

Results

The effects of R- and S-equol on cell viability in BSO-treated FRDA fibroblasts

To determine the effect of R- and S-equol (Figure 1) on cell viability, we first assessed their protective potential compared to 17β-estradiol (E2) at 100nM, a concentration previously shown to be very protective in this cell model [18]. At 100nM, both R- and S-equol provided statistically significant protection compared to the BSO-alone treated group, however the two groups did not differ significantly from each other (Figure 2a). E2 also provided significantly more protection than either of these two compounds (Figure 2a). A dose–response assessment showed that R- and S-equol have almost identical cytoprotective profiles at all concentrations (Figure 2b), and EC_{50} evaluation demonstrated that the two have statistically equivalent EC_{50} values (Table 1), indicating that the cytoprotective effect is not due to stimulation of ERβ.

The effects of R- and S-equol on BSO-induced reactive oxygen species (ROS) formation

To determine the effects of R- and S-equol on ROS attenuation, these two compounds were again compared to E2 (Figure 3a). BSO induced a 2-fold increase of ROS, which was prevented by 100nM concentrations of E2, R-equol and S-equol. None of these groups differed from each other. In addition, a dose response curve for R- and S-equol shows that there is no significant difference in the ROS attenuation profiles of these two

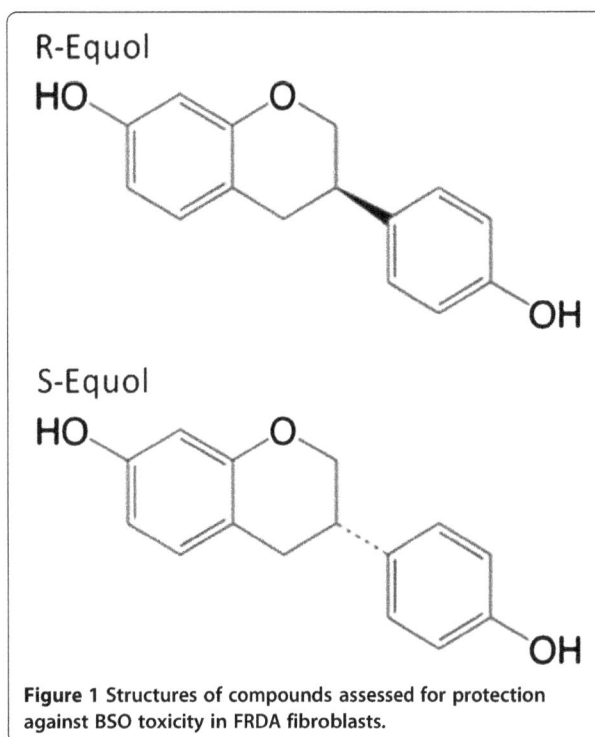

Figure 1 Structures of compounds assessed for protection against BSO toxicity in FRDA fibroblasts.

compounds at any concentration (Figure 3b), and the EC_{50} values do not differ significantly (Table 1).

Discussion

FRDA is the most common of the inherited ataxias world wide, affecting an estimated 1:50,000 to 1:20,000 people [2,4]. With the effective loss of functional frataxin throughout all organ systems, and the resulting ROS proliferation and mitochondrial respiration impairment, cells in organs most dependent on ATP production begin to degenerate [4,20]. This results in the loss of cells in the posterior columns and spinocerebellar tracts of the spinal cord, resulting in tremor and ataxia, as well as lateral and kyphoscoliosis, weakness, speech problems, pes cavitus, an increased incidence of diabetes mellitus and glucose intolerance and cardiac disorders, such as hypertrophic cardiomyopathy with interstitial fibrosis [4]. Disease onset

Table 1 EC_{50} values for R- and S-equol with respect to cell viability and ROS attenuation

Cell Viability		
Compound	EC50 (nM)	Standard Error (nM)
R-Equol	440.5	21.11
S-Equol	459.9	12.75
Reactive Oxygen species		
Compound	EC50 (nM)	Standard Error (nM)
R-Equol	413.9	34.91
S-Equol	439.1	33.77

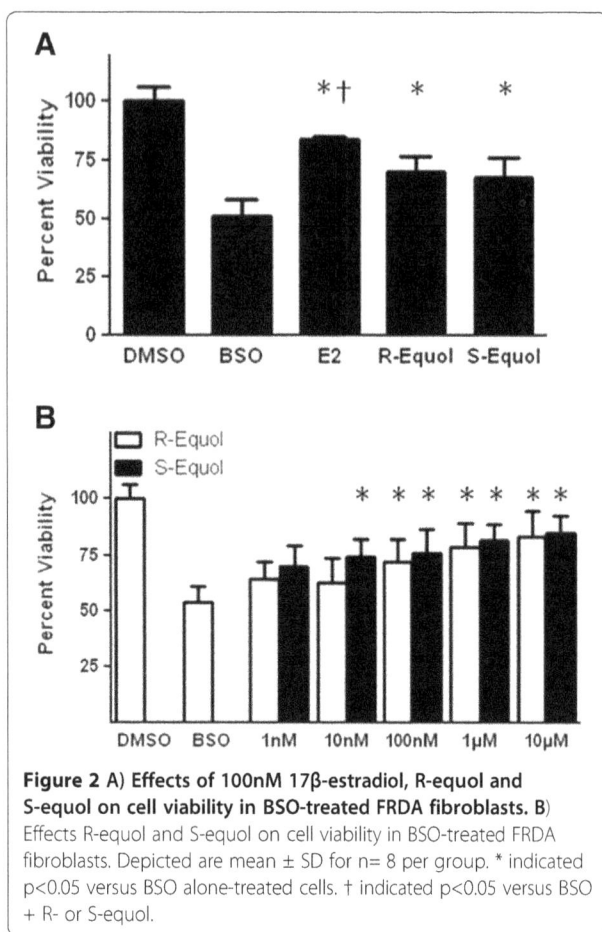

Figure 2 A) Effects of 100nM 17β-estradiol, R-equol and S-equol on cell viability in BSO-treated FRDA fibroblasts. B) Effects R-equol and S-equol on cell viability in BSO-treated FRDA fibroblasts. Depicted are mean ± SD for n= 8 per group. * indicated $p<0.05$ versus BSO alone-treated cells. † indicated $p<0.05$ versus BSO + R- or S-equol.

and severity is variable depending on the number of GAA trinucleotide repeats present in the first intron of the *FXN* gene, although this alone is not able to account for the full course of the disease process [21]. There is little difference between males and females in terms of disease onset, progress and severity as this is inherited in an autosomal recessive manner and symptoms begin in the first 2 decades of life, before hormone level changes in puberty [22].

Estrogen and non-feminizing estrogens have been shown to be potently cytoprotective in many different cell and animal models of disease states [23,24], including a FRDA cell model [18]. Previous observations have demonstrated that antioxidants, especially mitochondrially targeted antioxidants [25,26], including estrogen receptor agonists and non-feminizing estrogens [18] are protective against FRDA. These effects have been shown to be ER independent and are instead based in the antioxidant properties of phenolic estrogens [27,28].

Estrogens exert both genomic and non-genomic effects on redox status of cells for reviews see [29-34]. Unfortunately, no studies on the genomic effects of estrogens has been published using FRDA cells, but we have reported that these cells respond to estrogens even in the presence of a pan-estrogen receptor inhibitors, ICI 182780 [18], have no detectable ERα

and low levels of ERβ [19], and exhibit these effects at concentrations in excess of the ED_{50} for 17β-estradiol [18]. Nonetheless, genomic effects of estrogens on antioxidant enzymes have been reported, which could contribute to estrogen's antioxidant effects. For example, tamoxifen is reported to up-regulated the quinine reductase, NQO1 [29], and estrogens up-regulate expression of peroxidase-1 and MnSOD [30]. In contrast, Pajovic and Saicic [31] have reported that MnSOD, glutathione peroxidase, glutathione-S-transferase and glutathione reductase are decreased by estradiol, whereas catalase is increased. The extent to which the non-genomic effects of estrogens influence these paradoxical decreases in antioxidant enzyme expression is not known.

Estrogens are highly lipid soluble (the logarithm of the octanol/water partition coefficient, $\log P$, is 3.35) and largely reside in the membrane component of cells [35] where they are ideally suited to affect oxidation of unsaturated bonds in phospholipids. Indeed, estrogens appear to intercalate into the membrane with their phenolic A ring situated near the site of lipid peroxidation [36]. We reasoned that estrogens may interrupt lipid peroxidation chain reactions via oxidation in a manner that could be redox-cycled back to the parent estrogen, using a plentiful and regenerable source of cellular reducing potential, such as glutathione or NADPH. We discovered that estrogens were converted via hydroxyl radical exposure to a quinol product that was, in turn, enzymatically reduced back to the parent estrogen in the presence of NAD(P)H as a co-factor [27,28]. This estrogen redox cycle is operative in the central nervous system [27] where it serves, together with the "classical" antioxidant mechanism for phenolic compounds, as a defense mechanism against ROS.

Equol is a naturally derived biphenolic (Figure 1) product of soy digestion in a substantial percentage of the American population [5]. It is created by intestinal flora as a racemic mixture of the R- and S-forms, with the S-form being very selective for ERβ, the only ER present in FRDA fibroblasts [19] while the R-form is only a very weak agonist at this receptor [16,17]. Our results indicate that, while not as potent or efficacious as E2 (Figure 2a and 3a) [18], the R- and S-forms of equol are equally effective in attenuating ROS (Figure 3b, Table 1) and preventing cell death (Figure 2b, Table 1). These data indicate that equol, specifically the non-feminizing R-equol, could potentially be used to prevent or delay cell death and pathologic symptoms in FRDA and supports our previous hypothesis that estrogen-like compounds are acting in a manner unrelated to any known ER [18,19].

Conclusions

Because the biphenolic compounds R- and S-equol have statistically equal cytoprotective profiles despite

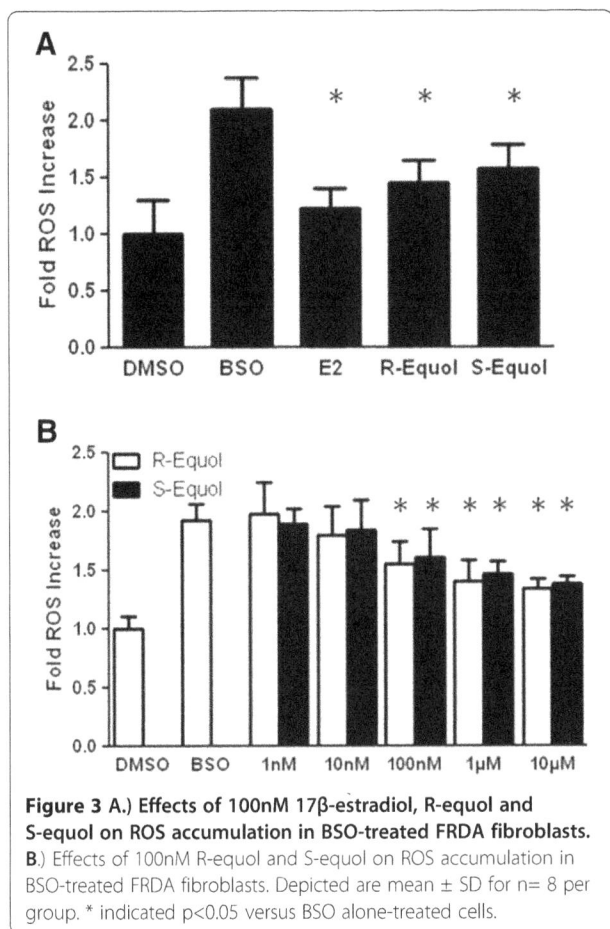

Figure 3 A.) Effects of 100nM 17β-estradiol, R-equol and S-equol on ROS accumulation in BSO-treated FRDA fibroblasts. **B.**) Effects of 100nM R-equol and S-equol on ROS accumulation in BSO-treated FRDA fibroblasts. Depicted are mean ± SD for n= 8 per group. * indicated p<0.05 versus BSO alone-treated cells.

penicillin-streptomycin (Invitrogen, Carlsbad, CA, USA) at 37°C in 90% humidity and 5% CO_2. At the time of treatment, the FRDA fibroblast media was changed to phenol red- and sodium pyruvate-free DMEM (ThermoScientific, Waltham, MA, USA) and 1% penicillin-streptomycin. Experiments were conducted using cell passages 15–19.

Chemicals & reagents

17β-Estradiol (E2) was acquired from Steraloids, Inc. (Newport, RI, USA). L-buthionine (S,R)-sulfoximine (BSO) was obtained from Sigma-Aldrich (St Louis, MO, USA). R- and S- Equol were obtained from the laboratory of Dr Robert J Handa at The University of Arizona.

Treatment paradigm

FRDA fibroblasts were removed from culture with 0.25% Trypsin-EDTA (Invitrogen, Carlsbad, CA, USA) and plated on 96-well plates at a density of 3000 cells per well in DMEM with 10% CSFBS, 1% GlutaMAX and 1% penicillin-streptomycin. After 24 hours the media was removed and replaced with phenol red- and sodium pyruvate-free DMEM with 1% penicillin-streptomycin. The cells were then treated for 12 to 48 hours with either dimethyl sulfoxide vehicle control (DMSO; Sigma-Aldrich, St Louis, MO, USA) or 1mM BSO in the presence of E2, R-equol or S-equol ((3S)-3-(4-Hydroxyphenyl)-7-chromanol). This duration of exposure was chosen based on our observation of BSO-induced enhancement of ROS at 12 hours and cell death at 48 hours [18].

Calcein AM cell viability assay

Cells were plated on a 96-well plate at a density of 5,000 cells per well, then treated with vehicle or 1mM BSO. After 48 hours of BSO treatment, the media was removed, and 1 µg/mL Calcein AM (CalBiochem, San Diego, CA, USA) in phosphate buffer pH 7.2 (PBS; Fisher Scientific, Pittsburg, PA, USA) was added to each well and the plate was incubated for 10 minutes at 37°C. Cell viability was determined with a Tecan Infinite M200 (Tecan Systems, Inc., San Jose, CA) plate reader with an excitation of 490nm and emission of 520nm at 48 hours.

Reactive oxygen species assay

After 12 hours of treatment the media was removed from each well of the 96-well plate, and 100µL of a 1µM 2',7'-Dichlorodihydrofluorescein diacetate (DCFDA; AnaSpec Inc., Fremont, CA, USA) in PBS was added to each well. The plates were returned to a 37°C incubator for 20 minutes, then each well was washed three times with PBS and the resulting reaction was read on a Tecan Infinite M200 plate reader with an absorbance of 495 nm and an emission of 529 nm.

extremely different ERβ binding profiles, these data confirm that ERβ is not involved in the protective effects of E2 seen previously in this FRDA fibroblast model [18,19]. Furthermore, this study demonstrates that estrogen and soy-derived equols are effective at reducing ROS and improving cell viability in FRDA fibroblasts and shows that naturally derived soy estrogens could have a beneficial effect in delaying the onset and decreasing the severity of symptoms in FRDA patients by an antioxidant mechanism. These data add more weight to the neuroprotective hypothesis of estrogen and provide evidence that E2 and other phenol ring-containing estrogens should be considered as candidate drugs for the treatment and prevention of the symptoms of FRDA.

Methods

Cell culture

Fibroblasts from a 30 year old Friedreich's Ataxia (FRDA) patient (Coriell Institute, Camden NJ, USA) were maintained in Dulbecco's Modified Eagle Medium (DMEM; ThermoScientific, Waltham, MA, USA) with 10% charcoal-stripped fetal bovine serum (CSFBS; ThermoScientific, Waltham, MA, USA), 1% GlutaMAX (ThermoScientific, Waltham, MA, USA) and 1%

Data and statistics

All data are displayed as mean ± 1 standard deviation. These data were analyzed using the ANOVA against an alpha level of 0.05. All bar graphs were made using GraphPad Prism 5 and EC_{50} calculations were made with GraphPad Prism 5. For all groups, n=8 wells and experiments were repeated three times to ensure consistency.

Abbreviations

BSO: L-buthionine (S,R)-sulfoximine; FRDA: Friedreich's Ataxia; E2: 17β-Estradiol; ROS: Reactive oxygen species; ER: Estrogen receptor; ERα: Estrogen receptor α; ERβ: Estrogen receptor β.

Competing interests

The authors declare that they have no competing interests.

Authors' contributions

TER carried out the experiments, performed statistical analysis and wrote the initial draft of the manuscript. JWS revised and approved the final manuscript. All authors were involved with the conception and design of the studies. Both authors read and approved the final manuscript.

Acknowledgements

The authors would like to thank Dr Robert J Handa for providing us with the R- and S-equol compounds. We would also like to thank Yogesh Mishra for help with ChemDraw software. Supported in part by NIH Grants P01 AG100485, P01 AG22550, and P01 AG027956 (to JWS) and NIA Grant T31 AG020494 (to TER).

Author details

[1]Institute for Aging and Alzheimer's Disease Research, Department of Pharmacology & Neuroscience, University of North Texas Health Science Center, Fort Worth, TX 76107, USA. [2]Texas College of Osteopathic Medicine, University of North Texas Health Science Center, Fort Worth, TX 76107, USA.

References

1. Friedreich N: Uber degenerative Atrophie der spinalen Hinterstrange. *Arch Pathol Anat Phys Klin Med* 1863, **26**:391–419.
2. Harding AE: Classification of the hereditary ataxias and paraplegias. *Lancet* 1983, **1**:1151–1155.
3. Campuzano V, Montermini L, Moltò MD, Pianese L, Cossée M, Cavalcanti F, Monros E, Rodius F, Duclos F, Monticelli A, Zara F, Cañizares J, Koutnikova H, Bidichandani SI, Gellera C, Brice A, Trouillas P, De Michele G, Filla A, De Frutos R, Palau F, Patel PI, Di Donato S, Mandel JL, Cocazza S, Koenig M, Pandolfo M: Friedreich's ataxia: autosomal recessive disease caused by an intronic GAA triplet repeat expansion. *Science* 1996, **271**:1423–1427.
4. Santos R, Lefevre S, Sliwa D, Seguin A, Camadro JM, Lesuisse E: Friedreich ataxia: molecular mechanisms, redox considerations and therapeutic opportunities. *Antioxid Redox Signal* 2010, **13**:651–690.
5. Axelson M, Kirk DN, Farrant RD, Cooley G, Lawson AM, Setchell KD: The identification of the weak oestrogen equol [7-hydroxy-3-(4′-hydroxyphenyl)chroman] in human urine. *Biochem J* 1982, **201**:353–357.
6. Wang XL, Hur HG, Lee JH, Kim KT, Kim SI: Enantioselective synthesis of S-equol from dihyrodaidzein by a newly isolated anaerobic human intestinal bacterium. *Appl Environ Microbiol* 2005, **71**:214–219.
7. Price KR, Fenwick GR: Naturally occurring oestrogens in foods – a review. *Food Addit Contam* 1985, **2**:73–106.
8. Kelly GE, Nelson C, Waring MA, Joannou GE, Reeder AY: Metabolites of dietary (soya) isoflavones in human urine. *Clin Chim Acta* 1993, **223**:9–22.
9. Akaza H, Miyanaga N, Takashima N, Naito S, Hirao Y, Tsukamoto T, Fujioka T, Mori M, Kim WJ, Song JM, Pantuck AJ: Comparisons of percent equol producers between prostate cancer patients and controls: case-controlled studies of isoflavones in Japanese, Korean and American residents. *Jpn J Clin Oncol* 2004, **34**:86–89.
10. Pereboom D, Gilaberte Y, Sinues B, Escanero J, Alda JO: Antioxidant intracellular activity of genistein and equol. *J Med Food* 1999, **2**:253–256.
11. Mitchell JH, Gardner PT, McPhail DB, Morrice PC, Collins AR, Duthie GG: Antioxidant efficacy of phytoestrogens in chemical and biological model systems. *Arch Biochem Biophys* 1998, **360**:142–148.
12. Duncan AM, Merz-Demlow BE, Xu X, Phipps WR, Kurzer MS: Premenopausal equol excretors show plasma hormone profiles associated with lowered risk of breast cancer. *Cancer Epidemiol Biomarkers Prev* 2000, **9**:581–586.
13. Lund TD, Munson DJ, Haldy ME, Setchell KD, Lephart ED, Handa RJ: Equol is a novel anti-androgen that inhibits prostate growth and hormone feedback. *Biol Reprod* 2004, **70**:1188–1195.
14. Mitchell JH, Duthie SJ, Collins AR: Effects of phytoestrogens on growth and DNA integrity in human prostate tumor cell lines: PC-3 and LNCaP. *Nutr Cancer* 2000, **38**:223–228.
15. Frankenfeld CL, McTiernan A, Aiello EJ, Thomas WK, LaCroix K, Schramm J, Schwartz SM, Holt VL, Lampe JW: Mammographic density in relation to daidzein-metabolizing phenotypes in overweight, postmenopausal women. *Cancer Epidemiol Biomarkers Prev* 2004, **13**:1156–1162.
16. Muthyala RS, Ju YH, Sheng S, Williams LD, Doerge DR, Katzenellenbogen BS, Helferich WG, Katzenellenbogen JA: Equol, a natural estrogenic metabolite from soy isoflavones: convenient preparation and resolution of R- and S-equols and their differing binding and biological activity through estrogen receptors alpha and beta. *Bioorg Med Chem* 2004, **12**:1559–1567.
17. Setchell KD, Clerici C, Lephart ED, Cole SJ, Heenan C, Castellani D, Wolfe BE, Nechemias-Zimmer L, Brown NM, Lund TD, Handa RJ, Heubi JE: S-Equol, a potent ligand for estrogen receptor {beta}, is the exclusive enantiomeric form of the soy isoflavone metabolite produced by human intestinal bacterial flora. *Am J Clin Nutr* 2005, **81**:1072–1079.
18. Richardson TE, Yang SH, Wen Y, Simpkins JW: Estrogen protection in Friedreich's ataxia skin fibroblasts. *Endocrinology* 2011, **152**:2742–2749.
19. Richardson TE, Yu AE, Wen Y, Yang SH, Simpkins JW: Estrogen prevents oxidative damage to the mitochondria in Friedreich's ataxia skin fibroblasts. *PLoS One* 2012, **7**:e13600.
20. Marmolino D: Friedreich's ataxia: past, present and future. *Brain Res Rev* 2011, **67**:311–330.
21. Klopstock T, Chahrokh-Zadeh S, Holinski-Feder E, Meindl A, Gasser T, Pongratz D, Müller-Felber W: Markedly different course of Friedreich's ataxia in sib pairs with similar GAA repeat expansions in the frataxin gene. *Acta Neuropathol* 1999, **97**:139–142.
22. Leone M, Brignolio F, Rosso MG, Curtoni ES, Moroni A, Tribolo A, Schiffer D: Friedreich's ataxia: a descriptive epidemiological study in an Italian population. *Clin Genet* 1990, **38**:161–169.
23. Simpkins JW, Green PS, Gridley KE, Singh M, de Fiebre NC G, Rajakumar G: Role of estrogen replacement therapy in memory enhancement and the prevention of neuronal loss associated with Alzheimer's disease. *Am J Medicine* 1997, **103**:195–255.
24. Behl C: Oestrogen as a neuroprotective hormone. *Nat Rev Neurosci* 2002, **3**:433–442.
25. Jauslin ML, Wirth T, Meier T, Shoumacher F: A cellular model for Friedreich Ataxia reveals small-molecule glutathione peroxidase mimetics as novel treatment strategy. *Hum Mol Genet* 2002, **13**:3055–63.
26. Jauslin ML, Meier T, Smith RA, Murphy MP: Mitochondria-targeted antioxidants protect Friedreich Ataxia fibroblasts from endogenous oxidative stress more effectively than untargeted antioxidants. *FASEB J* 2003, **17**:1972–4.
27. Prokai L, Prokai-Tatrai K, Perjesi P, Simpkins JW: Mechanistic insights into the direct antioxidant effects of estrogens. *Drug Dev Res* 2006, **66**:118–125.
28. Prokai L, Prokai-Tatrai K, Perjesi P, Zharikova AD, Perez EJ, Liu R, Simpkins JW: Quinol-based cyclic antioxidant mechanism in estrogen neuroprotection. *Proc Natl Acad Sci USA* 2003, **100**:11741–11746.
29. Montano MM, Bianco NR, Deng H, Wittmann BM, Chaplin LC, Katzenellenbogen BS: Estrogen receptor regulation of quinone reductase in breast cancer: implications for estrogen-induced breast tumor growth and therapeutic uses of tamoxifen. *Front Biosci* 2005, **10**:1440–1461.
30. Viña J, Sastre J, Pallardó FV, Gambini J, Borrás C: Role of mitochondrial oxidative stress to explain the different longevity between genders: protective effect of estrogens. *Free Radic Res* 2006, **40**:1359–1365.
31. Pajović SB, Saicić ZS: Modulation of antioxidant enzyme activities by sexual steroid hormones. *Physiol Res* 2008, **57**:801–811.

32. Simpkins JW, Dykens JA: **Mitochondrial mechanisms of estrogen neuroprotection.** *Brain Res Rev* 2008, **57**:421–430.

33. Duckles SP, Miller VM: **Hormonal modulation of endothelial NO production.** *Pflugers Arch* 2010, **459**:841–851.

34. White RE, Gerrity R, Barman SA, Han G: **Estrogen and oxidative stress: a novel mechanism that may increase the risk for cardiovascular disease in women.** *Steroids* 2010, **75**:788–793.

35. Liang Y, Belford S, Tang F, Prokai L, Simpkins JW, Hughes JA: **Membrane fluidity effects of estratrienes.** *Brain Res Bull* 2001, **54**:661–668.

36. Cegelski L, Rice CV, O'Connor RD, Caruano AL, Tochtrop GP, Cai ZY, Covey DF, Schaefer J: **Mapping the locations of estradiol and potent neuroprotective analogues in phospholipid bilayers by REDOR NMR.** *Drug Dev Res* 2006, **66**:93–102.

5

Vascular disrupting agent for neóvascular age related macular degeneration: a pilot study of the safety and efficacy of intravenous combretastatin a-4 phosphate

Mohamed A Ibrahim[1], Diana V Do[1,6], Yasir J Sepah[1], Syed M Shah[1], Elizabeth Van Anden[1], Gulnar Hafiz[1], J Kevin Donahue[2,3], Richard Rivers[4], Jai Balkissoon[5], James T Handa[1], Peter A Campochiaro[1] and Quan Dong Nguyen[1,6*]

Abstract

Background: This study was designed to assess the safety, tolerability, and efficacy of intravenous infusion of CA4P in patients with neovascular age-related macular degeneration (AMD).

Methods: Prospective, interventional, dose-escalation clinical trial. Eight patients with neovascular AMD refractory to at least 2 sessions of photodynamic therapy received CA4P at a dose of 27 or 36 mg/m^2 as weekly intravenous infusion for 4 consecutive weeks. Safety was monitored by vital signs, ocular and physical examinations, electrocardiogram, routine laboratory tests, and collection of adverse events. Efficacy was assessed using retinal fluorescein angiography, optical coherence tomography, and best corrected visual acuity (BCVA).

Results: The most common adverse events were elevated blood pressure (46.7%), QTc prolongation (23.3%), elevated temperature (13.3%), and headache (10%), followed by nausea and eye injection (6.7%). There were no adverse events that were considered severe in intensity and none resulted in discontinuation of treatment. There was reduction of the excess foveal thickness by 24.15% at end of treatment period and by 43.75% at end of the two-month follow-up (p = 0.674 and 0.161, respectively). BCVA remained stable throughout the treatment and follow-up periods.

Conclusions: The safety profile of intravenous CA4P was consistent with that reported in oncology trials of CA4P and with the class effects of vascular disruptive agents; however, the frequency of adverse events was different. There are evidences to suggest potential efficacy of CA4P in neovascular AMD. However, the level of systemic safety and efficacy indicates that systemic CA4P may not be suitable as an alternative monotherapy to current standard-of-care therapy.

Trial registration: ClinicalTrials.gov NCT01570790.

Keywords: Angiogenesis, Neovascularization, Ocular pharmacology, Retinal degeneration, Combretastatin A-4 Phosphate, CA4P, Vascular disrupting agents, VDA

* Correspondence: qnguyen4@jhmi.edu
[1]Wilmer Eye Institute, Johns Hopkins University School of Medicine, 600 North Wolfe Street, Maumenee 745, Baltimore, MD 21287, USA
[6]Stanley M. Truhlsen Eye Institute, University of Nebraska Medical Center, Omaha, NE, USA
Full list of author information is available at the end of the article

Background

Combretastatin-A4-phosphate (CA4P) is a vascular disrupting agent (VDA), a class of experimental medications that lead to collapse or occlusion of abnormal vascular structures. CA4P is a synthetic phosphorylated pro-drug of CA4, a naturally occurring derivative of the South African willow tree, *combretum caffrum*, which reversibly binds tubulin at the colchicine-binding site to inhibit microtubule assembly. The mechanism by which CA4P and CA4 act on pathologic neovasculature is not completely understood; although it appears that through its reversible binding to tubulin, CA4P causes distortion and detachment of immature proliferating endothelial cells in abnormal vasculature (mature endothelial cell shape is maintained by the secondary scaffolding protein actin). Because of its reversible effects and the short half-life of about 10-27 min, as demonstrated in animal studies, CA4P does not display the side effects typical of tubulin binding inhibitors [1]. Although it is a vascular targeted agent, its specific mechanism of action and side effect profile differ from those of vascular endothelial growth factor (VEGF) inhibitors [2].

CA4P has been shown to disrupt tumor neovasculature and decrease tumor blood flow in both animals and humans [3]. Multiple human studies have demonstrated significant decrease in tumor blood flow within a few hours of CA4P administration, whether examined with dynamic contrast enhanced (DCE), MRI, PET scan or perfusion CT scan. The safety profile of CA4P in oncology patients suggests that adverse effects are generally mild to moderate and mostly occur in the few hours following an infusion. Consistent with its vascular activity, the most typical adverse effects in descending order are nausea, headache, tumor pain, fatigue, vomiting, sinus tachycardia and bradycardia, paresthesia, diarrhea, sweating, and transient hypertension and QTc prolongation [4].

CA4P was reported to decrease neovascularization in mice with laser-induced disruption of Bruch's membrane, in VEGF overexpressing mice, and in a model of retinopathy of prematurity (ROP) induced by excessive oxygen [5,6]. In the ROP model, CA4P demonstrated specificity for abnormal vasculature with sparing of normal angiogenesis required to support growth of the developing eye. The dose of CA4P required in the laser burn model was approximately *30-fold* higher than that required in the other two models, suggesting greater potency on abnormal vascular structures in contrast to normal wound healing [6].

These preclinical observations along with the apparent tolerability of systemic CA4P in oncology patients [7-10] provided the rationale for the pilot study of intravenous CA4P in patients with neovascular AMD. The index study is the first clinical trial of CA4P in patients with an ophthalmic disorder, and is the first trial of systemic CA4P in a population of patients without malignancy. Therefore, the study may contribute unique safety and biological activity data to the VDA literature.

Methods

Selection criteria

A prospective, open-label, dose-escalation phase 1 study was conducted to assess the safety, tolerability, and potential efficacy of CA4P in patients with choroidal neovascularization (CNV) secondary to AMD. The clinical trial was approved by the Johns Hopkins Medicine Institutional Review Board (IRB). Prior to determination of eligibility for enrollment, patients provided informed written consent to participate in the Study and to allow the information about them such as their eye, gender, and age (but not their names and other specific identifiable information) to be published in scientific literature so that others can be educated and learn from the trial.

Fluorescein angiography (FA) was employed to document presence of active subfoveal CNV. Patients with conditions that might contribute to CNV, such as pathologic myopia, histoplasmosis, and others were excluded. The CNV lesion size was limited to ≤12 Macular Photocoagulation Study (MPS) disc areas, of which at least 50% had to be active CNV. Subretinal hemorrhage was limited to <50% of total lesion size and scarring or atrophy to <25% of lesion size.

All major types of CNV were eligible. However, in patients with minimally classic or purely occult CNV, there has to be a documented evidence of two or more lines of vision loss during the previous 12 weeks. Eyes with best corrected visual acuity (BCVA) equivalent to 20/40 or worse, as measured by ETDRS charts, were eligible provided BCVA in the fellow eye is equivalent to 20/800 or better. When both eyes were eligible, the eye with better vision was selected.

Patients with any therapy for neovascular AMD within 12 weeks of screening or with prior subfoveal thermal laser therapy were excluded. There were specific exclusions for history of hemorrhagic or bleeding disorders and for cardiac disease, including angina, myocardial infarction, congestive heart failure or diagnostic tests showing an ejection fraction less than 50%, atrial fibrillation, clinically significant arrhythmias, and syncope. Conditions or medications associated with QTc prolongation were excluded. A normal 12-lead electrocardiogram (ECG) showing a QTc < 440 ms was required within 4 weeks prior to enrollment. Patients were also required to have a normal cardiac stress test of any type within 2 months prior to study entry. Laboratory tests obtained prior to enrollment were required to demonstrate adequate bone marrow, hepatic and renal functions, and normal blood coagulation profile. Uncontrolled hypertension (defined as blood pressure consistently greater than 150/100 mmHg irrespective of medication) or uncontrolled hypokalemia unresponsive to supplementation and/or hypomagnesaemia were exclusion criteria.

Treatment plan and study design

Patients received CA4P (OxiGene Inc., South San Francisco, CA) at a dose of 27 or 36 mg/m^2 as a 10-minute intravenous infusion weekly for 4 weeks. Vital signs were obtained every 15 minutes for two hours and then hourly for five hours after infusion. ECGs were collected hourly for five hours after completion of the infusion. Adverse events (AEs) were collected and graded using The NCI Common Terminology Criteria for Adverse Events (CTCAE) v 3.0. Subjects were reassessed and had to continue to meet inclusion/exclusion criteria for hematologic, hepatic, and renal functions prior to each scheduled dose. No further CA4P would be administered to any subjects who experienced AEs of Grade-2 or greater: ventricular arrhythmia, second or third degree AV block, severe sinus bradycardia less than 45 bpm or tachycardia >120 bpm not due to other causes (e.g. fever), persistent supraventricular arrhythmia [e.g. *atrial fibrillation, flutter, atrioventricular nodal tachycardia (AVNRT)]* lasting more than 24 hours, ventricular tachycardia defined as >9 beats in a row, or any length of torsades de pointes (polymorphic ventricular tachycardia with long QTc), or unexplained recurrent syncope), QTc prolongation in which the interval exceeds 500 msec on any two consecutive ECGs, Grade-2 or greater myocardial infarction, or ocular toxicities deemed by the investigator not acceptable for the patients to receive further treatments. A cardiac electrophysiologist (JKD) reviewed the ECGs and made recommendations pertaining to the conduct of the study. In addition, an anesthesiologist participated in taking care for the patients during the study, including the management of hypertension.

The study was designed as a single escalating dose with cohorts of five subjects. Escalation to the next cohort was based on the presence of no more than one subject with a dose limiting toxicity (DLT). DLTs were defined as specific events that are considered to be probably or definitely related to CA4P. Major DLTs included QTc interval ≥ 500 msec *(based on measurements provided by the core laboratory for ECG analysis),* Grade-2 or greater ventricular arrhythmia, unexplained syncope, Grade-3 or greater toxicity, delayed recovery postponing re-treatment by >14 days, and ocular toxicity such as keratopathy, uveitis, optic neuropathy, and retinopathy, at the discretion of the investigator.

Prior to each treatment, patients had ocular and physical examinations, ECG, complete blood count, and serum chemistry determinations. These safety tests were also performed 1 and 2 months following the last administration of CA4P. Ocular examination included slit-lamp biomicroscopy, indirect ophthalmoscopy, intraocular pressure (IOP) measurements, and BCVA. Assessment of CNV was performed using FA and OCT at screening, 1 hour after the first infusion, and immediately prior to the second, third, and fourth infusions, and at 4-week and 8-week visits. BCVA was assessed at all the visits prior to infusion.

Statistical methods

Descriptive statistical summaries were performed for safety and efficacy parameters. There were no predictive statistical designs used in this pilot study.

Results

Patient characteristics

Between August 2003 and May 2005, 15 patients with AMD were screened at a single center, the Wilmer Eye Institute at the Johns Hopkins University. Seven subjects were not eligible; eight subjects were enrolled; five subjects received 27 mg/m^2 and three subjects received 36 mg/m^2. The age of the enrolled patients ranged from 57 to 84 years (Table 1). BCVA in the study eyes ranged from 25 to 73 letters and in the fellow eyes ranged from zero to 80 letters. At baseline, all patients had active subfoveal CNV: occult in 6 patients and minimally classic in two. In the fellow eyes, 5 patients had active CNV at baseline, one patient had history of CNV resolved with disciform scarring and light-perception vision, and two patients had no history of CNV. None of our patients was naïve to treatment at baseline with all of them receiving at least 2 sessions of photodynamic therapy (PDT) prior to the study (Table 1).

Systemic safety

The majority of the adverse events were encountered during infusion and within the following 5 hours. The most common AEs were transient elevated blood pressure (46.7%), transient QTc prolongation (23.3%), elevated temperature (13.3%), and headache (10%), followed by nausea, and eye injection (6.7% each). Other noted AEs included T-wave inversion, tachycardia, premature ventricular contractions, and chest pain. All AEs resolved before dismissal of the patient no later than 5 hours post-infusion. There were no AEs that were considered serious or severe (Grade-3 or 4) and none resulted in discontinuation of treatment. One patient did not receive all four administrations of CA4P secondary to non-specific gastrointestinal symptoms that were not considered grade-3 or 4.

Systolic and diastolic blood pressure changes following the first infusion of CA4P in each subject are shown in Figure 1. Prior to treatment, one subject was normotensive (systolic ≤120 mmHg), three were borderline hypertensive (systolic >120 and ≤140 mmHg), and four were hypertensive. The changes in the mean systolic blood

Table 1 Demographics of the study subjects who were treated with intravenous combretastatin A-4 phosphate and characteristics of study and fellow eyes at baseline

Patient	Age	Gender	Race	Previous treatment	CNV SE	CNV FE	BCVA		FTH	
							SE	FE	SE	FE
1	81	F	White	PDT × 3	Subfoveal occult	Disciform Scar*	60	25	187	127
2	82	F	Hispanic	PDT × 2	Subfoveal occult	Subfoveal occult disciform scar*	73	4	204	573
3	84	F	White	PDT × 2	Subfoveal occult	No CNV	64	80	404	183
4	57	M	White	PDT × 3	Subfoveal minimally classic	Extrafoveal active occult foveal disciform scar *	67	73	346	236
5	64	F	White	PDT × 4	Subfoveal occult with disciform scar	Disciform scar	30	PL	519	x
6	70	M	White	PDT × 2	Subfoveal minimally	Subfoveal occult*	72	47	366	256
7	75	F	White	PDT × 2	Subfoveal occult	No CNV	25	72	292	238
8	79	F	White	PDT × 3	Subfoveal occult	Subfoveal occult*	64	48	450	393
Mean (±SD)	74 (±9.6)						56.9 (18.7±)	49.9 (±27.9)	346.0 (±115.2)	286.6(±150.2)

The asterisks indicate the fellow eyes that had active CNV at baseline. CNV = Choroidal neovascular membrane; SE = Study Eye; FE = Fellow Eye, BCVA = Best corrected visual acuity; FTH = central foveal thickness; PDT = photodynamic therapy; M = Male; F = Female; SD = Standard deviation.

pressure were similar following each of the four infusions (Table 2). The average systolic blood pressure at baseline was 145 mmHg and the average diastolic pressure was 74 mmHg. Six patients (75%) showed either worsening of the pre-existing systolic blood pressure (an increase of >20 mmHg) or development of hypertension (elevation of systolic blood pressure >140mgHg). The elevation in systolic blood pressure was transient and resolved spontaneously within the post-infusion period. Diastolic blood pressure did not show any significant change in any patient either after the infusion or during the course of the study. The average systolic blood pressure at the end of the study was 142 mmHg and the average diastolic blood pressure was 72 mmHg.

One subject had a baseline pressure of 156/82 mmHg despite prescriptions of lisinopril, atenolol and hydrochlorothiazide. Following the first administration of CA4P, her blood pressure climbed to 216/102 mmHg 45 minutes post infusion and returned to baseline level two hours post-infusion. Prior to the planned second treatment, blood pressure was 176/84 mmHg, so CA4P was withheld and lisinopril dose was increased. Prior to next infusion, blood pressure was 164/75 mmHg and peaked to 226/102 mmHg one hour post-treatment. The subject complained of chest heaviness that was not accompanied by ECG changes. Two doses of nitroglycerine were administered without relief; however, an oral antacid relieved the symptoms. The absence of ECG changes and the resolution of heartburn with antacid/belching suggested the symptoms to be of gastrointestinal origin. Due to the adverse experiences, the

patient did not receive any further administration of CA4P.

Baseline QTc was normal for all patients (median 409 ms, range 396-426 ms). QTc increased in all patients after infusion of CA4P, with a peak QTc significantly higher than baseline (median 438 ms, range 418–474 ms, $p < 0.05$). The changes in QTc interval following first infusion of CA4P are shown in Figure 2. The time-to-peak QTc was a median of 2 hours post-infusion (range 1–5 hours). Two female patients had grade-1 prolongation of QTc ≥450 ms *(3/4 infusions; patients 3 and 5)*, and one had a grade-2 complication of QTc peak ≥ 470 ms *(1/4 infusions: patient 5)*. The relative increase in QTc did not correlate with baseline QTc *(linear regression r = 0.15, p = 0.49)*. Mean changes in QTc are summarized in Table 2.

Ocular safety

Two of the eight patients experienced unilateral conjunctival injection during one of their treatments; another patient reported flashes and floaters in one eye. Both observations were transient and resolved without sequelae. Both observations were judged to be related to the study drug but were not serious adverse events. Since no DLTs were observed, a maximal tolerated dose (MTD) was not defined in this study.

Ocular efficacy
Study eyes
The mean foveal thickness of the central 1 mm of the retina (FTH) in the study eyes was 346 μm at baseline

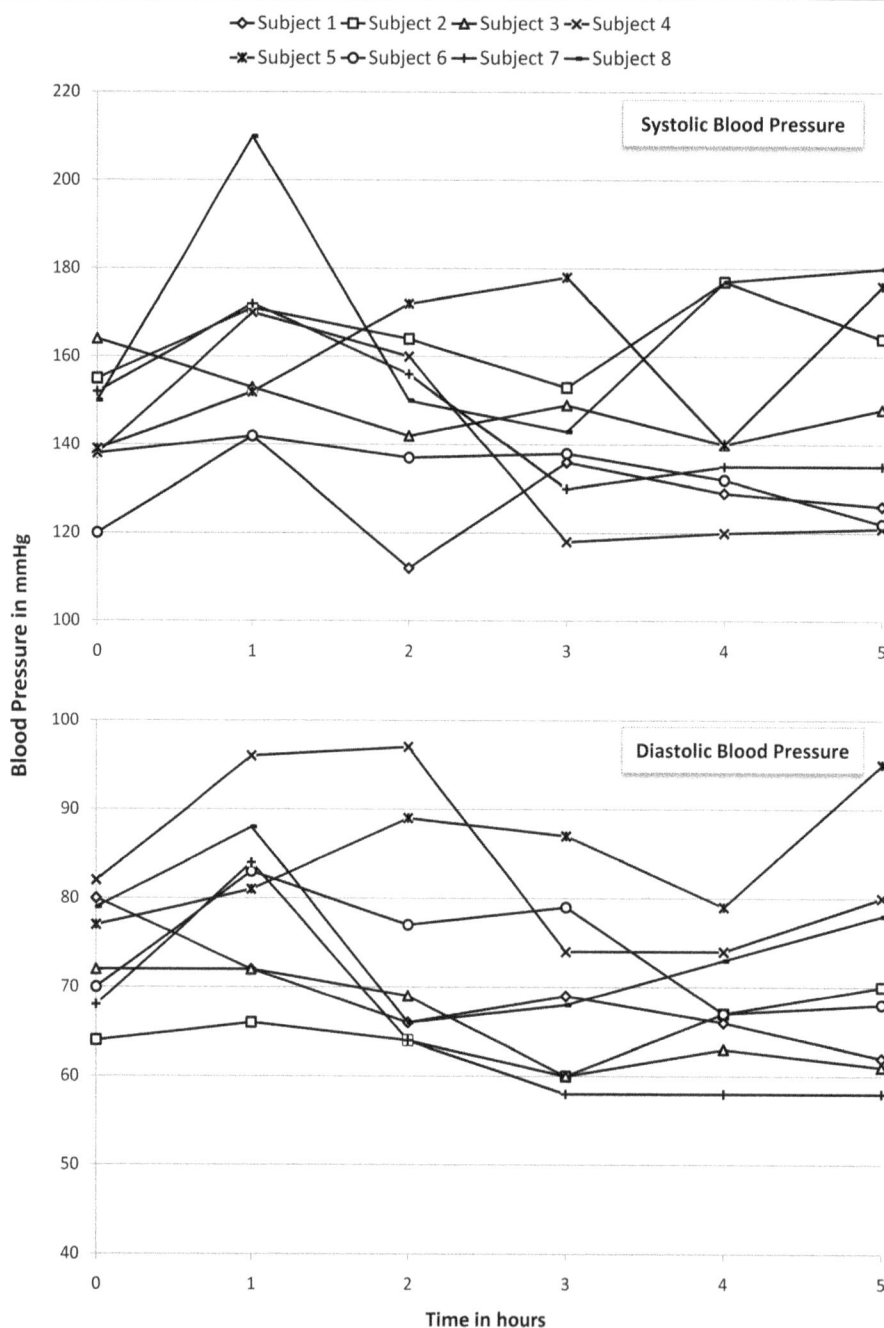

Figure 1 Changes in systolic (top) and diastolic (bottom) blood pressure in the study subjects following the first infusion of combretastatin A-4 phosphate.

(Figure 3 top), with an excess FTH of 134 μm *[normal FTH = 212 μm as measured by OCT2 (Carl Zeiss Meditec, Inc.)]*. After the 4th infusion *(end of treatment period)*, the mean FTH showed a 32.37 μm reduction (313.63 μm), representing 24.15% decrease in excess FTH. The change in FTH was not statistically significant when assessed using Wilcoxon signed rank test *(P = 0.674)*. FTH continued however to decrease during the follow-up period with thickness values of 294 μm and 287.38 μm, one and two

months after the last treatment, respectively. The total reduction in FTH at the end of follow-up period (8 weeks after last infusion) represented 43.75% of the excess FTH at baseline *(p =0.161)*.

Despite the reduction in the central foveal thickness, BCVA remained mainly unchanged throughout the study. At baseline, mean BCVA in the study eyes was 57.75 letters (20/80-20/63). During the treatment period, the maximum mean BCVA was 57.63 letters, reached at

Table 2 Changes in the mean systolic blood pressure and QTc interval following each infusion of combretastatin A-4 phosphate (SE = Standard error)

	1st infusion		2nd infusion		3rd infusion		4th infusion	
	mmHg (SE)	QTc in µm (SE)	mmHg (SE)	QTc in µm (SE)	mmHg (SE)	QTc in µm (SE)	mmHg (SE)	QTc in µm (SE)
Prior to Infusion	145 (4.8)	411 (3.51)	131 (3.38)	406 (3.25)	136 (4.78)	412 (3.58)	132 (7.11)	415 (6.14)
Hour 1	164 (7.9)	419 (4.41)	165 (5)	405 (4.75)	163 (9.48)	416 (3.44)	154 (4.84)	417 (4.82)
Hour 2	149 (6.66)	430 (10.12)	148 (5.53)	427 (8.09)	148 (5.32)	428 (6.62)	139 (6.56)	425 (8.75)
Hour 3	143 (6.31)	424 (7.23)	141 (2.95)	422 (4.78)	139 (5.33)	428 (6.01)	136 (7.8)	424 (7.47)
Hour 4	144 (7.6)	426 (4.93)	137 (4.5)	426 (4.78)	131 (5.75)	424 (5.09)	128 (6.63)	423 (7.35)
Hour 5	148 (9.7)	423 (7.55)	137 (5.08)	429 (12.83)	142 (3.62)	423 (6.61)	138 (5.72)	421 (7.65)

week 3 *(before 3rd infusion)* and week 4 *(the end of treatment period, before 4th infusion,* i.e. *the patients only received 3 treatments at the time of the VA measurements)*, and the minimum was 55.5 letters reached at week 2 *(before 2nd infusion)*. During follow-up period, the mean BCVA was 55.5 letters at week 8 *(p =0.128)* and 56.13 (20/80) letters at week 12 *(p = 0.398)*, losing 1.63 letters when compared to the baseline visual acuity.

Fluorescein angiography images of the study eyes at baseline showed that six study eyes had macular leakage of 1 to 2 MPS disc areas. Two eyes had large CNV lesions with leakage of 10 to 12 MPS disc areas. Of these two eyes, one eye had extensive hemorrhage and the other eye showed disciform scarring. At the end of the treatment period (after 4th infusion), the FA images from five patients did not show any changes in the size of leakage area. Of the other three eyes, one eye showed mild reduction and two eyes showed mild increase in leakage.

Fellow eyes
Five of the fellow eyes had neovascular AMD with mean FTH of 318.67 µm at baseline (an excess FTH of 106.67 µm) (Figure 3 bottom). At the end of the treatment period (after 4th infusion), the mean FTH showed a 31.92 µm reduction (286.75 µm) representing 30% of excess FTH at baseline. The fellow eyes maintained the reduced FTH during the follow-up period with FTH of 284.5 µm and 287 µm, one and two months after the last infusion of CA4P, respectively. The change in foveal thickness was not statistically significant when assessed using non-parametric testing with Wilcoxon signed rank test with *p >0.5* at every visit.

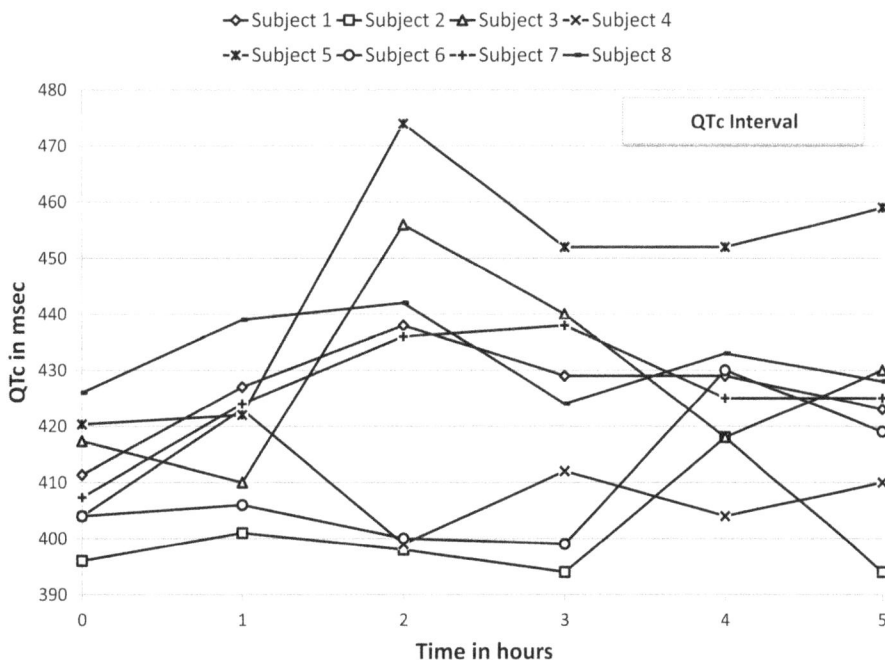

Figure 2 Changes in the QTc interval in the study subjects following the first infusion of combretastatin A-4 phosphate.

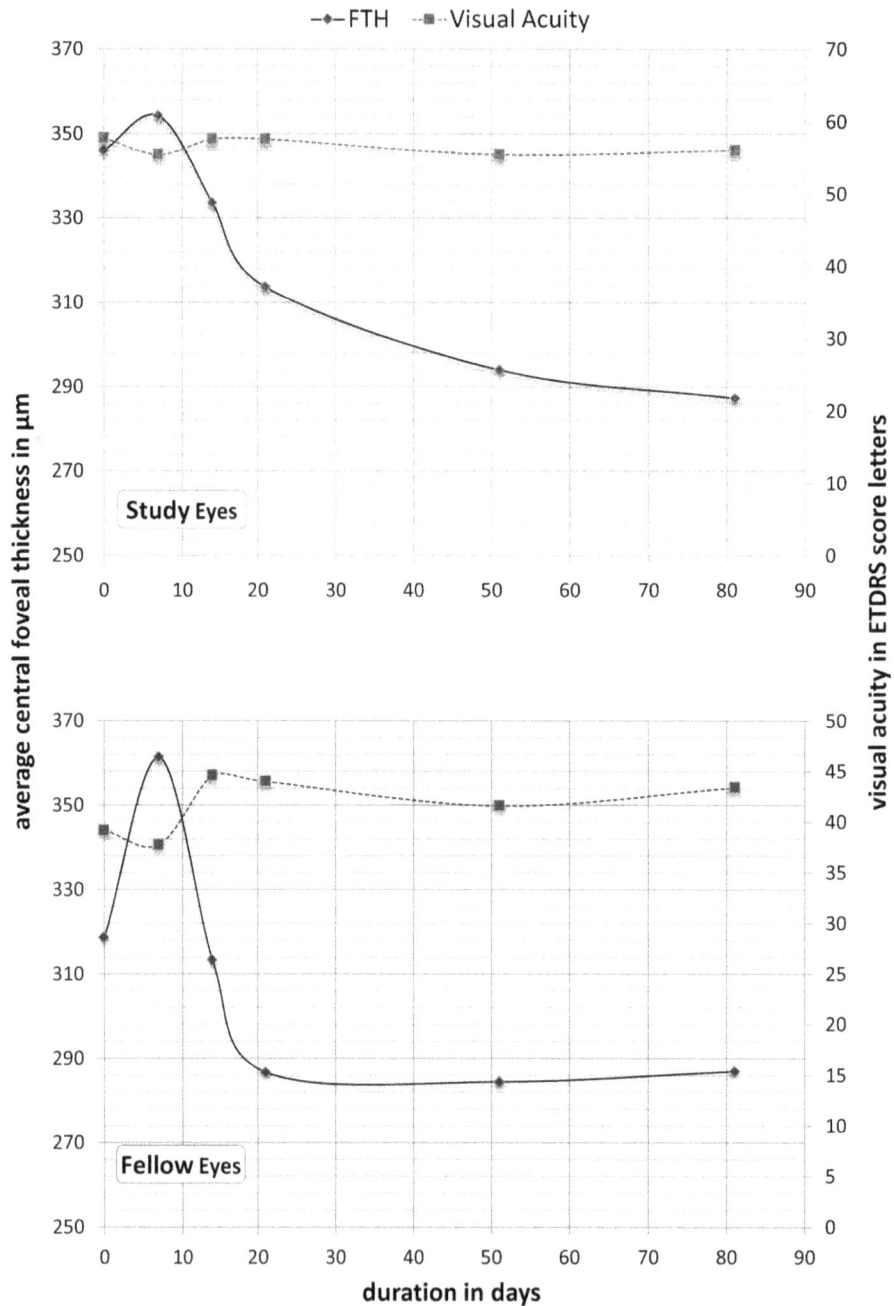

Figure 3 Mean changes in visual acuity and central retinal thickness during the study period in the study eyes (top) and the fellow eyes (bottom).

At baseline, the mean BCVA in the fellow eyes was 39.2 ETDRS letters (20/160). At the end of the treatment period, there was a gain of 4.8 ETDRS letters (44 letters = 20/125). The fellow eyes maintained the improvement in BCVA. At the end of the follow-up period (8 weeks after last infusion), BCVA remained at 43.4 ETDRS letters (20/125). However, the improvement of BCVA was not statistically significant following third infusion (p = 0.39) and at the end of the study (p = 0.38).

Discussion

Targeting the growth factors and signaling pathways involved in endothelial cell proliferation has led to the development and approval of the antiangiogenic therapies, pegaptanib and ranibizumab in neovascular AMD. The primary goal of these agents is to suppress the growth of new vessels underneath the retina. CA4P represents a lead compound in a separate group of agents known as VDAs that, unlike anti-VEGFs, are designed to selectively and rapidly compromise abnormal neovasculature. CA4P has been administered to patients with refractory solid tumors in multiple Phase 1, 2 and 3 trials [4,7,9,10].

Our study represents the first study of CA4P for an ophthalmic disease in humans. Clinical experience with CA4P consists of 18 completed and ongoing clinical trials in oncology and ophthalmology, together comprising more than 350 patients [4]. CA4P is currently being studied in patients with non-small cell lung cancer (NSCLC), anaplastic thyroid cancer (ATC) and platinum-resistant ovarian cancer. However, CA4P has not been investigated in patients without systemic malignancies until this study. As a VDA, it is expected that CA4P will have some vascular activities and that potential cardiovascular adverse events could be seen. In general, cardiovascular events have been observed at lesser frequency in doses of CA4P < 50 mg/m^2. In our study, negative cardiac stress was an inclusion criterion; however, current studies with CA4P in oncology and ophthalmology do not require such testing as part of the screening procedures.

The class side effects of VDA encountered in oncology studies [7,9,10] were observed in our study population as well. However, CA4P was tolerated in our study without experiencing severe adverse effects of Grade-3 or 4 (CTCAE v.3.0). The most commonly encountered adverse event in our study was transient hypertension. Tubulin depolymerization is believed to be responsible of this transient elevation of blood pressure. Depolymerization of endothelial microtubules makes vessels more sensitive to vasoconstriction and, consequently, hypertension [4]. Elevation of blood pressure is of particular concern in our study population giving the susceptibility and high prevalence of hypertension in the age group of neovascular AMD. The majority of our study patients had either a pre-existing or a borderline hypertension, which, along with other factors such as the presence of higher risk factors of cardiovascular disease in our study's age group, may be responsible for the higher incidence of post-infusion hypertension in our study (75%) when compared with the reported rates in oncology (30%) [11]. In support of our explanation, the SANA study [12] have demonstrated that when bevacizumab was administered intravenously in patients with neovascular AMD it resulted in an incidence of hypertension (78%), which is comparable to our study results. The BEAT-AMD Study has reported a mean elevation of systolic blood pressure from 140 mmHg to 150 mmHg in patients who received bevacizumab intravenously [13]. In another study, Geitzenauer et al. reported comparable (to ours) elevation in blood pressure following intravenous administration of bevacizumab in patients with neovascular AMD, which has peaked in the second day post infusion. In all previous studies that evaluated intravenous bevacizumab, the investigators have

concluded that the elevated blood pressure is insignificant [14]. However, despite having generally comparable results, our study cannot be directly compared with the previous studies due to the different methodologies employed and different patient characteristics. For example, it is not known from the BEAT-AMD Study, whether blood pressure has or has not elevated in the immediate post-infusion hours, which was when we noticed the transient hypertension in our patients [13]. In addition, while our study has allowed patients with high blood pressure to participate, Geitzenauer et al., have excluded patients with blood pressure >140/90 mmHg and patients taking more than one drug to control their blood pressure; they also did not allow bevacizumab infusion if pretreatment blood pressure is >140/90 mmHg [14]. Therefore, our results should be taken within their own context and any comparison with previous studies that utilized other intravenous agents should be interpreted with caution.

Angiotensin converting enzyme (ACE) inhibitors were used to manage the elevated blood pressure in our study. However, experiences from more recent studies suggest that management guidelines using nitrates and calcium channel blockers can result in a decrease in cardiovascular toxicity [4,15]. Giving the short-lived duration of elevated pressure, which can be explained by the short plasma half-life of CA4P, the control of hypertension may only be required for few hours following the infusion. Routine prophylaxis with a calcium channel blocker could also become part of the treatment in high-risk patients [4].

Similar to the elevation in blood pressure, the changes in QTc were generally mild and confined to the post-infusion period. QTc could not be predicted from baseline values. Current clinical trials, in both oncology and ophthalmology, implement guidelines with magnesium and potassium supplementation to decrease or prevent episodes of QTc prolongation.

Consistent with previous studies [8,16,17], intravenous CA4P did not show any cytotoxic side effects, and also did not demonstrate adverse effects previously reported with intravenous anti-VEGF agents, such as proteinuria, hemorrhage or thrombosis; however, our pilot study sample was too small to uncover all potential AEs associated with CA4P.

There were no serious ocular AEs associated with CA4P therapy. Such result should be interpreted with caution giving the small sample size and the non-randomized open label design of this pilot study.

The observations in our study further extend the reported effects of CA4P in animal models of ocular disease [5,6] with suggestive evidence of biological activity in human subjects with neovascular AMD. Such effect is evidenced by the reduction of the excess foveal thickness in the study eyes by 24.15% and 43.75% at the end of the treatment and follow-up periods, respectively. A similar sustainable reduction was also observed at the end of the treatment period in the fellow eyes that had CNV. The results need to be taken with caution giving the limitations of the OCT technology utilized in our study. Other studies utilizing the newly emergent spectral domain technology may shed different light on the anatomical outcome of CA4P therapy in neovascular AMD. The fact that the FTH reduction in our study is much less pronounced than with anti-VEGF as demonstrated in some studies [12,14] can be explained in part by the advanced disease of our study sample. It is also possible that a vascular disrupting agent does not have as significant effect in reducing retinal edema as an anti-VEGF agent.

At the functional level, BCVA remained stable in the study eye for the 12-week duration of the study, which may be attributed to either the nature of the disease or the bioactivity of CA4P. As the number of study subjects was small, it would not be appropriate to generate conclusions regarding the bioactivity of the drug. However, the visual gain in the fellow eye and the stability of BCVA in the study eye, in addition to the observed reduction of the retinal thickness in both study and fellow eyes, may warrant further exploration of the potential beneficial effects of CA4P in eyes with neovascular AMD. Significant visual gain has been reported in patients who received intravenous bevacizumab [12,14]. In the SANA study patients gained a median of 8 letters over 12 weeks [12]. Nevertheless, all studies were non-controlled, non-randomized, open-labeled, and small sampled; hence, no directed comparison can be accurately drawn between both studies. In the only controlled study, the BEAT-AMD Study did not demonstrate significant change in BCVA in patients with neovascular AMD when treated with intravenous bevacizumab, which seems consistent with our results [13]. All patients enrolled in our study presented at baseline with active disease despite at least two sessions of PDT, which perhaps indicate a level of severity that may not be present in many of the anti-VEGF studies.

No maximal tolerated dose (MTD) was determined in this study. The dose levels employed, 27 to 36 mg/m^2, are below the MTD (approximately 60 mg/m^2) that was independently determined in three separate oncology studies [9,10]. The dose level of 27 mg/m^2 was approximately the threshold dose for inhibition of blood flow in oncology studies. Investigators concluded that significant impact on tumor blood flow was observed in a higher proportion of patients when dose levels of 40 to 60 mg/m^2 were administered [4,7,9,18]. Further assessment of the dose dependency of CA4P for CNV might be of interest due to the potential for greater biological effect with higher doses,

provided no additional or more severe adverse events are noted.

Compared with the current intraocular treatment options that are available for patients with neovascular AMD, agents administered intravenously, especially those with potential systemic effects, are admittedly less appealing to patients and ophthalmologists. However, the novelty of mechanisms though which CA4P exerts its biological activity may add to the expanding arsenal of therapeutic options available today for patients with neovascular AMD. Furthermore, recent studies in rabbits and primates have suggested that topical administration of CA4P allows sufficient penetration of the drug to the choroid [19]; hence, localized ocular therapy with CA4P may be feasible and available in the future. In addition, further study of systemically administered CA4P in AMD may be warranted, especially if the associated side effects are known and can be controlled with proper therapy and monitoring.

Although CA4P is an anti-vascular agent, its mechanism of action and side effect profile differs from that of anti-angiogenic VEGF inhibitors. Synergetic inhibitory effects of CA4P and bevacizumab on blood flow have been demonstrated in recent studies in both xenograft models and in patients with refractory solid tumors. CA4P may, therefore, have potential role in the management of neovascular AMD and other retinal vascular diseases, either as monotherapy or in combination with anti-VEGF treatments, especially if topical or intravitreal or other local formulation/s are developed.

Conclusion

The safety profile of intravenous CA4P was consistent with that reported in oncology patients and with the class effects of vascular disruptive agents. There are evidences to suggest efficacy of CA4P in neovascular AMD. However, the level of systemic safety and efficacy indicates that systemic CA4P may not be suitable as an alternative monotherapy for neovascular AMD, especially when compared to the overall safe and very effective intravitreal anti-VEGF therapy today. There might be a role for CA4P as an adjunctive therapy, to be used in combination approach, when delivered intravitreally/topically. Further studies of CA4P in AMD and other ophthalmic disorders are indicated to investigate the potential role of vascular disrupting agents in the management of angiogenic retinal vascular diseases.

Competing interests

Jai Balkissoon is the Vice President, Clinical Research and Clinical Operations, OXIGENE, Inc.

Authors' contributions

MI has contributed in data analysis and interpretation, have been involved in drafting and critical revision of the manuscript, and have given final approval of the version to be published; DVD has contributed in the concept and design of this study, have been involved in data interpretation and in critical revision of the manuscript, and have given final approval of the version to be published; YJS has contributed in data analysis and interpretation, have been involved in drafting and critical revision of the manuscript and have given final approval to this version to be published; SMS has contributed in the concept and design of this study, have been involved in data collection and critical revision of the manuscript, and have given final approval of the version to be published; EVA has contributed in data collection and critical revision of the manuscript and have given final approval to of the version to be published; GH has contributed in data collection and critical revision of the manuscript and have given final approval to of the version to be published; JKD has contributed in data analysis and interpretation, have been involved in data collection and in drafting and critical revision of the manuscript, and have given final approval to of the version to be published; RR has contributed in data analysis and interpretation, have been involved in data collection and in drafting and critical revision of the manuscript, and have given final approval to of the version to be published; JB has contributed in the concept and design of this study, have been involved in critical revision of the manuscript, and have given final approval of the version to be published, JTH has contributed in the concept and design of this study, have been involved in data collection and critical revision of the manuscript, and have given final approval of the version to be published; PAC has contributed in the concept and design of this study, have been involved in data collection and critical revision of the manuscript, and have given final approval of the version to be published; QDN has contributed in the concept and design of this study, has been involved in data collection and critical revision of the manuscript, and has given final approval of the version to be published. All authors read and approved the final manuscript.

Acknowledgements
The study was supported by the Foundation Fighting Blindness with the study drug provided by OxiGene, Inc.

Author details
[1]Wilmer Eye Institute, Johns Hopkins University School of Medicine, 600 North Wolfe Street, Maumenee 745, Baltimore, MD 21287, USA. [2]Division of Cardiology, Department of Medicine, Johns Hopkins University School of Medicine, Baltimore, MD, USA. [3]Department of Medicine, Case Western Reserve University School of Medicine, Cleveland, OH, USA. [4]Department of Anesthesia, Johns Hopkins University School of Medicine, Baltimore, MD, USA. [5]OxiGene, Inc., South San Francisco, California, CA, USA. [6]Stanley M. Truhlsen Eye Institute, University of Nebraska Medical Center, Omaha, NE, USA.

References
1. Hu E, Ko R, Koda R, Rosen P, Jeffers S, Scholtz M, Muggia F: **Phase I toxicity and pharmacology study of trimethylcolchicinic acid in patients with advanced malignancies.** *Cancer Chemother Pharmacol* 1990, **26**(5):359–364.
2. Siemann DW, Bibby MC, Dark GG, Dicker AP, Eskens FA, Horsman MR, Marme D, Lorusso PM: **Differentiation and definition of vascular-targeted therapies.** *Clin Cancer Res* 2005, **11**(2 Pt 1):416–420.
3. Duncan DD, Lemaillet P, Ibrahim M, Nguyen QD, Hiller M, Ramella-Roman J: **Absolute blood velocity measured with a modified fundus camera.** *J Biomed Opt* 2010, **15**(5):056014.
4. Siemann DW, Chaplin DJ, Walicke PA: **A review and update of the current status of the vasculature-disabling agent combretastatin-A4 phosphate (CA4P).** *Expert Opin Investig Drugs* 2009, **18**(2):189–197.
5. Griggs J, Skepper JN, Smith GA, Brindle KM, Metcalfe JC, Hesketh R: **Inhibition of proliferative retinopathy by the anti-vascular agent combretastatin-A4.** *Am J Pathol* 2002, **160**(3):1097–1103.
6. Nambu H, Nambu R, Melia M, Campochiaro PA: **Combretastatin A-4 phosphate suppresses development and induces regression of choroidal neovascularization.** *Invest Ophthalmol Vis Sci* 2003, **44**(8):3650–3655.
7. Cooney MM, Savvides P, Agarwala S, Wang D, Flick S, Bergant S, Bhakta S, Lavertu P, Ortiz J, Remick S: **Phase II study of combretastatin A4 phosphate (CA4P) in patients with advanced anaplastic thyroid carcinoma (ATC).** *J Clin Oncol (Meet Abstracts)* 2006, **24**(18_suppl):5580.
8. Dowlati A, Robertson K, Cooney M, Petros WP, Stratford M, Jesberger J, Rafie N, Overmoyer B, Makkar V, Stambler B, *et al*: **A phase I pharmacokinetic and translational study of the novel vascular targeting agent combretastatin a-4 phosphate on a single-dose intravenous schedule in patients with advanced cancer.** *Cancer Res* 2002, **62**(12):3408–3416.
9. Stevenson JP, Rosen M, Sun W, Gallagher M, Haller DG, Vaughn D, Giantonio B, Zimmer R, Petros WP, Stratford M, *et al*: **Phase I trial of the antivascular agent combretastatin A4 phosphate on a 5-day schedule to patients with cancer: magnetic resonance imaging evidence for altered tumor blood flow.** *J Clin Oncol* 2003, **21**(23):4428–4438.
10. Rustin GJ, Galbraith SM, Anderson H, Stratford M, Folkes LK, Sena L, Gumbrell L, Price PM: **Phase I clinical trial of weekly combretastatin A4 phosphate: clinical and pharmacokinetic results.** *J Clin Oncol* 2003, **21**(15):2815–2822.
11. Martel CL, Ebrahimi B, Horns RC, Upadhyaya GH, Vakil MJ, Yeon CH, Bosserman LD, Presant CA: **Incidence of bevacizumab (BE) related toxicities: Association of hypertension (HTN) and proteinuria (PTN), a BE toxicity syndrome (BETS).** *J Clin Oncol* 2005, **23**(16):744s.
12. Michels S, Rosenfeld PJ, Puliafito CA, Marcus EN, Venkatraman AS: **Systemic bevacizumab (Avastin) therapy for neovascular age-related macular degeneration twelve-week results of an uncontrolled open-label clinical study.** *Ophthalmology* 2005, **112**(6):1035–1047.
13. Schmid-Kubista KE, Krebs I, Gruenberger B, Zeiler F, Schueller J, Binder S: **Systemic bevacizumab (avastin) therapy for exudative neovascular age-related macular degeneration. The BEAT-AMD-study.** *Br J Ophthalmol* 2009, **93**(7):914–919.
14. Geitzenauer W, Michels S, Prager F, Rosenfeld PJ, Kornek G, Vormittag L, Schmidt-Erfurth U: **Comparison of 2.5 mg/kg and 5 mg/kg systemic bevacizumab in neovascular age-related macular degeneration: twenty-four week results of an uncontrolled, prospective cohort study.** *Retina* 2008, **28**(10):1375–1386.
15. Spaide RF, Koizumi H, Freund KB: **Photoreceptor outer segment abnormalities as a cause of blind spot enlargement in acute zonal occult outer retinopathy–complex diseases.** *Am J Ophthalmol* 2008, **146**(1):111–120.
16. Cooney MM, Radivoyevitch T, Dowlati A, Overmoyer B, Levitan N, Robertson K, Levine SL, DeCaro K, Buchter C, Taylor A, *et al*: **Cardiovascular safety profile of combretastatin A4 phosphate in a single-dose phase I study in patients with advanced cancer.** *Clin Cancer Res* 2004, **10**(1):96–100.
17. Griggs J, Metcalfe JC, Hesketh R: **Targeting tumour vasculature: the development of combretastatin A4.** *Lancet Oncol* 2001, **2**(2):82–87.
18. Koh DM, Blackledge M, Collins DJ, Padhani AR, Wallace T, Wilton B, Taylor NJ, Stirling JJ, Sinha R, Walicke P, *et al*: **Reproducibility and changes in the apparent diffusion coefficients of solid tumours treated with combretastatin A4 phosphate and bevacizumab in a two-centre phase I clinical trial.** *Eur Radiol* 2009, **19**(11):2728–2738.
19. Patterson DMRGJS, Serradell N, Rosa E, Bolos J: **Combretastatin A-4 phosphate: Vascular disrupting agent oncolytic treatment of age-related macular degeneration.** *Drugs future* 2007, **32**(12):1025–1032.

6

Immunogenicity of panitumumab in combination chemotherapy clinical trials

Dohan Weeraratne, Alin Chen, Jason J Pennucci, Chi-Yuan Wu, Kathy Zhang, Jacqueline Wright, Juan José Pérez-Ruixo, Bing-Bing Yang, Arunan Kaliyaperumal, Shalini Gupta, Steven J Swanson, Narendra Chirmule and Marta Starcevic*

Abstract

Background: Panitumumab is a fully human antibody against the epidermal growth factor receptor that is indicated for the treatment of metastatic colorectal cancer (mCRC) after disease progression on standard chemotherapy. The purpose of this analysis was to examine the immunogenicity of panitumumab and to evaluate the effect of anti-panitumumab antibodies on pharmacokinetic and safety profiles in patients with mCRC receiving panitumumab in combination with oxaliplatin- or irinotecan-based chemotherapies.

Methods: Three validated assays (two screening immunoassays and a neutralizing antibody bioassay) were used to detect the presence of anti-panitumumab antibodies in serum samples collected from patients enrolled in four panitumumab combination chemotherapy clinical trials. The impact of anti-panitumumab antibodies on pharmacokinetic and safety profiles was analyzed using population pharmacokinetic analysis and descriptive statistics, respectively.

Results: Of 1124 patients treated with panitumumab in combination with oxaliplatin- or irinotecan-based chemotherapy with postbaseline samples available for testing, 20 (1.8%) patients developed binding antibodies and 2 (0.2%) developed neutralizing antibodies. The incidence of anti-panitumumab antibodies was similar in patients with tumors expressing wild-type or mutant *KRAS* and in patients receiving oxaliplatin- or irinotecan-based chemotherapies. No evidence of an altered pharmacokinetic or safety profile was found in patients who tested positive for anti-panitumumab antibodies.

Conclusions: The immunogenicity of panitumumab in the combination chemotherapy setting was infrequent and similar to the immunogenicity observed in the monotherapy setting. Panitumumab immunogenicity did not appear to alter pharmacokinetic or safety profiles. This low rate of immunogenicity may be attributed to the fully human nature of panitumumab.

Trial registration: ClinicalTrials.gov: NCT00339183 (study 20050181), NCT00411450 (study 20060277), NCT00332163 (study 20050184), and NCT00364013 (study 20050203).

Background

Panitumumab is a high affinity ($K_d = 5 \times 10^{11}$ M) fully human IgG2 monoclonal antibody (mAb) directed against human epidermal growth factor receptor (EGFR). Panitumumab is indicated as monotherapy for the treatment of metastatic colorectal cancer (mCRC) after disease progression on fluoropyrimidine, oxaliplatin, and irinotecan chemotherapy regimens in the United States (US) and European Union (EU) [1,2]. In the US,

treatment of patients whose tumors have *KRAS* mutations in codon 12 or 13 is not recommended [1]. In the EU, panitumumab is indicated for patients whose tumors express EGFR and wild-type *KRAS* [2]. Panitumumab has been shown to significantly improve progression-free survival as first-line therapy with FOLFOX4 [3] and as second-line therapy with FOLFIRI [4] in patients with mCRC tumors expressing wild-type *KRAS*.

An important concern with the administration of therapeutic proteins is the potential to induce an immune response. Immune responses against biologics can affect

* Correspondence: mstarcev@amgen.com
Amgen Inc., One Amgen Center Drive, Thousand Oaks, CA 91320, USA

their pharmacokinetics (eg, alter serum concentrations), safety (by eliciting injection-site reactions or hypersensitivity), or reduce efficacy [5]. Therefore, one of the considerations for mAb therapeutic development has been to reduce the risk of undesirable immunogenicity [6]. Based on the premise that humanized or fully human mAbs would be less likely to induce an immune response than chimeric or murine-derived mAbs, engineering technologies have focused on decreasing or eliminating the presence of nonhuman sequences within the molecule. The comparison of immunogenicity rates between mAb therapeutics is challenging because of differences in dosing regimens, patient populations, and methods used to detect anti-drug antibodies. Nevertheless, it appears that the reduction in mouse sequence content has generally resulted in improved immunogenicity profiles [7], with only a few examples of fully human mAbs with high incidences of anti-drug antibody development [8,9]. Despite these advances, the immunogenic potential of a molecule is difficult to predict based on the protein sequence alone. Various additional factors may contribute to the overall immunogenicity risk, including other product characteristics (impurity profile, formulation, post-translational modifications), patient characteristics (eg, pre-existing immunodeficiency, concurrent illness), and drug administration characteristics (frequency, route, and duration) [5].

Cetuximab, an anti-EGFR chimeric mouse-human monoclonal antibody, had a reportedly low incidence of anti-chimeric antibodies as measured by a radiometric assay in early phase clinical trials [10,11]. However, a high incidence of hypersensitivity reactions consistent with IgE-mediated anaphylaxis has been observed in patients treated for mCRC in some areas of the US [12]. These hypersensitivity reactions appeared to be caused by pre-existing IgE antibodies to galactose-α-1,3-galactose, an oligosaccharide component added during the production of cetuximab in a mouse cell line by a murine-specific enzyme [13]. As expected from the apparent absence of this post-translational modification on panitumumab, hypersensitivity reactions resembling anaphylactic reactions to galactose-α-1,3-galactose have not been seen in clinical trials or postmarketing reports of patients receiving panitumumab. Additionally, the presence of murine-derived N-glycolylneuraminic acid has been demonstrated on cetuximab, which is introduced by the manufacturing process [14]. Most or all humans make antibodies to this sialic acid; these antibodies have been shown to form immune complexes with cetuximab, but not panitumumab, in vitro [14].

The fully human nature of panitumumab was expected to decrease the rate of immunogenicity compared with therapeutic antibodies containing nonhuman coding sequences [15]. However, unique sequences in the complementarity determining regions (CDRs) and potential

manufacturing-related modifications still provide the potential for panitumumab to be recognized as nonself by the human immune system, which could result in the development of anti-panitumumab antibody responses. As it is not known whether these immune responses could lead to clinically serious outcomes, the monitoring of patients who participated in clinical trials for the development of antibodies and an assessment of the impact of anti-panitumumab antibodies on pharmacokinetics and safety was a critical component of the panitumumab clinical development program.

The immunogenicity of panitumumab when administered as monotherapy was evaluated in clinical trials of patients with mCRC and other solid tumors. The incidence of binding antibodies to panitumumab (excluding predose and transient positive patients) was < 1% as detected by the acid dissociation enzyme-linked immunosorbent assay (ELISA) [16] and 4.6% as detected by the Biacore® assay [1,16]. The incidence of neutralizing antibodies was 1.6%. The analysis described here examined the immunogenicity of panitumumab when administered as combination therapy with oxaliplatin- or irinotecan-based chemotherapy regimens in patients with refractory mCRC and explored the relationship between panitumumab immunogenicity and pharmacokinetic and safety profiles.

Methods
Patients and sample collection
Serum samples for anti-panitumumab antibody testing were collected from mCRC patients enrolled in 4 panitumumab clinical trials (20050184, 20060277, 20050181, and 20050203). Patients in these studies received irinotecan-based (including FOLFIRI) or oxaliplatin-based (FOLFOX) chemotherapies with or without panitumumab. Study 20050184 (STEPP) was a phase 2, open-label, randomized trial to compare pre-emptive skin toxicity therapy with reactive treatment in patients with mCRC receiving panitumumab plus irinotecan or FOLFIRI [17]. Study 20060277 (PRECEPT) was a phase 2, open-label, single-arm trial that estimated the effect of tumor *KRAS* status (wild-type or mutant) on efficacy endpoints in patients receiving panitumumab plus FOLFIRI as second-line therapy for mCRC [18]. Study 20050181 was a phase 3 randomized trial to evaluate panitumumab plus FOLFIRI combination therapy versus FOLFIRI alone as second-line therapy for mCRC [4]. Study 20050203 (PRIME) was a phase 3, randomized trial to evaluate the efficacy and safety of panitumumab in combination with FOLFOX4 versus FOLFOX4 alone as first-line therapy for mCRC [3]. Panitumumab was administered at 6.0 mg/kg every 2 weeks (Q2W) in all studies; patients in one arm of study 20050184 received panitumumab at 9.0 mg/kg every 3 weeks.

Per the study protocols, serum samples for immunogenicity assessments were collected from all panitumumab-treated patients prior to study treatment (baseline samples) and from all patients at the safety follow-up visit (postbaseline samples, obtained 30 ± 3 days after the administration of the last study treatment). Serum samples used for the measurement of panitumumab concentration (pharmacokinetic assessments) were collected from patients enrolled in study 20050181 before dosing on cycle 1 day 1 and cycle 2 day 1, every 8 weeks starting at week 8, and at the safety follow-up visit (30 ± 3 days after administration of the last dose).

KRAS mutation status was determined using DNA isolated from fixed tumor samples. Mutations in *KRAS* were detected using a *KRAS* mutation kit (DxS Ltd, Manchester, UK) as previously described [19]. *KRAS* status was available from 87 (95%) patients in study 20050184, 109 (95%) patients in study 20060277, 1083 (91%) patients in study 20050181, and 1096 (93%) patients in study 20050203.

Patients receiving both doses of panitumumab (6.0 mg/kg Q2W and 9.0 mg/kg Q3W) were included in the immunogenicity and safety analyses.

These studies were conducted in accordance with the principles for human experimentation as defined in the International Conference on Harmonization Good Clinical Practice guidelines and the principles of the Declaration of Helsinki. All studies were approved by the corresponding Investigational Review Boards, and informed consent was obtained from each patient after being advised of the potential risks and benefits as well as the investigational nature of the study.

Anti-panitumumab antibody detection assays

Antibody samples were evaluated for the presence of anti-panitumumab antibodies according to the testing strategy depicted in Figure 1. The screening assays used to detect antibodies capable of binding to panitumumab, an ELISA and a Biacore assay, have been previously described [16]. All samples confirmed to be positive in either screening assay were further tested for antibodies capable of neutralizing the activity of panitumumab in vitro in a cell-based EGFR phosphorylation bioassay as previously described [16]. Immunogenicity assay characteristics are shown in Table 1. Developing antibodies were defined as antibodies that were observed only at a postbaseline time point(s) but not at the baseline time point. Pre-existing antibodies were defined as antibodies that were observed at the baseline time point.

The assays and sample collection strategy were optimized to reduce drug interference with antibody detection. The performance of the immunogenicity assays was monitored by implementing a trending process utilizing Westgard multirules that tracked negative control and positive control values for each assay performed [20].

The observed low incidences of trending alarms and assay failures in the screening immunoassays and bioassay were indicative of assay stability.

Serum panitumumab concentration immunoassay

Panitumumab concentrations in human serum were measured by a validated ELISA. Briefly, panitumumab was captured in microplate wells precoated with mouse anti-panitumumab antibody (Amgen Inc., Thousand Oaks, CA, USA). Horseradish peroxidase-labeled rabbit polyclonal anti-panitumumab antibody (Amgen Inc.) was added to the wells and allowed to react with the captured panitumumab. A colorimetric signal was produced after the addition of tetramethylbenzidine-peroxidase substrate solution. The optical density (OD) of the signal, measured at 450-650 nm, was proportional to the amount of captured panitumumab. The conversion of OD units to concentrations for the assay quality controls and samples was achieved through a computer software-mediated comparison to a standard curve on the same assay run, which was regressed according to a 5 PL (Auto Estimate) regression model with a weighting factor of $1/Y$. The lower limit of quantitation was 400 ng/mL in human serum.

Impact of immunogenicity on panitumumab pharmacokinetics

A population pharmacokinetic (PopPK) modeling and simulation approach was performed to evaluate the impact of immunogenicity on panitumumab pharmacokinetics by comparing the observed panitumumab concentrations of antibody-positive patients from study 20050181 with the predicted pharmacokinetic profiles based on PopPK parameters for antibody-negative patients.

A 2-compartment model with parallel linear and nonlinear (Michaelis-Menten) elimination pathways has been used to describe the disposition of panitumumab [21,22]. A previously developed and validated PopPK model [21] was updated by including the pharmacokinetic data from antibody-negative patients in study 20050181. The predictive check [23] was used to evaluate the validity of the updated PopPK model before subsequent analyses were performed. Using the updated PopPK parameters for antibody-negative patients, 1000 pharmacokinetic profiles were simulated for each antibody-positive patient according to the actual individual dosing history. The observed concentrations from each antibody-positive patient were superimposed with the model-predicted distribution. The pharmacokinetics of panitumumab in antibody-positive patients would be considered similar to antibody-negative patients if the proportions of the observed concentrations from antibody-positive patients falling within and outside the 90% prediction interval were not statistically different (chi-square test; $\alpha < 0.05$) from hypothesized proportions, ie, 5% above, 5% below, and 90% within the interval. A

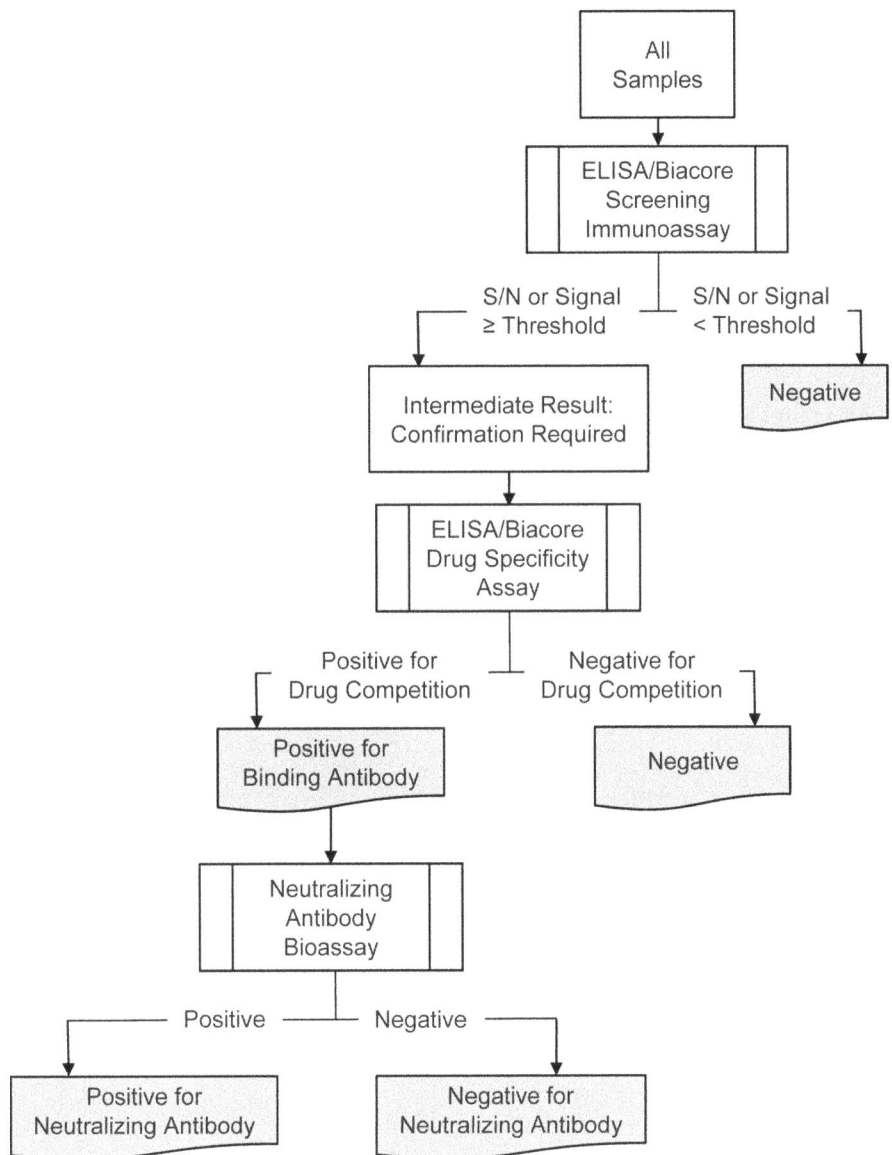

Figure 1 Panitumumab immunogenicity testing strategy. Three validated assays were used to detect the presence of anti-panitumumab antibodies. All clinical study samples were tested in two screening immunoassays (an acid-dissociation ELISA and a Biacore-based biosensor assay) to detect antibodies capable of binding to panitumumab. Samples that tested above the assay threshold and demonstrated reduction in response in the drug-competition specificity assay were reported as positive for binding antibodies and tested further in a cell-based neutralizing antibody bioassay. Assay thresholds were based on the upper bound of a one-sided 95% reference interval for the distribution of signals generated by serum samples from healthy subjects or cancer patients. S/N, signal-to-noise ratio.

sensitivity analysis was conducted to evaluate the minimum difference in panitumumab concentration between antibody-positive and antibody-negative patients that, given the available sample size, could be statistically significant.

Impact of immunogenicity on panitumumab safety

The impact of immunogenicity on safety was evaluated through the review and assessment of the incidence of adverse events, potential infusion reactions, reasons for discontinuation from therapy, and total number of doses received while on study for panitumumab-treated antibody-positive patients and anti-panitumumab antibody-negative patients.

Results
Patients

A total of 1325 patients were tested for anti-panitumumab antibodies, including 558 patients who were treated with panitumumab plus oxaliplatin-based chemotherapy

Table 1 Immunogenicity assay characteristics

Assay	Assay Sensitivity*	LLRD	Drug Tolerance[†]	
			Anti-panitumumab	Panitumumab
ELISA	10 ng/mL	60 ng/mL	60 ng/mL 500 ng/mL	9 μg/mL 81 μg/mL
Biacore	1.8 μg/mL	1.8 μg/mL	4 μg/mL 20 μg/mL	1.9 μg/mL 7.8 μg/mL
Bioassay	~62.5 ng/mL	~125 ng/mL	~1 μg/mL	~2.5 μg/mL

*Intersection of the assay threshold with the rabbit polyclonal anti-panitumumab antibody dose-response curve.

[†]Level of anti-panitumumab antibodies that can be detected in the presence of the amount of panitumumab in the adjacent column.

LLRD, lower limit of reliable detection, the lowest concentration of the rabbit polyclonal anti-panitumumab antibody that could be reliably detected as positive when spiked into neat serum from multiple donors.

(study 20050203) and 767 patients treated with panitumumab plus irinotecan-based chemotherapy (studies 20050181, 20050184, and 20060277). Of these, 1225 patients (511 treated with panitumumab plus oxaliplatin and 714 treated with panitumumab plus irinotecan) had baseline samples available and 1124 patients (480 treated with panitumumab plus oxaliplatin and 664 treated with panitumumab plus irinotecan) had postbaseline samples available for testing. Over half of the patients were men and the population was predominantly white. Overall, 53% of the patients had tumors expressing wild-type *KRAS* (39% had mutant *KRAS* and 8% were unevaluable).

Anti-panitumumab antibodies

The development of anti-panitumumab antibodies in patients receiving panitumumab in combination with chemotherapy (oxaliplatin- or irinotecan-based) occurred infrequently: 1.8% of patients developed binding antibodies and 0.2% of patients developed neutralizing antibodies (Table 2). The incidence of developing antibodies was low

Table 2 Incidence of anti-panitumumab antibodies

	Wild-Type *KRAS*		Mutant *KRAS*		All Patients*	
	Either Biacore or ELISA	Bioassay	Either Biacore or ELISA	Bioassay	Either Biacore or ELISA	Bioassay
Total Antibody Incidence, n_1/n_2 (%)						
20050184	6/48 (12.5)	1/48 (2.1)	0/37 (0)	0/37 (0)	6/93 (6.5)	1/93 (1.1)
20060277	0/64 (0)	0/64 (0)	1/45 (2.2)	1/45 (2.2)	1/115 (0.9)	1/115 (0.9)
20050181	11/288 (3.8)	0/288 (0)	9/223 (4.0)	1/223 (0.4)	22/559 (3.9)	1/559 (0.2)
20050203 (Pmab + OX)	21/308 (6.8)	3/308 (1.0)	10/206 (4.9)	1/206 (0.5)	36/558 (6.5)	4/558 (0.7)
Pmab + IRI	17/400 (4.3)	1/400 (0.3)	10/305 (3.3)	2/305 (3.3)	29/767 (3.8)	3/767 (0.4)
Pmab + IRI or OX	38/708 (5.4)	4/708 (0.6)	20/511 (3.9)	3/511 (0.6)	65/1325 (4.9)	7/1325 (0.5)
Pre-existing Antibody Incidence, n_3/n_4 (%)						
20050184	4/48 (8.3)	1/48 (2.1)	0/37 (0)	0/37 (0)	4/93 (4.3)	1/93 (1.1)
20060277	0/64 (0)	0/64 (0)	1/45 (2.2)	1/45 (2.2)	1/115 (0.9)	1/115 (0.9)
20050181	11/252 (4.4)	0/252 (0)	7/210 (3.3)	1/210 (0.5)	19/506 (3.8)	1/506 (0.2)
20050203 (Pmab + OX)	11/282 (3.9)	2/282 (0.7)	7/188 (3.7)	0/188 (0)	22/511 (4.3)	2/511 (0.4)
Pmab + IRI	15/364 (4.1)	1/364 (0.3)	8/292 (2.7)	2/292 (0.7)	24/714 (3.4)	3/714 (0.4)
Pmab + IRI or OX	26/646 (4.0)	3/646 (0.5)	15/480 (3.1)	2/480 (0.4)	46/1225 (3.8)	5/1225 (0.4)
Developing Antibody Incidence, n_5/n_6 (%)						
20050184	2/37 (5.4)	0/37 (0)	0/26 (0)	0/26 (0)	2/68 (2.9)	0/68 (0)
20060277	0/42 (0)	0/42 (0)	0/30 (0)	0/30 (0)	0/75 (0)	0/75 (0)
20050181	0/255 (0)	0/255 (0)	3/205 (1.5)	0/205 (0)	4/501 (0.8)	0/501 (0)
20050203 (Pmab + OX)	10/264 (3.8)	1/264 (0.4)	3/178 (1.7)	1/178 (0.6)	14/480 (2.9)	2/480 (0.4)
Pmab + IRI	2/334 (0.6)	0/334 (0)	3/261 (1.1)	0/261 (0)	6/644 (0.9)	0/644 (0)
Pmab + IRI or OX	12/598 (2.0)	1/598 (0.2)	6/439 (1.4)	1/439 (0.2)	20/1124 (1.8)	2/1124 (0.2)

*All Patients includes patients with wild-type, mutant, and unknown *KRAS* status.

Pmab, panitumumab; IRI, irinotecan-based chemotherapy; OX, oxaliplatin-based chemotherapy; n_1, number of patients with a positive antibody result at any time point; n_2, number of patients with at least one immunoassay result; n_3, number of patients with a positive antibody result at or before baseline; n_4, number of patients with an immunoassay antibody result at or before baseline; n_5, number of patients with negative or no antibody result at or before baseline and a positive antibody result at a postbaseline time point; n_6, number of patients with at least one postbaseline immunoassay antibody result in patients with tumors expressing wild-type and mutant *KRAS* (2.0% and 1.4% binding antibodies and 0.2% and 0.2% neutralizing antibodies, respectively). The incidence of developing antibodies was low in patients treated with oxaliplatin-based chemotherapy (2.9% binding antibodies and 0.4% neutralizing antibodies) and in patients treated with irinotecan-based chemotherapy (0.9% binding antibodies and 0% neutralizing antibodies). Pre-existing binding and neutralizing antibodies were detected in 3.8% and 0.4% of all patients before the start of any investigational product, respectively.

Impact of immunogenicity on panitumumab pharmacokinetics

Of the 22 patients with pre-existing and post-treatment developing anti-panitumumab antibodies in study 20050181, 38 samples from 11 patients were available for evaluation of panitumumab concentration. In addition, 68 samples from 53 antibody-negative patients in study 20050181 were analyzed for panitumumab concentration. Because of the low rate of immunogenicity in study 20050181 and limited availability of pharmacokinetic samples, the concentration data from patients with pre-existing and post-treatment developing antibody responses were combined for analysis.

Among 38 observed concentrations from the antibody-positive patients, 2 (5%) were below, 5 (13%) were above, and 31 (82%) were within the 90% prediction interval derived from pharmacokinetic profiles of antibody-negative patients. The proportions were not statistically different ($P = 0.0685$) from the hypothesized proportions (Table 3) and were similar to those for the antibody-negative patients ($P = 0.8807$), suggesting that no marked difference in the observed panitumumab concentrations was observed between the antibody-positive and antibody-negative patients.

Results of the sensitivity analysis showed that a statistically significant effect of immunogenicity would have been observed if the serum concentrations of antibody-positive patients were at least 55% lower than the current observed values given the current sample size. To further evaluate the impact of the sample size on the analysis, additional analyses were performed and the results showed that 200 and 650 samples would be needed to detect a 38% and

20% difference in panitumumab serum concentration, respectively (Figure 2).

Impact of immunogenicity on panitumumab safety profiles

No apparent difference in the rate of grade 3 and grade 4 adverse events (as graded per National Cancer Institute Common Terminology Criteria for Adverse Events [NCI CTCAE] version 3.0) was observed between patients who tested positive for anti-panitumumab antibodies and those who tested negative (Table 4). Although the incidence of grade 5 events was higher in patients testing positive for developing antibodies (n = 4; 19%) than in antibody-negative patients (n = 82; 6%), following a medical review of these cases, all were reported in the setting of progression of the underlying disease. The number of chemotherapy cycles received varied among patients; no apparent relationship between antibody status and number of cycles received was observed. Three patients experienced infusion reactions deemed related to panitumumab. Two patients (1 predose-positive and 1 developing antibody-positive) experienced grade 1 (mild) infusion reactions reported as vomiting and fever. One patient (predose-positive) had a grade 2 (moderate) infusion reaction of hypersensitivity, which was reported on study day 272 following multiple administrations of panitumumab. The event of hypersensitivity was confounded by the coadministration of oxaliplatin. Although the analysis of the impact of immunogenicity on safety was limited by the small number of antibody-positive patients, there was no evidence of an altered safety profile found in patients who tested positive for pre-existing or post-treatment developing anti-panitumumab antibodies compared to the safety profile of those patients who tested negative.

Discussion

The panitumumab immunogenicity testing strategy utilized two validated screening immunoassays to detect the presence of all antibodies capable of binding to panitumumab. The screening immunoassays were chosen to provide the optimal combination of sensitivity and drug tolerance (ELISA) and the ability to detect antibodies of various affinities (Biacore) [16]. A cell-based bioassay was used to detect antibodies with neutralizing activity.

Table 3 Distribution of the observed concentrations of panitumumab relative to the 90% predictive interval

Distribution in Relation to 90% Prediction Interval	Antibody-Positive Patients				Antibody-Negative Patients				P-value†
	N	%	95% CI	P-value*	N	%	95% CI	P-value*	
Below	2	5.3	0.6 -17.8	0.07	3	4.4	0.9 - 12.4	0.13	0.88
Above	5	13.2	4.4 - 28.1		7	10.3	4.2 - 20.1		
Within	31	81.6	65.7 - 92.3		58	85.3	74.6 - 92.7		

*Chi-square test with hypothesized proportions (5% below, 5% above, 90% within).
†Chi-square test of antibody-positive proportion vs antibody-negative proportion.

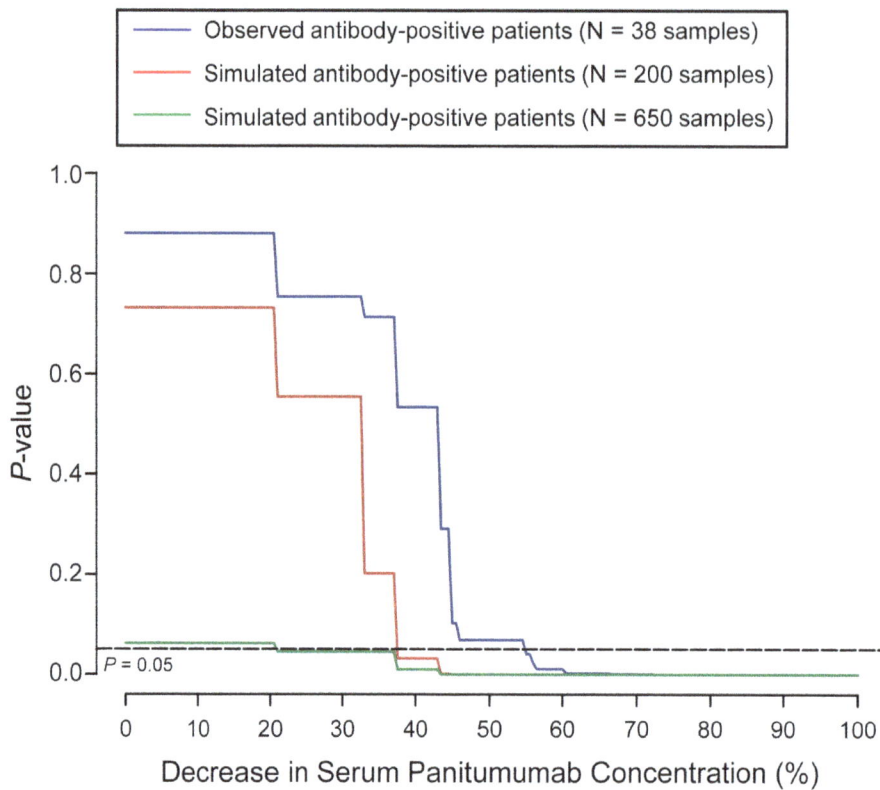

Figure 2 Sensitivity analysis. The sensitivity analysis estimated the minimum difference in panitumumab concentration between antibody-positive and antibody-negative samples that could be statistically significant ($P < 0.05$) with respect to the model prediction. Results show that the current observed sample size for pharmacokinetic testing (n = 38) from antibody-positive patients was only adequate to detect a difference of > 55%. Approximately 200 and 650 samples from antibody-positive patients would be required to detect differences of 38% and 20%, respectively.

Despite the use of these validated and sensitive assays, the development of anti-panitumumab antibodies in combination chemotherapy patients was detected infrequently. Developing antibody incidences did not appear to be affected by tumor *KRAS* status (wild-type or mutant) or combination chemotherapy regimen (oxaliplatin- or irinotecan-based).

Pre-existing binding and neutralizing antibodies were detected prior to the administration of panitumumab in 3.8% and 0.4% of patients, respectively. Positive results from these baseline samples may be due to the presence of cross-reacting antibodies generated against antigens that share a similar epitope with panitumumab. The presence of pre-existing antibodies in panitumumab-treated patients did not appear to affect the postdose antibody state of these patients. In addition, patients who tested positive for pre-existing antibodies did not appear to have altered safety profiles.

The broad, nonspecific cytotoxic effects of chemotherapy have the potential to impair the immune system, which could reduce the incidence of anti-panitumumab antibodies in patients receiving panitumumab in combination with chemotherapy. Both oxaliplatin and irinotecan have gastrointestinal toxicities [24,25], and have the potential to affect local and systemic immunity. The effects of chemotherapy on acquired immunity may have affected the development of anti-panitumumab antibodies in patients receiving chemotherapy plus panitumumab. The incidence of binding antibodies in the monotherapy setting (excluding predose and transient positive patients) was 3/613 (< 1%) as detected by the acid dissociation ELISA and 28/613 (4.6%) as detected by the Biacore assay [1], and neutralizing antibodies were detected in 10/613 (1.6%) of the patients [1]. The incidence of developing binding and neutralizing antibodies in the combination chemotherapy setting described here was similar but slightly lower (1.0% as detected by the ELISA, 0.8% as detected by the Biacore assay and 0.2% as detected by the neutralizing assay).

Based on available pharmacokinetic data from study 20050181, the phase 3 study of panitumumab plus FOL-FIRI for second-line treatment of mCRC, no evidence of an altered panitumumab pharmacokinetic profile was found in patients who received panitumumab 6.0 mg/kg

Table 4 Summary of adverse events (safety analysis set*)

	Antibody Negative (N = 1317)	Antibody Positive (N = 65)	Predose Positive (N = 46)	Developing Antibody Positive (N = 21)
Patients with any adverse event[†], n (%)	1312 (100)	65 (100)	46 (100)	21 (100)
Worst grade of 3[‡]	716 (54)	26 (40)	18 (39)	8 (38)
Worst grade of 4[‡]	264 (20)	18 (28)	15 (33)	4 (19)
Worst grade of 5[‡]	82 (6)	6 (9)	2 (4)	4 (19)
Any serious adverse event	544 (41)	32 (49)	23 (50)	10 (48)
Patients with any adverse event leading to permanent discontinuation of any study drug, n (%)	299 (23)	16 (25)	8 (17)	8 (38)
Not serious	217 (16)	12 (18)	6 (13)	6 (29)
Serious	108 (8)	6 (9)	3 (7)	3 (14)
Patients with any treatment-related adverse event[§], n (%)	1298 (99)	65 (100)	46 (100)	21 (100)
Worst grade of 3[‡]	739 (56)	30 (46)	20 (43)	11 (52)
Worst grade of 4[‡]	204 (15)	15 (23)	13 (28)	2 (10)
Worst grade of 5[‡]	13 (1)	1 (2)	0	1 (5)
Any serious adverse event	314 (24)	20 (31)	14 (30)	6 (29)
Patients with any adverse event leading to permanent discontinuation of any study drug, n (%)	251 (19)	11 (17)	5 (11)	6 (29)
Not serious	200 (15)	9 (14)	4 (9)	5 (24)
Serious	64 (5)	2 (3)	1 (2)	1 (5)

*The safety analysis set included all patients who were enrolled, randomized, and received at least one dose of study treatment in studies 20050203, 20050181, 20050184, and 20060277. Patients not testing positive by ELISA, Biacore, and bioassay or with all antibody results missing were included.

[†]Adverse events were coded using the Medical Dictionary for Regulatory Activities (MedDRA) version 12.0.

[‡]Severity was graded using the Common Terminology Criteria for Adverse Events (CTCAE) version 3.0, with the exception of some dermatology/skin adverse events, which were graded using CTCAE version 3.0 with modifications. Fatal adverse events were classified as grade 5.

[§]The investigator considered there to be a reasonable possibility that the event may have been caused by study drug.

Q2W and tested positive for pre-existing or developing anti-panitumumab antibodies. The results from study 20050181 were in agreement with previously published observations that there were no apparent differences in steady-state AUC, C_{max}, and C_{min} between patients who developed anti-panitumumab antibodies and those who did not [21,22]. A sensitivity analysis was conducted to show that even though the pharmacokinetic data were limited, a statistically significant effect of immunogenicity would have been observed if the difference in serum concentrations between antibody-positive and antibody-negative patients was greater than 55%. Therefore, this analysis ruled out the possibility that immunogenicity would cause a > 55% decrease in the panitumumab serum concentrations. Since the relationship between pharmacokinetics and efficacy has not been established, it is unclear what level of decrease in panitumumab serum concentration would result in a change in efficacy. By assuming a < 20% difference would be biologically unimportant, additional simulations were conducted to understand the sample size required to detect that level of difference. The result suggested that approximately 650 samples from antibody-positive patients would be required to detect a 20% difference in pharmacokinetics. To obtain this larger number of samples, it would require either fewer samples (ie, sparse sampling) from a larger antibody-positive population or

more samples (ie, intensive sampling) from a smaller antibody-positive population, both of which would be challenging, considering the low rate of immunogenicity for panitumumab.

Overall, there did not appear to be an association between the development of antibodies and safety outcomes. Higher incidences of adverse events observed in patients who were antibody negative at baseline and developed antibodies during the conduct of the study (n = 21) compared with those who were antibody negative throughout the study (n = 1317) may be related to the small sample size. Grade 5 events in antibody-positive patients occurred in the setting of disease progression, and serious adverse events were similar in type and nature to those reported in patients who did not develop anti-panitumumab antibodies.

Although panitumumab was expected to have a low rate of immunogenicity compared to therapeutic antibodies containing nonhuman coding sequences, unique sequences in the CDRs could still be immunogenic. An in silico analysis to evaluate the potential risk of panitumumab sequence-associated immunogenicity suggested that panitumumab light and heavy chains do not contain any non-tolerant agretopes predicted to be able to bind to the eight most common HLA-DRB1 alleles. The low risk of panitumumab immunogenicity was confirmed by the results of antibody testing in combination chemotherapy clinical trials, which indicated that patients treated with panitumumab in combination with irinotecan- or oxaliplatin-based chemotherapy infrequently developed antibodies against panitumumab.

Conclusions

In summary, the immunogenicity of panitumumab in the combination chemotherapy setting was infrequent and was similar to the immunogenicity observed in the monotherapy setting. This low rate of immunogenicity may be attributed to the fully human nature of panitumumab. Additionally, the presence of anti-panitumumab antibodies did not appear to alter pharmacokinetic or safety profiles of panitumumab.

Acknowledgements and Funding

We thank Julia R. Gage, PhD, whose work was funded by Amgen Inc. for assistance with writing the manuscript. We also thank Theresa Goletz of Amgen for performing the in silico analysis to evaluate the potential risk of panitumumab sequence-associated immunogenicity.

Support for the study and preparation of the manuscript was provided by Amgen Inc. All authors are employees of the study sponsor and were collectively responsible for the analysis plan; the collection, analysis, and interpretation of data; writing of the manuscript; and the decision to submit the manuscript for publication.

Authors' contributions

DW and JJP developed the methods and coordinated the implementation of binding and neutralizing antibody testing. AC performed the PopPK analysis and interpreted results. CYW, JJPR, and BBY made substantial contributions to the PopPK analysis planning and interpreted the results. KZ performed the statistical analysis of the antibody data. JW performed the analysis of the impact of immunogenicity on safety. AK and SG supervised development and implementation of the neutralizing antibody testing method. SJS contributed to the interpretation of antibody data. NC and MS developed and implemented the immunogenicity testing strategy and made substantial contributions to data interpretation. All authors contributed to the writing of the manuscript or critically reviewing the manuscript for technical and intellectual content. All authors approved the final draft of the manuscript.

Competing interests

All authors are employees and shareholders of Amgen Inc.

References

1. Vectibix® (panitumumab) prescribing information. Amgen Inc, Thousand Oaks, CA; 2011.
2. EPARs for authorised medicinal products for human use. [http://www.emea.europa.eu/humandocs/Humans/EPAR/vectibix/vectibix.htm].
3. Douillard JY, Siena S, Cassidy J, Tabernero J, Burkes R, Barugel M, Humblet Y, Bodoky G, Cunningham D, Jassem J, et al: Randomized, phase III trial of panitumumab with infusional fluorouracil, leucovorin, and oxaliplatin (FOLFOX4) versus FOLFOX4 alone as first-line treatment in patients with previously untreated metastatic colorectal cancer: the PRIME study. J Clin Oncol 2010, 28(31):4697-4705.
4. Peeters M, Price TJ, Cervantes A, Sobrero AF, Ducreux M, Hotko Y, Andre T, Chan E, Lordick F, Punt CJ, et al: Randomized phase III study of panitumumab with fluorouracil, leucovorin, and irinotecan (FOLFIRI) compared with FOLFIRI alone as second-line treatment in patients with metastatic colorectal cancer. J Clin Oncol 2010, 28(31):4706-4713.
5. Shankar G, Pendley C, Stein KE: A risk-based bioanalytical strategy for the assessment of antibody immune responses against biological drugs. Nat Biotechnol 2007, 25(5):555-561.
6. Nelson AL, Dhimolea E, Reichert JM: Development trends for human monoclonal antibody therapeutics. Nat Rev Drug Discov 2010, 9(10):767-774.
7. Hwang WY, Foote J: Immunogenicity of engineered antibodies. Methods 2005, 36(1):3-10.
8. Bartelds GM, Wijbrandts CA, Nurmohamed MT, Stapel S, Lems WF, Aarden L, Dijkmans BA, Tak PP, Wolbink GJ: Clinical response to adalimumab: relationship to anti-adalimumab antibodies and serum adalimumab concentrations in rheumatoid arthritis. Ann Rheum Dis 2007, 66(7):921-926.
9. Bender NK, Heilig CE, Droll B, Wohlgemuth J, Armbruster FP, Heilig B: Immunogenicity, efficacy and adverse events of adalimumab in RA patients. Rheumatol Int 2007, 27(3):269-274.
10. Khazaeli M, LoBuglio A, Falcey J, Paulter V, Fetzer M, Waksal H: Low immunogenicity of a chimeric monoclonal antibody (MoAb), IM-C225, used to treat epidermal growth factor receptor-positive tumor [abstract]. Proc Am Soc Clin Oncol 2000, 19:Abst 808.
11. Fracasso PM, Burris H, Arquette MA, Govindan R, Gao F, Wright LP, Goodner SA, Greco FA, Jones SF, Willcut N, et al: A phase 1 escalating single-dose and weekly fixed-dose study of cetuximab: pharmacokinetic and pharmacodynamic rationale for dosing. Clin Cancer Res 2007, 13(3):986-993.
12. O'Neil BH, Allen R, Spigel DR, Stinchcombe TE, Moore DT, Berlin JD, Goldberg RM: High incidence of cetuximab-related infusion reactions in Tennessee and North Carolina and the association with atopic history. J Clin Oncol 2007, 25(24):3644-3648.
13. Chung CH, Mirakhur B, Chan E, Le QT, Berlin J, Morse M, Murphy BA, Satinover SM, Hosen J, Mauro D, et al: Cetuximab-induced anaphylaxis and IgE specific for galactose-alpha-1,3-galactose. N Engl J Med 2008, 358(11):1109-1117.
14. Ghaderi D, Taylor RE, Padler-Karavani V, Diaz S, Varki A: Implications of the presence of N-glycolylneuraminic acid in recombinant therapeutic glycoproteins. Nat Biotechnol 2010, 28(8):863-867.
15. Weiner LM: Fully human therapeutic monoclonal antibodies. J Immunother 2006, 29(1):1-9.
16. Lofgren JA, Dhandapani S, Pennucci JJ, Abbott CM, Mytych DT, Kaliyaperumal A, Swanson SJ, Mullenix MC: Comparing ELISA and surface plasmon resonance for assessing clinical immunogenicity of panitumumab. J Immunol 2007, 178(11):7467-7472.
17. Lacouture ME, Mitchell EP, Piperdi B, Pillai MV, Shearer H, Iannotti N, Xu F, Yassine M: Skin toxicity evaluation protocol with panitumumab (STEPP), a phase II, open-label, randomized trial evaluating the impact of a pre-emptive skin treatment regimen on skin toxicities and quality of life in patients with metastatic colorectal cancer. J Clin Oncol 2010, 28(8):1351-1357.
18. Cohn AL, Shumaker GC, Khandelwal P, Smith DA, Neubauer MA, Mehta N, Richards D, Watkins DL, Zhang K, Yassine MR: An open-label, single-arm, phase 2 trial of panitumumab plus FOLFIRI as second-line therapy in patients with metastatic colorectal cancer. Clin Colorectal Cancer 2011, 10(3):171-177.
19. Amado RG, Wolf M, Peeters M, Van Cutsem E, Siena S, Freeman DJ, Juan T, Sikorski R, Suggs S, Radinsky R, et al: Wild-type KRAS is required for panitumumab efficacy in patients with metastatic colorectal cancer. J Clin Oncol 2008, 26:1626-1634.
20. Barger TE, Zhou L, Hale M, Moxness M, Swanson SJ, Chirmule N: Comparing exponentially weighted moving average and run rules in process control of semiquantitative immunogenicity immunoassays. AAPS J 2010, 12(1):79-86.
21. Ma P, Yang BB, Wang YM, Peterson M, Narayanan A, Sutjandra L, Rodriguez R, Chow A: Population pharmacokinetic analysis of panitumumab in patients with advanced solid tumors. J Clin Pharmacol 2009, 49(10):1142-1156.
22. Yang BB, Lum P, Chen A, Arends R, Roskos L, Smith B, Perez Ruixo JJ: Pharmacokinetic and pharmacodynamic perspectives on the clinical drug development of panitumumab. Clin Pharmacokinet 2010, 49(11):729-740.
23. Yano Y, Beal SL, Sheiner LB: Evaluating pharmacokinetic/pharmacodynamic models using the posterior predictive check. J Pharmacokinet Pharmacodyn 2001, 28(2):171-192.

24. Eloxatin® (oxaliplatin) prescribing information. sanofi aventis, Bridgewater, NJ; 2009.
25. Camptosar® (irinotecan hydrochloride) prescribing information. Pharmacia & Upjohn Co. Division of Pfizer Inc., New York, NY; 2010.

7

Anvirzel™ in combination with cisplatin in breast, colon, lung, prostate, melanoma and pancreatic cancer cell lines

Panagiotis Apostolou[1], Maria Toloudi[1], Marina Chatziioannou[1], Eleni Ioannou[1], Dennis R Knocke[2], Joe Nester[2], Dimitrios Komiotis[3] and Ioannis Papasotiriou[1*]

Abstract

Background: Platinum derivatives are used widely for the treatment of many cancers. However, the toxicity that is observed makes imperative the need for new drugs, or new combinations. Anvirzel™ is an extract which has been demonstrated with experimental data that displays anticancer activity. The aim of the present study is to determine whether the combination of Cisplatin and Anvirzel™ has a synergistic effect against different types of cancer.

Materials and methods: To measure the efficacy of treatment with Cisplatin and Anvirzel™, methyl-tetrazolium dye (MTT) chemosensitivity assays were used incorporating established human cancer cell lines. Measurements were performed in triplicates, three times, using different incubation times and different concentrations of the two formulations in combination or on their own. t-test was used for statistical analysis.

Results: In the majority of the cell lines tested, lower concentrations of Anvirzel™ induced a synergistic effect when combined with low concentrations of Cisplatin after an incubation period of 48 to 72 h. The combination of Anvirzel™/Cisplatin showed anti-proliferative effects against a wide range of tumours.

Conclusion: The results showed that the combination of Anvirzel™ and Cisplatin is more effective than monotherapy, even when administered at low concentrations; thus, undesirable toxic effects can be avoided.

Keywords: Anvirzel™, Cisplatin, Viability assays, Cancer cell lines, Methyl-tetrazolium dye

Background

Many studies demonstrate the anti-proliferative activity of Oleandrin. These properties make it attractive for use as a treatment for cancer [1-5]; however, a major problem is that Oleandrin is toxic to normal cells and tissues [6,7]. Anvirzel™ is an extract of *Nerium oleander* comprised primarily of Oleandrin and Oleandrigenin [8]. Recent studies demonstrate that Anvirzel™ decreases viability in prostate cancer cell lines as well as a wide range of other human cancer cell lines [9-12]. Cisplatin (CDDP) is a platinum-based chemotherapy drug used to treat various types of cancer [13,14]. Because it is highly toxic, and because of primary and secondary resistance of cancer cells to Cisplatin [15], it is commonly used in combination with other drugs [16,17]. A recent study reported that the combination of Anvirzel™, Carboplatin and Docetaxel is more effective than monotherapy [18]. Therefore, the aim of the current study was to determine whether the combination of Anvirzel™ and Cisplatin was more effective than the use of either drug alone using MTT chemosensitivity assays based on human cancer cell lines [19-23].

Methods

The human carcinoma cell lines used were obtained from the ECACC-HPA (European Collection of Cell Cultures - Health Protective Agency, UK). PC3, LNCaP and 22Rv1 are human prostate cancer cell lines, MDA-MB 231, T47D, and MCF-7 are human breast cancer lines, CALU-1, COLO699N and COR-L 105 are non-small cell lung carcinoma lines (NSCLC), HCT-116, HT55 and HCT-15 are colorectal cancer lines, and A375 and PANC-1 are melanoma and pancreatic cancer cells

* Correspondence: papasotiriou.ioannis@rgcc-genlab.com
[1]Research Genetic Cancer Centre Ltd (R.G.C.C. Ltd), Filotas, Florina, Greece
Full list of author information is available at the end of the article

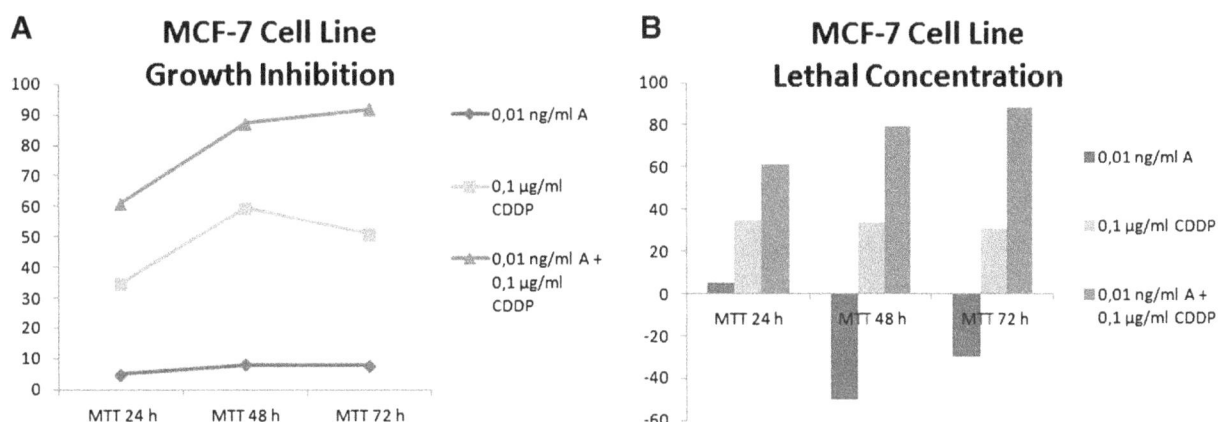

Figure 1 A. The illustration shows the effect of Anvirzel™ and Cisplatin, and their combination compared with the growth rate of cells in cell line MCF-7 which represents breast cancer. **B.** The effect of the above drugs in monotherapy as well their combination compared with the lethality of cells.

lines, respectively. MTT chemosensitivity assays were used to determine the efficacy of combined treatment compared with that each drug alone. The incubation times used in the study were 24, 48 and 72 h at concentrations ranging from 0.01 ng/ml to 10 ng/ml for Anvirzel™ and from 0.1 µg/ml to 100 µg/ml for Cisplatin.

Cell lines
Cells were cultured in 75 cm² flasks (Orange Scientific, 5520200) in the recommended media supplemented with the appropriate amount of heat inactivated Fetal Bovine Serum (FBS, Invitrogen, 10106–169, California) and 2 mM L-Glutamine (Sigma, G5792, Germany). The cells were maintained at 37°C in a 5% CO_2 atmosphere.

Viability assays
Cells were detached by trypsinisation (Trypsin-0.25% EDTA, Invitrogen, 25200–072) during the logarithmic

phase of growth and plated in 96-well plates (Corning, Costar 3595) at a density of 18,000 cells/well in a final volume of 200 µl medium per well. When the cells reached 70–80% confluence, the medium was removed and Anvirzel™ (Salud Integral; diluted in water) and Cisplatin (Sigma, P4394; diluted in N, N-dimethylformamide; Fluka, 40255) were added to the cells at different concentrations. Absorbance was measured after 24, 48 and 72 h of incubation.

MTT assay
For the MTT assay, methyl-tetrazolium dye (Sigma, M2128) was added to each well at a concentration of 5 mg/ml (diluted in PBS) and the plates incubated for 3 h at 37°C. The medium was then discarded and the cells rinsed with PBS. Finally, the formazan crystals were dissolved in dimethylsulphoxide (Sigma, D4540).

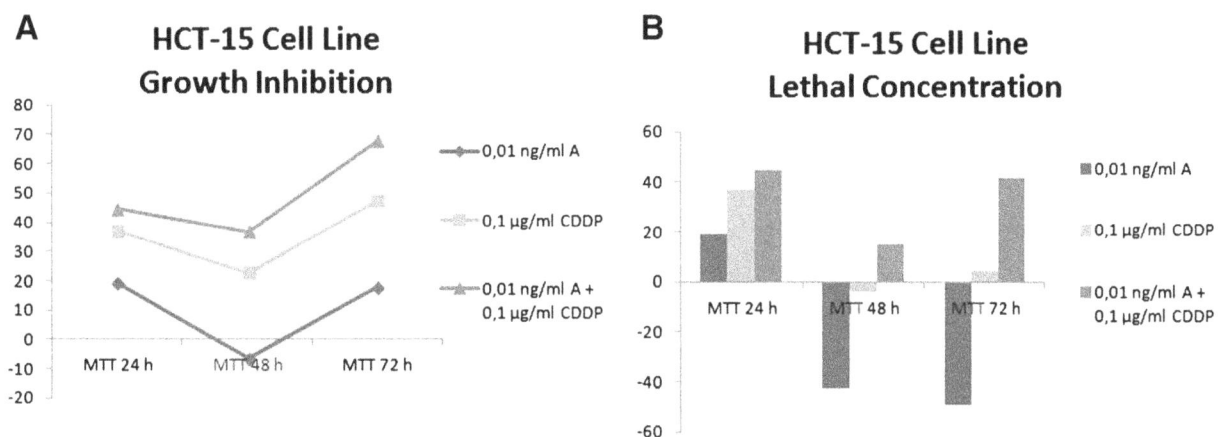

Figure 2 A. The illustration shows the effect of Anvirzel™ and Cisplatin, and their combination compared with the growth rate of cells in cell line HCT-15 which represents colorectal cancer. **B.** The effect of the above drugs in monotherapy as well their combination compared with the lethality of cells.

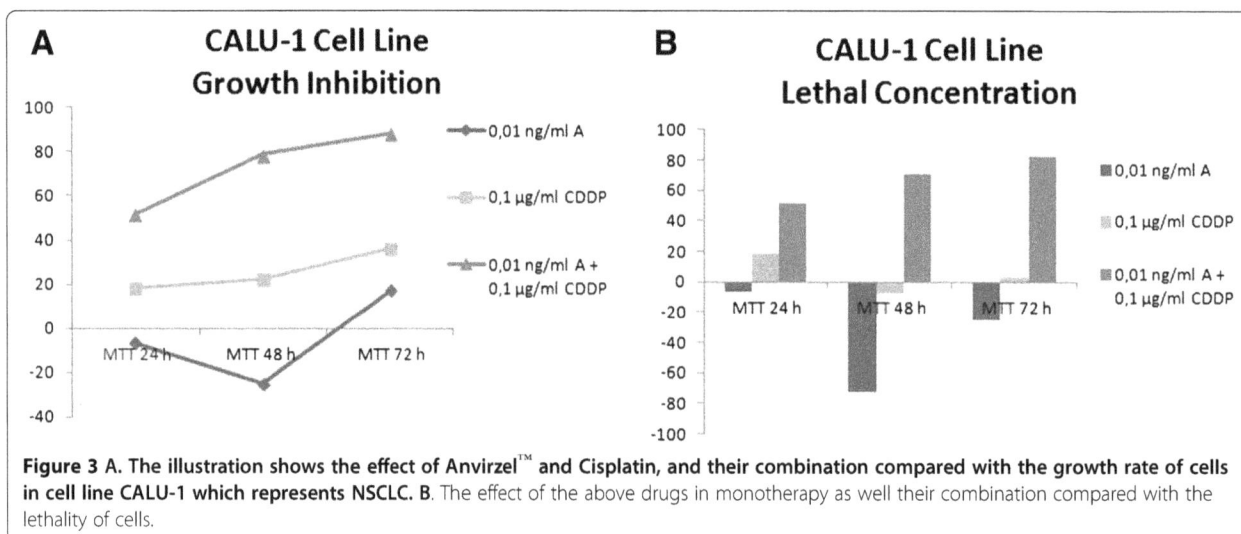

Figure 3 A. The illustration shows the effect of Anvirzel™ and Cisplatin, and their combination compared with the growth rate of cells in cell line CALU-1 which represents NSCLC. **B**. The effect of the above drugs in monotherapy as well their combination compared with the lethality of cells.

To calculate the fold-decrease in staining the absorbance was calculated using the Beer-Lambert law: $A = \varepsilon c l$, where "A" is the absorbance, "ε" is an extinction coefficient, "l" is the distance the light travels through the material, and "c" is the concentration of the absorbing species [24].

The optical density of the plate was measured using a μQuant spectrophotometer (μQuant Biomolecular Spectrophotometer MQX200) and the data analysed with Gen5 software (Gen5™ Microplate Data Collection & Analysis software, BioTek® Instruments. Inc, April 2008). Absorbance was measured at 570 nm and a second wavelength at 630 nm was measured to subtract background "noise".

Statistical analysis

All treatments for each cell line were performed in triplicate, three times. The statistical significance of all effects was evaluated using the "difference of the means" test. A p value < 0.05 was considered significant.

Results

Different results were observed not only between each type of cancer but also between each cell line within the same carcinoma group. In all cell lines has been studied LC50 (lethal concentration 50), which is the concentration that kill half of the sample population, and GI50 (growth inhibition 50), which is the concentration required to inhibit growth by 50%. In all cell lines tested, administration of the combined formulation at lower concentrations was more effective than monotherapy. The formulation that elicited the most effective results in most of the cell lines was a combination of 0.01 ng/ml Anvirzel™ and 0.1 μg/ml Cisplatin, with incubation period of 48 h or 72 h. The combination of 0.01 ng/ml Anvirzel™ and 1 μg/ml Cisplatin was more effective in

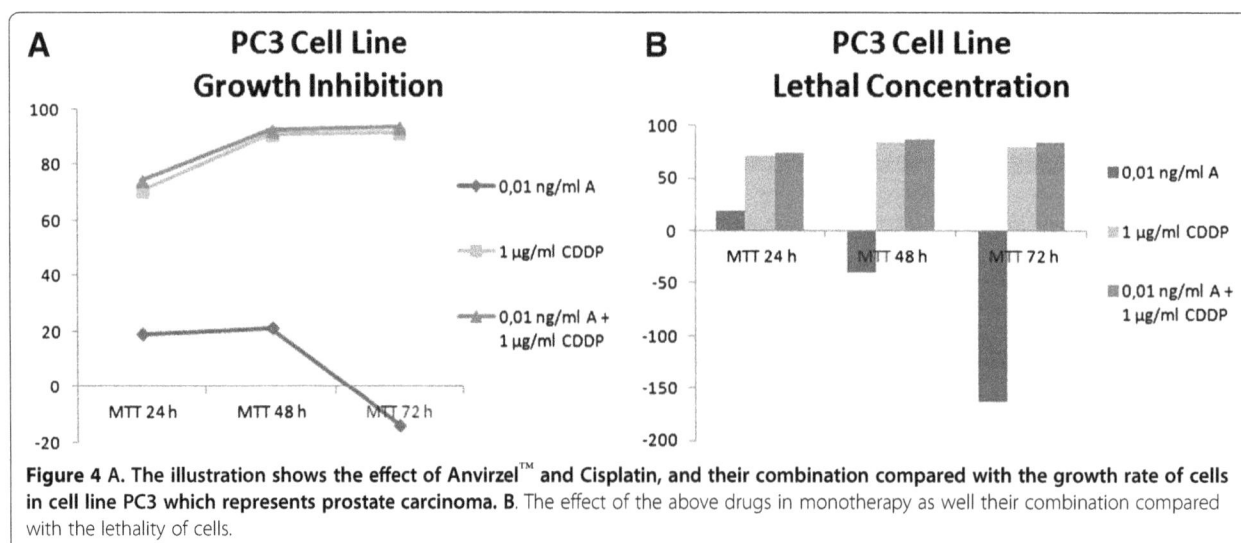

Figure 4 A. The illustration shows the effect of Anvirzel™ and Cisplatin, and their combination compared with the growth rate of cells in cell line PC3 which represents prostate carcinoma. **B**. The effect of the above drugs in monotherapy as well their combination compared with the lethality of cells.

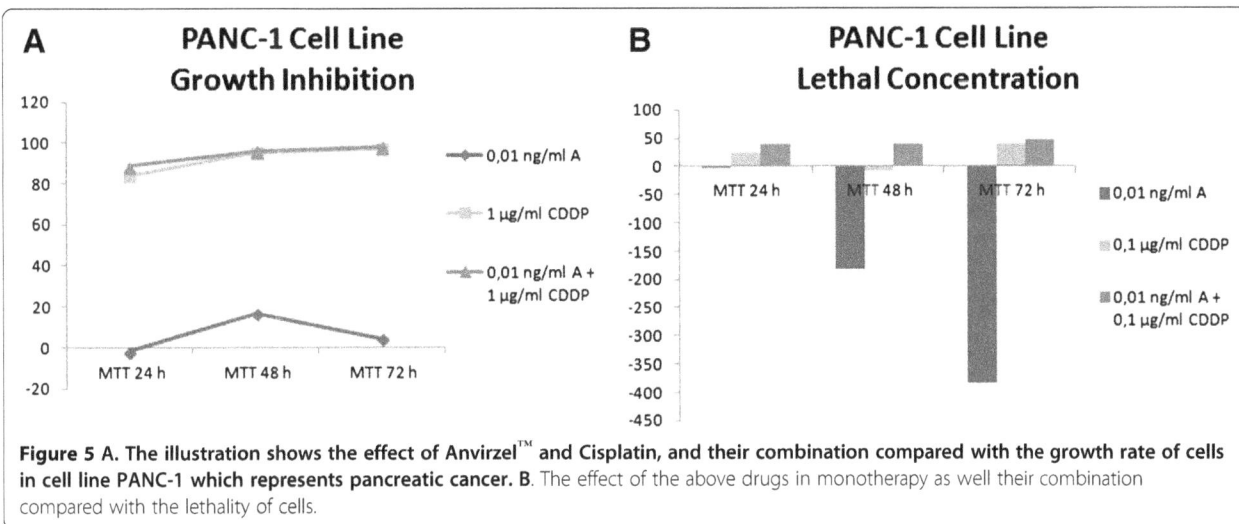

Figure 5 A. The illustration shows the effect of Anvirzel™ and Cisplatin, and their combination compared with the growth rate of cells in cell line PANC-1 which represents pancreatic cancer. B. The effect of the above drugs in monotherapy as well their combination compared with the lethality of cells.

pancreatic cancer cell line, as well in PC3 and MDA-MB231 cell lines. The Figures 1, 2, 3, 4, 5, 6 represent data from cell lines that were tested both for Growth inhibition and for Lethal Concentrations.

Discussion

Anvirzel™ is an extract of *Nerium oleander* (family Apocynaceae) that contains two toxic cardiac glycosides, Oleandrin and Oleandrigenin [8], which have anti-proliferative effects against various types of cancer. According to literature data, *Nerium oleander* is often used for its healing properties [25]. Oleandrin is used to treat heart failure, and alters the levels of intracellular K^+ and Ca^{2+} [26]. Other studies show that Oleandrin suppresses the activation of many transcription factors and enhances the radiosensitivity of tumours [27,28]. Oleandrin induces cell death through the activation of

caspases in a variety of human tumour cells, as well as by activating calcineurin and NF-AT via the Fas ligand [3]. Recent studies of Anvirzel™ in prostate cell lines show that it interacts with the membrane Na^+/K^+-ATPase and thus inhibits the export of FGF-2 [11,28]. Cisplatin is a platinum-based chemotherapy drug widely used to treat various types of cancer [13,14]. In high concentrations, Cisplatin is highly cytotoxic. In addition, tumour cells often develop resistance to treatment [15]. Many studies demonstrate that administration of Cisplatin in combination with other treatments is more effective and produces fewer toxic effects. The present study aimed the demonstrate the synergistic effect of Anvirzel™ and Cisplatin in a wide range of cell lines, which represent the most common types of cancer. It was used the methyl-tetrazolium dye assay, which is used to measure the activity of enzymes in the mitochondria.

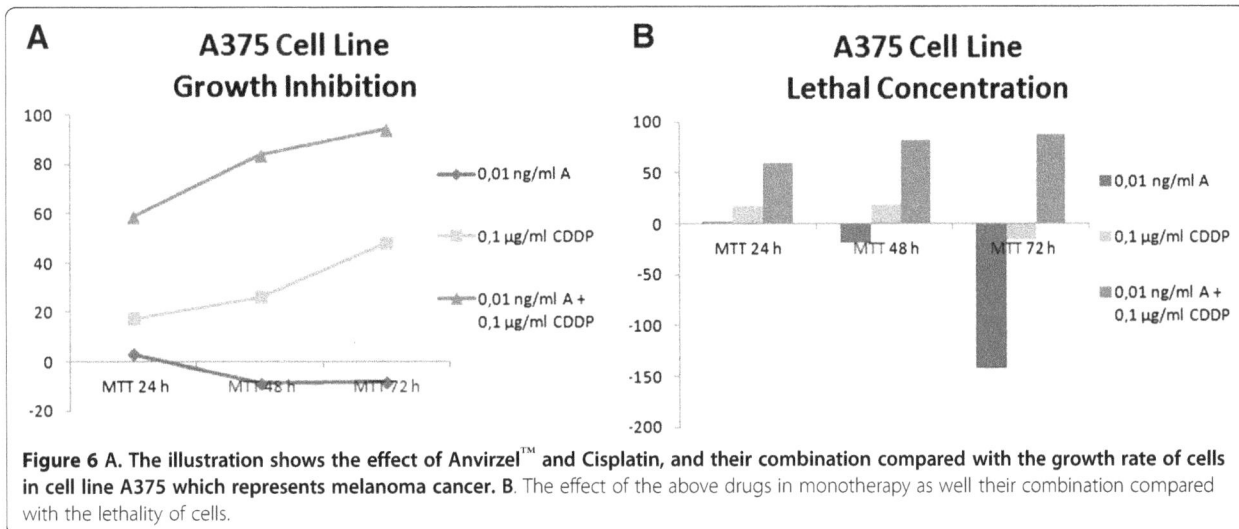

Figure 6 A. The illustration shows the effect of Anvirzel™ and Cisplatin, and their combination compared with the growth rate of cells in cell line A375 which represents melanoma cancer. B. The effect of the above drugs in monotherapy as well their combination compared with the lethality of cells.

During this assay, the dye is taken up by endocytosis and reduced by the mitochondrial enzymes to yield formazan, which is purple/blue [19,20].

It has been confirmed that Anvirzel™ has better activity at lower concentrations in many cancer cell lines, after 48 or 72 h of incubation. In contrast, low Cisplatin concentrations (<1 μg/ml), do not indicate activity in the same cells. The effect of platinum is evident at concentrations greater than 10 μg/ml. However, these concentrations have high cytotoxicity effects. The combination of the two formulations at very low concentrations is able to inhibit cell growth by more than 50% in an exposure time of 72 hours. The same concentration may also reduce the number of live cells at rates up to 85% in the same time of exposure. Lowered effect observed in cell lines that are hormone-dependent, cases such as breast and prostate cancer.

Conclusions

The MTT viability assays were used to test the hypothesis that combined treatment with Cisplatin and Anvirzel™ would be more effective than either drug alone. The results of all three assays were both concentration and cell line-dependent. It is noteworthy that increased efficacy was observed at lower concentrations of both substances, 0.01 ng/ml for Anvirzel™ and 0.1 μg/ml for Cisplatin, than of either drug alone. The results were neither reliable nor reproducible at higher concentrations of Anvirzel™ and Cisplatin. The results were also time-dependent: treatment was effective after 48 h and 72 h of incubation, but not after 24 h.

The present study contributes to demonstrate an effective interaction between Anvirzel™ and another widely used drug with cytostatic effects. Based on these data, it is crucial to perform further studies to identify and characterize the interaction between Anvirzel™ and other drugs currently used to treat cancer.

Abbreviations
CDDP: Cisplatin; MTT: 3-(4,5-Dimethylthiazol-2-yl)-2,3-diphenyltetrazolium bromide; NSCLC: Non-small cell lung cancer.

Competing interests
The authors declare that they have no competing interests.

Authors' contributions
PA carried out the chemosensitivity assays, drafted the manuscript and performed the statistical analysis. MT participated in the chemosensitivity assays. MC participated in the chemosensitivity assays. EI carried out the cell lines culture. DK participated in the design of the study and coordination. JN participated in the design of the study and coordination. DK participated in the design of the study. IP supervised the assays and the manuscript. All authors read and approved the final manuscript.

Acknowledgements
The authors thank the two anonymous referees whose valuable commentary allowed us to improve the manuscript.

Author details
[1]Research Genetic Cancer Centre Ltd (R.G.C.C. Ltd), Filotas, Florina, Greece. [2]Nerium Biotechnology, Inc. San Antonio, Texas, USA. [3]Department of Biochemistry & Biotechnology, University of Thessaly, Larisa, Greece.

References
1. Sreenivasan YSA, Manna SK: Oleandrin suppresses activation of nuclear transcription factor-kappa B and activator protein-1 and potentiates apoptosis induced by ceramide. *Biochem Pharmacol* 2003, 66:2223–2239.
2. Newman RA, Kondo Y, Yokoyama T, *et al*: Autophagic cell death of human pancreatic tumor cells mediated by oleandrin, a lipid-soluble cardiac glycoside. *Integr Cancer Ther* 2007, 6:354–364.
3. Raghavendra PB, Sreenivasan Y, Ramesh GT, Manna SK: Cardiac glycoside induces cell death via FasL by activating calcineurin and NF-AT, but apoptosis initially proceeds through activation of caspases. *Apoptosis* 2007, 12:307–1318.
4. Frese SF-SM, Andres AC, Miescher D, Zumkehr B, Schmid RA: Cardiac glycosides initiate Apo2L/TRAIL-induced apoptosis in non-small cell lung cancer cells by up-regulation of death receptors 4 and 5. *Cancer Res* 2006, 66:5867–5874.
5. Raghavendra PB, Sreenivasan Y, Manna SK: Oleandrin induces apoptosis in human, but not in murine cells: dephosphorylation of Akt, expression of FasL, and alteration of membrane fluidity. *Mol Immunol* 2007, 44:2292–2302.
6. Stenkvist B: Cardenolides and cancer. *Anticancer Drugs* 2001, 12:635–638.
7. Langford SD, Boor PJ: Oleander toxicity: an examination of human and animal toxic exposures. *Toxicology* 1996, 109:1–13.
8. Wang X, Plomley JB, Newman RA, Cisneros A: LC/MS/MS analyses of an oleander extract for cancer treatment. *Anal Chem* 2000, 72:3547–52.
9. Pathak S, Multani AS, Narayan S, Kumar V, Newman RA: Anvirzel, an extract of Nerium oleander, induces cell death in human but not murine cancer cells. *Anticancer Drugs* 2000, 11:455–63.
10. McConkey DJ, Lin Y, Nutt LK, Ozel HZ, Newman RA: Cardiac glycosides stimulate Ca2+ increases and apoptosis in androgen-independent, metastatic human prostate adenocarcinoma cells. *Cancer Res* 2000, 60:3807–3812.
11. Smith JA, Madden T, Vijjeswarapu M, Newman RA: Inhibition of export of fibroblast growth factor-2 (FGF-2) from the prostate cancer cell lines PC3 and DU145 by Anvirzel and its cardiac glycoside component, oleandrin. *Biochem Pharmacol* 2001, 62:469–472.
12. Apostolou P, Toloudi M, Chatziioannou M, Papasotiriou I: Determination of efficacy of Anvirzel™ in 37 established cancer cell lines. *International Pharmaceutical Industry* 2011, 3:68–72.
13. Rosenberg B, VanCamp L, Trosko JE, Mansour VH: Platinum compounds: a new class of potent antitumour agents. *Nature* 1969, 222:385–386.
14. Trzaska S: The top pharmaceuticals that changed the world. *C&EN News* 2005, 83:3.
15. Stordal B, Davey M: Understanding cisplatin resistance using cellular models. *IUBMB Life* 2007, 59:696–699.
16. Chen XX, Lai MD, Zhang YL, Huang Q: Less cytotoxicity to combination therapy of 5-fluorouracil and cisplatin than 5-fluorouracil alone in human colon cancer cell lines. *World J Gastroenterol* 2002, 8:841–846.
17. Alshehri A, Beale P, Yu JQ, Huq F: Synergism from combination of cisplatin and a trans-platinum compound in ovarian cancer cell lines. *Anticancer Res* 2010, 30:4547–4553.
18. Apostolou P, Toloudi M, Chatziioannou M, Papasotiriou I: Studying the effect of Anvirzel™, Carboplatin and Docetaxel in NSCLC cell lines. *Journal for Clinical Studies* 2011, 3:32–34.
19. Liu Y, Peterson DA, Kimura H, Schubert D: Mechanism of cellular 3-(4,5-dimethylthiazol-2-yl)-2,5-diphenyltetrazolium bromide (MTT) reduction. *J Neurochem* 1997, 69:581–593.
20. Mosmann T: Rapid colorimetric assay for cellular growth and survival: application to proliferation and cytotoxicity assays. *J Immunol Methods* 1983, 65:55–63.
21. Mickisch G, Fajta S, Keilhauer G, Schlick E, Tschada R, Alken P: Chemosensitivity testing of primary human renal cell carcinoma by a tetrazolium based microculture assay (MTT). *Urol Res* 1990, 18:131–136.

22. Sargent JM: The use of the MTT assay to study drug resistance in fresh tumour samples. *Recent Results Cancer Res* 2003, **161**:13–25.
23. Twentyman PR, Luscombe M: A study of some variables in a tetrazolium dye (MTT) based assay for cell growth and chemosensitivity. *Br J Cancer* 1987, **56**:279–285.
24. Ingle JDJ, Crouch SR: *Spectrochemical Analysis*. New Jersey: Prentice Hall; 1988.
25. Leporatti ML, Posocco E, Pavesi A: Some new therapeutic uses of several medicinal plants in the province of Terni (Umbria, Central Italy). *J Ethnopharmacol* 1985, **14**:65–68.
26. Wolfred MM: The evaluation of the glycoside oleandrin, on the embryo chick heart. *J Am Pharm Assoc Am Pharm Assoc* 1949, **38**:581–584.
27. Manna SK, Sah NK, Newman RA, Cisneros A, Aggarwal BB: Oleandrin suppresses activation of nuclear transcription factor-kappaB, activator protein-1, and c-Jun NH2-terminal kinase. *Cancer Res* 2000, **60**:3838–3847.
28. Chen JQ, Contreras RG, Wang R, *et al*: Sodium/potassium ATPase (Na+, K + −ATPase) and ouabain/related cardiac glycosides: A new paradigm for development of anti- breast cancer drugs? *Breast Cancer Res Treat* 2006, **96**:1–15.

8

Glibenclamide inhibits cell growth by inducing G0/G1 arrest in the human breast cancer cell line MDA-MB-231

Mariel Núñez[1], Vanina Medina[1], Graciela Cricco[1], Máximo Croci[2], Claudia Cocca[1], Elena Rivera[1], Rosa Bergoc[1,3]* and Gabriela Martín[1]

Abstract

Background: Glibenclamide (Gli) binds to the sulphonylurea receptor (SUR) that is a regulatory subunit of ATP-sensitive potassium channels (K_{ATP} channels). Binding of Gli to SUR produces the closure of K_{ATP} channels and the inhibition of their activity. This drug is widely used for treatment of type 2-diabetes and it has been signaled as antiproliferative in several tumor cell lines. In previous experiments we demonstrated the antitumoral effect of Gli in mammary tumors induced in rats. The aim of the present work was to investigate the effect of Gli on MDA-MB-231 breast cancer cell proliferation and to examine the possible pathways involved in this action.

Results: The mRNA expression of the different subunits that compose the K_{ATP} channels was evaluated in MDA-MB-231 cells by reverse transcriptase-polymerase chain reaction. Results showed the expression of mRNA for both pore-forming isoforms Kir6.1 and Kir6.2 and for the regulatory isoform SUR2B in this cell line. Gli inhibited cell proliferation assessed by a clonogenic method in a dose dependent manner, with an increment in the population doubling time. The K_{ATP} channel opener minoxidil increased clonogenic proliferation, effect that was counteracted by Gli. When cell cycle analysis was performed by flow cytometry, Gli induced a significant cell-cycle arrest in G0/G1 phase, together with an up-regulation of p27 levels and a diminution in cyclin E expression, both evaluated by immunoblot. However, neither differentiation evaluated by neutral lipid accumulation nor apoptosis assessed by different methodologies were detected. The cytostatic, non toxic effect on cell proliferation was confirmed by removal of the drug.
Combination treatment of Gli with tamoxifen or doxorubicin showed an increment in the antiproliferative effect only for doxorubicin.

Conclusions: Our data clearly demonstrated a cytostatic effect of Gli in MDA-MB-231 cells that may be mediated through K_{ATP} channels, associated to the inhibition of the G1-S phase progression. In addition, an interesting observation about the effect of the combination of Gli with doxorubicin leads to future research for a potential novel role for Gli as an adjuvant in breast cancer treatment

Keywords: Glibenclamide, Potassium channels, MDA-MB-231, Cytostatic effect

* Correspondence: rmbergoc@gmail.com
[1]Radioisotopes Laboratory, School of Pharmacy and Biochemistry, University of Buenos Aires, Buenos Aires, Argentina
[3]Institute of Health Sciences Barceló, Buenos Aires, Argentina
Full list of author information is available at the end of the article

Background

Sulphonylureas are used to increase insulin secretion in patient with type 2-diabetes due to their direct action on pancreatic β cells. These drugs bind to the β cell sulphonylurea receptor (SUR) that is a regulatory subunit of ATP-sensitive potassium channels (K_{ATP} channels) [1-3]. K_{ATP} channels regulate the transport of potassium ions through cell membranes. A diverse group of compounds can bind to K_{ATP} channels causing them to open or close. The opening of potassium channels in the cell membrane produces a hyperpolarization of membrane potential. These channels are hetero-octameric complexes that consist of two rings: an inner ring of four inwardly rectifying K^+ channels (Kir6.X) that forms the pore through which potassium ions pass, and an outer ring that comprises four SUR subunits. Two isoforms have been described for Kir6.X (Kir6.1 and Kir6.2) and also for SUR (SUR1 and SUR2; SUR2 also has two splice variants, SUR2A and SUR2B) [4]. In pancreatic β cells binding of sulphonylureas to SURs produce the closure of K_{ATP} channels reducing cellular potassium efflux thus favoring membrane depolarization, the induction of Ca^{2+} influx, and insulin secretion [1-3].

Glibenclamide (Gli), a diarylsulphonilurea that blocks specifically K_{ATP} channels, is widely employed in the treatment of diabetic patients [5], but various reports also described its antiproliferative effect in different neoplastic cell lines [6,7]. Additionally, the inhibition of other classes of potassium channels also leads to a decrease of proliferation in normal and cancer cells [8,9].

Breast cancer is the neoplastic disease most frequently observed in women all over the world [10-12]. A high proportion of mammary tumors are positive for estrogen receptors α (ERα) and consequently antihormonal therapy is indicated. The selective estrogen receptor modulator tamoxifen continues to be the drug regularly used in patients harboring this kind of tumors due to its efficacy and low toxicity [13]. However, approximately 30% of ERα (+) tumors do not respond to tamoxifen or develop resistance in the course of the treatment. In addition, it is known that approximately 30% of tumors do not express ERα [14]. Although a large number of drugs have been developed for the treatment of ERα (−) tumors, most of them give rise to important toxic effects. In order to attain better therapeutic effectiveness, combination cytotoxic treatments for aggressive cancers have been employed in clinics. The simultaneous use of drugs with different molecular targets can delay the emergence of chemoresistance whereas when drugs are directed to the same cellular pathway they could work synergically for higher efficacy and selectivity. However, combination therapy may also increase toxicity [15]. Doxorubicin is considered a highly effective agent in the treatment of aggressive breast cancer patients sometimes combined with cyclophosphamide, taxanes and/or 5-fluorouracil; however, resistance to doxorubicin is common [16,17]. The search for effective drugs with low side effects is still a challenge to researchers.

MDA-MB-231 cell line derived from a human breast carcinoma that do not express ERα, is often used as an experimental non hormone-dependent tumor model [18,19]. The objective of the present work was to investigate the effect of Gli on MDA-MB-231 cells proliferation and to examine the possible pathways involved in this action.

Material and methods

Materials

MBA-MB-231 cells were obtained from American Type Culture Collection (ATCC). Gli was kindly provided by Investi-Farma SA, Buenos Aires, Argentina. Tamoxifen (Tam) was a gift from Gador Laboratories SA, Buenos Aires, Argentina. RPMI 1640 medium and fetal bovine serum (FBS) were purchased from GIBCO, Invitrogen, CA, USA. Ribonuclease, propidium iodine, 3,3′dihexyloxacarbocyanine iodide (DiOC6), saponine, FITC-labeled anti-rabbit, 5-bromo-2′-deoxyuridine (BrdU), mouse anti-BrdU monoclonal antibody, FITC-conjugated anti-mouse IgG, 4′,6-Diamidino-2-phenyindole, dilactate (DAPI), 5-bromo-4-chloro-3-indolyl-β-d-galactoside (X-gal), mouse anti-β-actin polyclonal antibody, p27^{Kip1} monoclonal antibody and Nile-red stain were purchased from Sigma, St Louis, MO, USA. Apoptag®PLUS Peroxidase In Situ Detection Kit S701 was from Chemicon International, CA, USA. Rabbit polyclonal antibodies against human Bax, Bcl-2 and Bcl-x$_{L/S}$ were from Santa Cruz Biotechnologies, Santa Cruz, CA, USA. Mouse anti-cyclin B1 monoclonal antibodies, mouse anti-cyclin E monoclonal antibodies, and rabbit anti-cyclin D1 monoclonal antibodies were from Cell Signaling Technology, Inc., Danvers, MA, USA. Annexin V-FITC was from Biosciences, USA. Chemiluminiscence system (ECL) was from Amersham Biosciences Argentina SS (Argentina). Nitrocellulose membranes were from Santa Cruz Biotechnologies, Santa Cruz, CA, USA. Multiwells were from TPP, Switzerland. All other reagents were of analytical grade.

Methods

Reverse transcriptase polymerase chain reaction (RT-PCR) analysis

Total cellular RNA was extracted using Trizol® according to the instructions of the manufacturer (GIBCO, Life Technologies, USA). Total RNA (2 μg) was added to the reverse transcription (RT) reaction mixture (20 μl) in the presence of oligo-dT primers and samples were incubated at 37°C for 60 minutes. The quality of each individual's cDNA was confirmed by PCR with primers for β-actin producing bands of the expected size (data not shown).The primers used were employed previously by other workers for Kir6.1, Kir6.2, SUR1 [4], SUR2A and SUR2B [20]. PCR conditions were as follows: Kir6.1 forward (5′-CATCTTTACCATGTCCTTCC-3′) and reverse (5′-GTGAGCCTGAGCTGTTTTCA-3′), 336 bp; Kir6.2 forward (5′-GCTTTGTGTCCAAGAAAGG1-3′) and reverse (5′-CCAAAGCCAATAGTCACTTG-3′), 301 bp; 5 min 95°C, 35 cycles of 95°C for 20 s, 52°C for 45 s, and 72°C for 1 min. SUR1 forward (5′-CGATGC CATCATCACAGAAG-3′) and reverse (5′-CTGAG CAGCTTCTCTGGCTT-3′), 291 bp; SUR2A foward (5′-ATGCGGTTGTCACTGAAGG-3′) and reverse (5′-AATAGAAGAGACACGGTGAGC-3′), 215 bp; SUR2B forward (5′-GATGCGGTTGTCACTGAAGG-3′) and reverse (5′-TCATCACAATAACCAGGTCTGC-3′), 244 bp; 5 min 95°C, 35 cycles of 95°C for 1 min, 55°C for 1 min, and 72°C for 2 min. Reactions were terminated by final elongation step of 7 min at 72°C (Gene Amp PCR System 2400, PerkinElmer, MA, USA). Negative controls were performed with water instead of cDNA. PCR products were subjected to gel electrophoresis and detected by gel documentation system LumiBis DNR (Bio-Imaging Systems, Jerusalem, Israel).

Cell culture

MBA-MB-231 cels were cultured in RPMI 1640 medium supplemented with 10% FBS, 0.3 g/l L-glutamine and 40 mg/l gentamicine and in the presence of Gli, Tam or vehicle. Cells were maintained at 37°C in a humidified atmosphere containing 5% CO_2.

Cell proliferation assay

For clonogenic assay, cells were seeded in 6-well plates (1.5×10^3 cells/well) and incubated in the presence or absence of drugs for 10 days. Cells were treated with 10 to 50 µM Gli, 0.005 to 5 µM minoxidil; 0.1 to 5 µM tamoxifen; 0.01 to 0.1 nM doxorubicin or with the concentration of Gli that inhibited the proliferation to the 50% (IC_{50}) plus different doses of minoxidil, tamoxifen or doxorubicin to assess the combined action of both drugs. Cells were then fixed with 10% formaldehyde in phosphate-buffered saline, PBS, stained with 1% toluidine blue in 70% ethanol. The clonogenic proliferation was evaluated by counting the colonies with 50 cells or more. The results are expressed as a percentage of control values.

Determination of doubling time

For doubling time determination cells were seeded in 6-well plates (4×10^4 cells/well), starved for 24 h and then incubated with IC_{50} Gli (25 µM) or vehicle for up to 96 h. Cells were trypsinized at 0, 1, 2, 3 and 4 days and counted using a hemocytometer. All experiments were performed in the logarithmic phase of cell growth. Triplicate plates were analyzed for each

treatment and each time. The following formula was used to calculate the doubling time: $N_t = N_0 \times e^{kxt}$, where N_0 was the initial number of cells that increased exponentially with a rate constant, k. The doubling time (T) was calculated as: $T = \ln 2/k$. The GraphPad Prism 5.0 software (GraphPad Software Inc., Philadelphia, U.S.A.) was employed.

Cell cycle analysis by flow cytometry

Cells were cultured for 24 h without FBS. Synchronized cells were then treated with IC_{50} Gli (25 µM) or vehicle immediately after release from the block and harvested for up to 72 h. Then cells were collected by trypsinization, fixed with ice cold methanol, centrifuged and resuspended in 0.5 ml of propidium iodide (PI) staining solution (50 µg/ml PI in PBS containing 0.2 mg/ml of DNase-free RNase A). After incubation for 30 min at 37°C, samples were evaluated by flow cytometry (Becton Dickinson, USA). Cell cycle distribution was analyzed using Cylchred 1.0.2 software (Cardiff University, UK).

Quantification of DNA synthesis

The quantification of cellular DNA synthesis was performed on cells by the addition of 30 µM BrdU for 2 h. Cells grown on sterile slides were washed with PBS and fixed with 10% formaldehyde in PBS. To denature the DNA into single-stranded molecules, cells were incubated with 3 N HCl for 30 min at room temperature. Then cells were washed in 1 ml of 0.1 M $Na_2B_4O_7$, pH 8.5 to neutralize the acid and were then incubated overnight at 4°C with mouse anti-BrdU monoclonal antibody (1:50). Then, cells were incubated for 2 h at 37°C with FITC-conjugated anti-mouse IgG (1:100). After washed with PBS, cells were stained with DAPI (1:8000). Fluorescence was further visualized by fluorescence microscope. At least 1000 cells were scored for each determination.

Apoptosis

Apoptotic MDA-MB-231 cells were detected after treatment with Gli or vehicle for 72 h. Phosphatidylserine exposure on the surface of apoptotic cells was detected by flow cytometry after staining with Annexin V-FITC and PI (50 µg/ml). Data were analyzed using WinMDI 2.8 software (Scripps Institute, CA, USA).

Mitochondrial transmembrane potential

Variations of the mitochondrial transmembrane potential of the cells, $\Delta\Psi_m$, were studied by means of the uptake of DiOC6, a specific fluorochrome that has been widely used in monitoring $\Delta\Psi_m$. Cells were plated and treated 24 h after with 25 µM Gli for different incubation periods (24, 48 and 72 hs). The diluted dye at a final concentration of 40 nM in PBS was applied to cells for

15 min at 37°C. Cells were then washed twice with PBS, harvested and then analyzed by flow cytometry (Becton Dickinson, USA). Results were expressed as the percentage of mean fluorescence of respective controls.

Determination of cell cycle and apoptosis related proteins
Flow cytometry

After treatment with Gli or vehicle for 72 h MDA-MB-231 cells were harvested, fixed with 4% formaldehyde and permeabilized with saponine. To evaluate intracellular protein content, cells were incubated with rabbit anti-Bcl-2 and rabbit anti-Bax antibodies. After washing, cells were incubated for 20 min with FITC-labeled anti-rabbit. The samples were analyzed with a FACScalibur flow cytometer (Becton Dickinson, USA). Data analysis was performed using WinMDI 2.8 software. For each sample 20,000 events were collected. The results are expressed as the percentage of respective control values.

Western blot assay

Cells were placed on ice and washed twice with cold PBS. Cells were then scraped into a lysis buffer (100 mM Tris/HCl buffer, pH 8, containing 1% Triton X-100 and protease inhibitors) and incubated for 15 min on ice. After centrifugation at 6000 rpm for 10 min, the supernatants were used for protein determination according to Bradford assay [21]. For Western blot, loading buffer (100 mM Tris/HCl buffer, pH 8, containing 1.7% sodium dodecyl sulfate (SDS), 0.02% bromophenol blue, 1.5% dithiotreitol, and 5% of glycerol) was added to samples and they were boiled for 3 minutes. Equal amounts of proteins (50 μg) were fractionated on SDS-polyacrylamide gels (12%) and transferred electrophoretically onto nitrocellulose membranes. Membranes were blocked and probed overnight with primary mouse anti-cyclin D_1 (1:100), mouse anti-cyclin E (1:500), mouse anti-cyclin B (1:200), mouse anti-p27^{Kip1} (1:200), rabbit anti-Bax (1:500), rabbit anti-Bcl-x$_{L/S}$ (1:500) and mouse anti-β-actin (1:1000) antibodies. Immunoreactivity was detected by using horseradish peroxidase-conjugated anti-mouse or anti-rabbit IgG, as appropriate, and visualized by enhanced chemiluminescence. Densitometric analyses were performed using the software Image J 1.32 J (NIH, USA).

Evaluation of senescence-like phenotype

Senescence-associated β-galactosidase (SA-β-Gal) activity was detected in cells as previously described by Dimri [22] with some modifications. Cells treated with Gli (25 μM) or vehicle for 72 hs were fixed in 3.0% formaldehyde for 5 min, washed in phosphate buffered solution (PBS) and stained in 1 mg/ml X-gal solution at pH 6.0 for 4 hs at 37°C. SA-β-Gal positive cells were stained in blue. To visualize the cell architecture, the slides were counter-stained by haematoxylin and quantified by optical microscopy. At least 1000 cells were scored for each determination.

Lipid accumulation

In order to examine the possible action of Gli in lipid accumulation, a classic terminal differentiation marker in mammary cells, the levels of neutral lipid were measured by flow cytometry using Nile-red staining [23]. Cells treated with Gli or vehicle for 2, 3 or 7 days were fixed and then incubated with Nile-red at a final concentration of 1 μg/ml in PBS for 20 min at room temperature. Cells were then analyzed by flow cytometry (Becton Dickinson, USA).

Data analysis was performed using WinMDI 2.8 software (Scripps Institute, CA, USA). The results were expressed as a percentage of control values.

Cytostatic effect of glibenclamide

MDA-MB-231 cells (1×10^4 cells/well) were plated into 6-well plates. After 24 h, cells were treated with 25 μM Gli or vehicle and detached with trypsin 3 or 7 days later. Cells were then counted and seeded in 6-well plates (1.2×10^3 cells/well) in triplicates. After 10 days in culture, colonies were fixed with 10% buffered formalin and stained with 1% toluidine blue in 70% ethanol. The number of colonies was determined and normalized to the number of colonies in controls.

Statistical analysis

In all cases the data shown are the means ± SEM of at least three independent experiments. Statistical analysis is indicated in each legend. Data were analyzed using the GraphPad Prism 5.0 (GraphPad Software Inc., Philadelphia, U.S.A.) and P values less than 0.05 were considered statistically significant.

Results
Expression of K$_{ATP}$ channels in MDA-MB-231 cells

Though many reports describe the presence of different potassium channels in diverse human cancer cell lines, at present there is little evidence about the expression of K$_{ATP}$ channels in breast cancer cells. Since Gli is a specific blocker of K$_{ATP}$ channels, the expression of mRNA for different subunits (Kir6.1, Kir6.2 and SURs) was examined by RT-PCR in MDA-MB-231 cells. As shown in Figure 1A bands of 336 and 301 bp for Kir6.1 and Kir6.2 respectively were detected after electrophoresis, indicating gene expression of pore components for at least two channel types in this cell line. Furthermore, a predicted band of 244 bp was found indicating the expression of SUR2B gene. The expression of SUR1 and SUR2A genes was not detected (291 bp and 215 bp, respectively). Altogether these results indicate that pore-forming and regulatory subunits are expressed in this

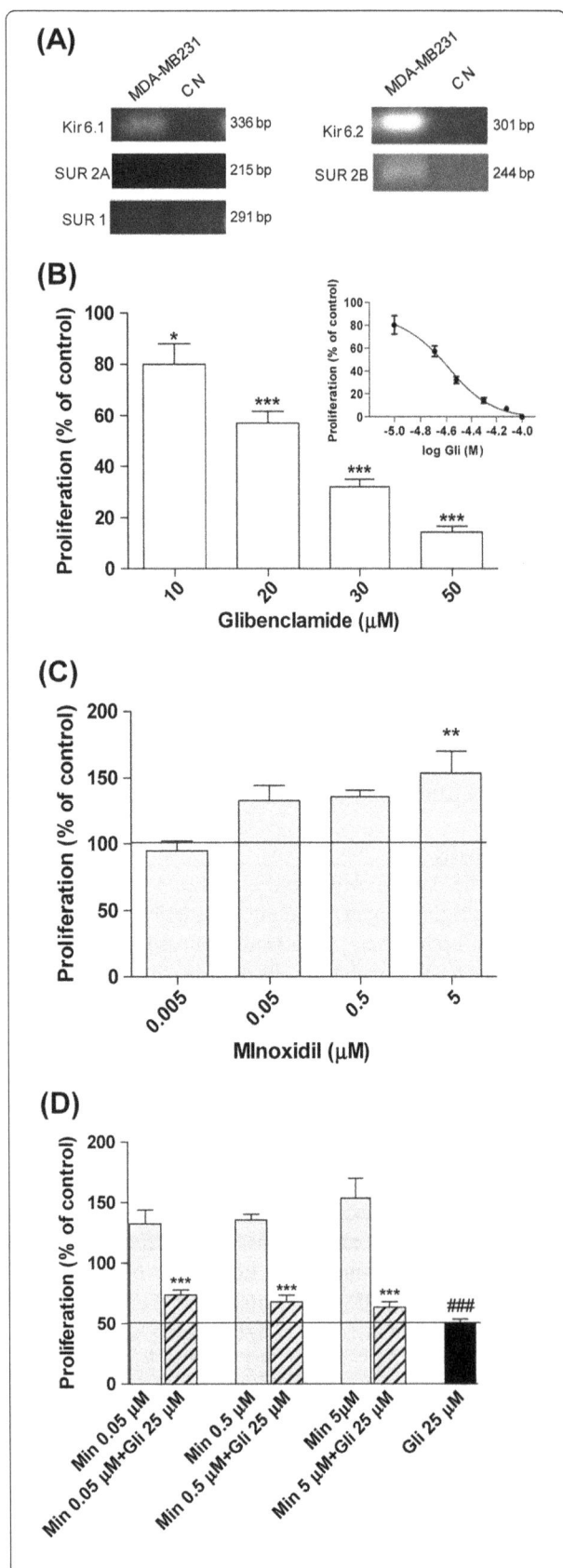

Figure 1 Effect of Glibenclamide, a specific blocker of the K_{ATP} channels, on cell growth. The figure shows the mRNA expression of K_{ATP} channels components and the effect of Gli and minoxidil (Min) on cell proliferation in MDA-MB-231 cells. Proliferation was evaluated by counting of colonies with 50 cells or more and expressed as percentage of values obtained with vehicle (means ± SEM of three experiments on parallel). Panel **A**: mRNA expression of K_{ATP} channels in MDA-MB-231 cells by RT-PCR analysis. Agarose gel electrophoresis of PCR products showed bands corresponding to: Kir6.1 (336 bp), Kir6.2 (301 bp), SUR2B (312 bp). No bands were detected for SUR2A (215 bp) or SUR1 (291 bp). CN: negative control Panel **B**: Inhibition of proliferation obtained with different concentrations of Gli (10, 20, 30 or 50 µM). Insert shows the dose–response curve used to determine IC_{50} (IC_{50} = 25 µM). Panel **C**: Increase of proliferation obtained with Min 0.05; 0.5 or 5 µM. Panel **D**: Results obtained with IC_{50} Gli plus different concentration of Min. Panel **B** and **C**: *p < 0.05 vs. control; **p < 0.01 vs control; ***p < 0.001 vs. control, One way ANOVA and Dunnet post test. Panel **D**: ***p < 0.01 vs. Min 0.05 µM; vs. Min 0.5 µM; vs. Min 5 µM. ###p < 0.001 vs. Min 0.05 µM; vs. Min 0.5 µM; vs. Min 5 µM. One way ANOVA and Tuckey post test.

cell line. ERα (+) MCF-7 breast cancer cells were also analyzed and Kir6.1, Kir6.2 and SUR1 were found expressed in this cell line (data not shown).

Effect of glibenclamide on cell proliferation

The effect of Gli on cell proliferation was tested by means of a clonogenic assay. A significant concentration dependent inhibition on cell growth was observed when Gli was added to cell cultures in concentrations over 10 µM; the IC_{50} value was 25.6 ± 3.2 µM (Figure 1B). The increased doubling time (T value, Table 1) obtained in the presence of 25 µM Gli is in concordance with the inhibition of proliferation previously demonstrated using the clonogenic assay.

In order to support the hypothesis of K_{ATP} channels involvement in MDA-MB-231 cell proliferation we used minoxidil, a well known specific opener of these channels. The results showed an increase in cell clonogenic growth for concentrations over 0.05 µM, which became significant at 5 µM (Figure 1C). Figure 1D shows that the increment in proliferation produced by the channel opener was totally reversed by 25 µM Gli.

The analysis of cell cycle phase distribution demonstrated that Gli produces a significant increase in the number of cells in G1 phase at 24, 48 and 72 h post treatment, clearly demonstrating a significant G0/G1 cell cycle arrest (Figure 2A). A consequent decrease in cells

Table 1 Determination of cell doubling time

Treatment	Duplication Time (hs)
Control	24.0 ± 4.3
Gli	34.6 ± 4.5 *

Gli: 25 µM glibenclamide. * p < 0.05 vs control, t test.

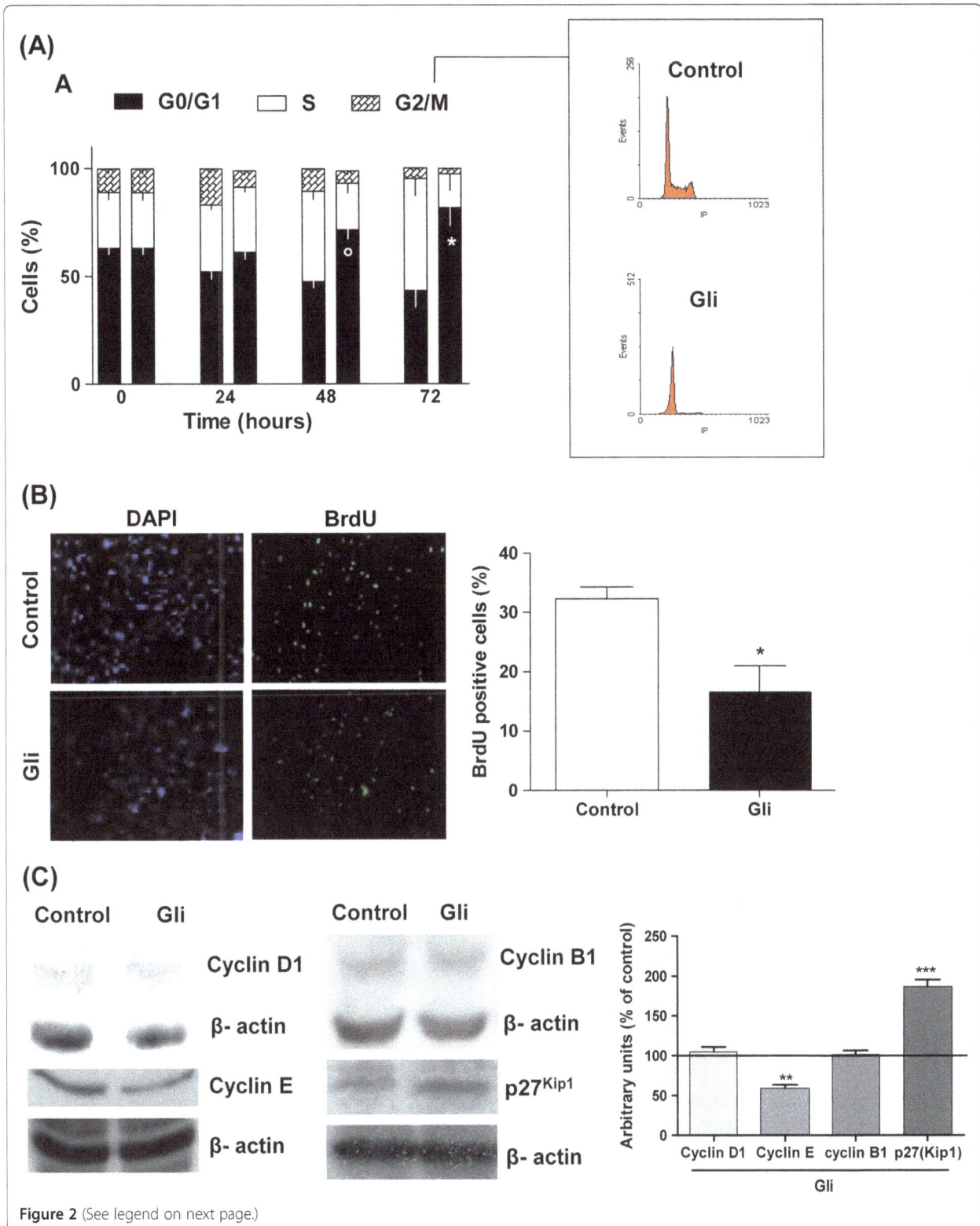

Figure 2 (See legend on next page.)

Figure 2 Effect of Glibenclamide on cell cycle progression. Panel **A**: Synchronized MDA-MB-231 cells were treated with IC_{50} Gli (25 μM) or vehicle for 24, 48 or 72 h and the fraction of cells in each phase of cell cycle was evaluated by flow citometry. Gli treatment clearly arrested cells at G0/G1 phase. Results are expressed as percentage of the value obtained with vehicle (means ± SEM of three experiments on parallel). °$p < 0.01$ vs control; *$p < 0.001$ vs control, t test. Left bars: control; right bars: Gli-treated cells. Panel **B**: A decrease in BrdU incorporation to DNA was observed when cells were treated with 25 μM Gli for 48 h. Results are expressed as the means ± SEM of three experiments on parallel. *$p < 0.05$ vs. control, t test. Panel **C**: Expression of G1-S regulatory proteins in MDA-MB-231 cells treated with Gli or vehicle for 72 h was analyzed by Western blot. Gli decreased the level of cyclin E and increased p27^{Kip1}. Representative immunoblot images of cyclins D1, B1, E and p27^{Kip1} are illustrated. Relative quantification was performed by densitometric analyses. Actin densitometric values were used to standardize for protein loading. Bars represent the mean ± SEM of three independent experiments. **$p < 0.01$ vs control; ***$p < 0.001$ vs control, t test.

in S and G2 phase versus control was also observed. Consistent with these observations, Gli inhibited the active DNA synthesis when it was evaluated by BrdU incorporation (Figure 2B).

The expression of proteins implicated in the control of different phases of the cell cycle was investigated by Western blot analysis. Studies of proteins specifically related with phase G1 of cell cycle demonstrated that 25 μM Gli reduced expression of cyclin E whereas cyclin D1 remained unchanged after 72 h of treatment. Furthermore, p27^{Kip1} levels were up-regulated in the same experimental conditions. In addition, the level of cyclin B1 expression, which is involved in the control of G2-M transition, was not modified by Gli treatment.

Effect of glibenclamide on cell death

To determine if the decrease in proliferation exerted by Gli could be due to an apoptotic effect, we assessed apoptosis by two different methodologies. Results showed that Gli did not increase the number of apoptotic cells by Annexin-V staining (3.66 ± 0.62% in control vs 3.70 ± 0.69%) after 72 h of treatment (Figure 3). In accordance, neither it produced the disruption of the

mitochondrial transmembrane potential ($\Delta\Psi_m$) that is associated with mitochondrial dysfunction and linked to cell death and loss of cell viability (Table 2).

It is known that the Bcl-2 family of mitochondrial proteins is strongly linked to the process of apoptotic cell death; some members of the family act as antiapoptotic proteins such as Bcl-2, Bcl-x$_L$, while others act as inductors of cell death as Bcl-x$_S$ and Bax [24-26]. We determined the expression of these proteins by flow cytometry and Western blot. By both methodologies we showed that 72 h after treatment with 25 μM Gli, the level of expression of pro-apoptotic protein Bax was slightly increased in relation to control at the same time, although this increase was not statistically significant (Figure 4A and 4B). On the other hand, antiapoptotic Bcl-2 protein did not modify its expression when cells were treated with Gli (Figure 4B). The pro-apoptotic isoform, Bcl-x$_S$, showed a very low expression while the antiapoptotic isoform Bcl-x$_L$ expression levels were higher but did not significantly change with Gli-treatment (Figure 4A).

We also evaluated the induction of cell senescence as a mechanism of cell death. To identify the senescent cells, senescence-associated β-galactosidase (SA-β-GAL)

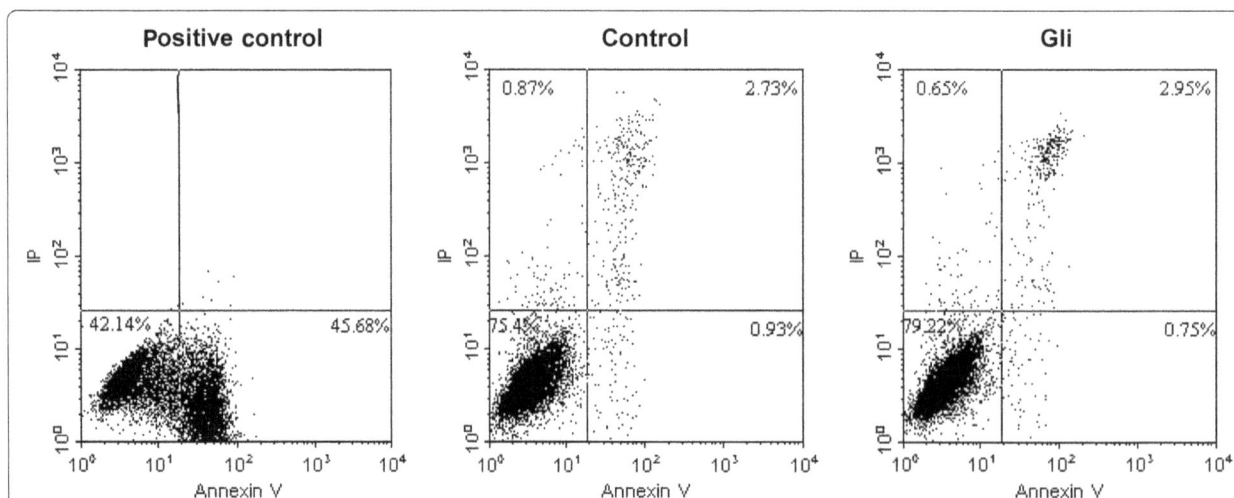

Figure 3 Evaluation of apoptosis by Annexin-V method. Apoptosis was assessed after incubating the cells with Gli or vehicle by 72 h. For positive control cells were treated with H_2O_2 (5 mM) for 30 minutes. Fluorescence was evaluated immediately after Annexin-V staining by flow cytometry. Gli (25 μM) did not induce an increment in apoptosis of MDA-MB-231 cells. Positive Annexin-V cells are shown in both right quadrants.

Table 2 Effect of Gli on mitochondrial transmembrane potential ($\Delta\Psi_m$)

Time (hs)	$\Delta\Psi$m (% of control)
24	99.7 ± 7.3
48	97.0 ± 3.9
72	94.3 ± 12.7

Gli: 25 µM glibenclamide. p:NS vs. control, One way ANOVA.

activity was assessed. MDA-MB-231 cells treated with 25 µM Gli showed an increase in the percentage of senescent cells versus those treated with vehicle ($3.5 \pm 0.4\%$ vs $1.2 \pm 0.2\%$; Figure 5).

Effect of glibenclamide on cell differentiation

Differentiation is one possible mechanism involved in the loss of cell proliferative ability. In mammary cells the accumulation of neutral lipids in cytoplasm is a specific marker of this process. We evaluated by flow cytometry the content of neutral lipids using Nile-red staining and results demonstrated no differences between control and 25 µM Gli treated cells up to 7 days (Table 3). Sodium butyrate, an effective differentiation agent in ERα (+) and ERα (−) breast cancer cells [27], was used as positive control.

Cytostatic effect of glibenclamide

To determine whether the growth inhibitory effect was reversible, a characteristic of cytostatic agents, cells were treated with 25 µM Gli or vehicle for 3 or 7 days and then they were trypsinized and re-plated at low density in the absence of any treatment to assess clonogenic proliferation. Results in Figure 6 showed that there is no significant difference between Gli-pretreated cells for different time periods and control cells, suggesting that the antiproliferative effect of Gli is elicited only when the drug is present and it does not involve cell toxicity.

Combination treatments

We assayed the combination of Gli with tamoxifen or doxorubicin to explore a possible increase in efficacy. The growth of MDA-MB-231 cells was inhibited by tamoxifen with an IC_{50} equal to 5 µM (Figure 7A). The concentration of Gli that inhibited cell growth in a 50% (25 µM) was used to evaluate the combined action of Gli plus tamoxifen. The inhibitory effect exerted by the combination of Gli plus tamoxifen was similar to that observed for Gli alone (Figure 7B).

Doxorubicin also inhibited cell proliferation in a concentration dependent manner (Figure 7C). The combination of 25 µM Gli plus doxorubicin in doses over 0.05 nM was more effective to inhibit cell proliferation than single treatments (Figure 7D).

Discussion

Different subtypes of potassium channels have been shown to be directly implicated in normal and malignant cell proliferation [9]. Some of these channels are overexpressed in tumors and therefore they are potential targets for anticancer therapies [28].

We have previously demonstrated that Gli exerts an antitumoral action on NMU-induced mammary tumors in rats, which is an experimental model similar in ER expression and hormone-dependence to human breast cancer [29,30]. In these tumors Gli action was potentiated by the combination with tamoxifen [31]. In this paper we analyzed the effect of Gli in MDA-MB-231 ERα (−) breast cancer cell proliferation.

We studied the expression of mRNA for the different subunits that constitute K_{ATP} channels in MDA-MB-231 cells and determined that these cells express both pore forming subunits, Kir6.1 and Kir6.2, and the regulatory subunit SUR2B. Coincidently, Bondestine et al. have recently reported the expression of SUR2 protein in MDA-MB-231 cells, while SUR1 could not be detected in this cell line [32]. In consequence two whole octameric functional channels could be present in MDA-MB-231 cells. In specific tissues different subunit combinations have been detected, e.g., pancreatic β cells and neurons have Kir6.2/SUR1 channels, whereas skeletal muscle expresses Kir6.2/SUR2A channels. These differences imply that drugs may have distinct abilities to affect K_{ATP} channels in diverse tissues depending on the type of SUR expressed [20]. Gli binds to every type of SUR and therefore inhibits the activity of all known K_{ATP} channels [33]. When we assayed the effect of Gli on MDA-MB-231 cell proliferation, results showed that Gli inhibits clonogenic ability in a concentration-dependent way, with an increment in population doubling time. It has been reported that the potassium-dependent changes in membrane potential play a crucial role in the proliferation of many types of normal and tumor cells. The opening of potassium channels in the cell membrane produces a hyperpolarization of membrane potential which is required for the progression through the cell cycle. As a consequence in the presence of potassium channel blockers cell proliferation is inhibited [34,35]. Woodfort et al. early determined that different potassium channel antagonists, as Gli, produce a concentration-dependent growth inhibition on MCF-7 cells with a significant arrest of cells in G0/G1 phase [36]. Diverse drugs signaled as specific K_{ATP} channel openers which include minoxidil, pinacidil and diazoxide augment DNA synthesis and proliferation of normal and tumor cells [37-39]. In the experiments using minoxidil

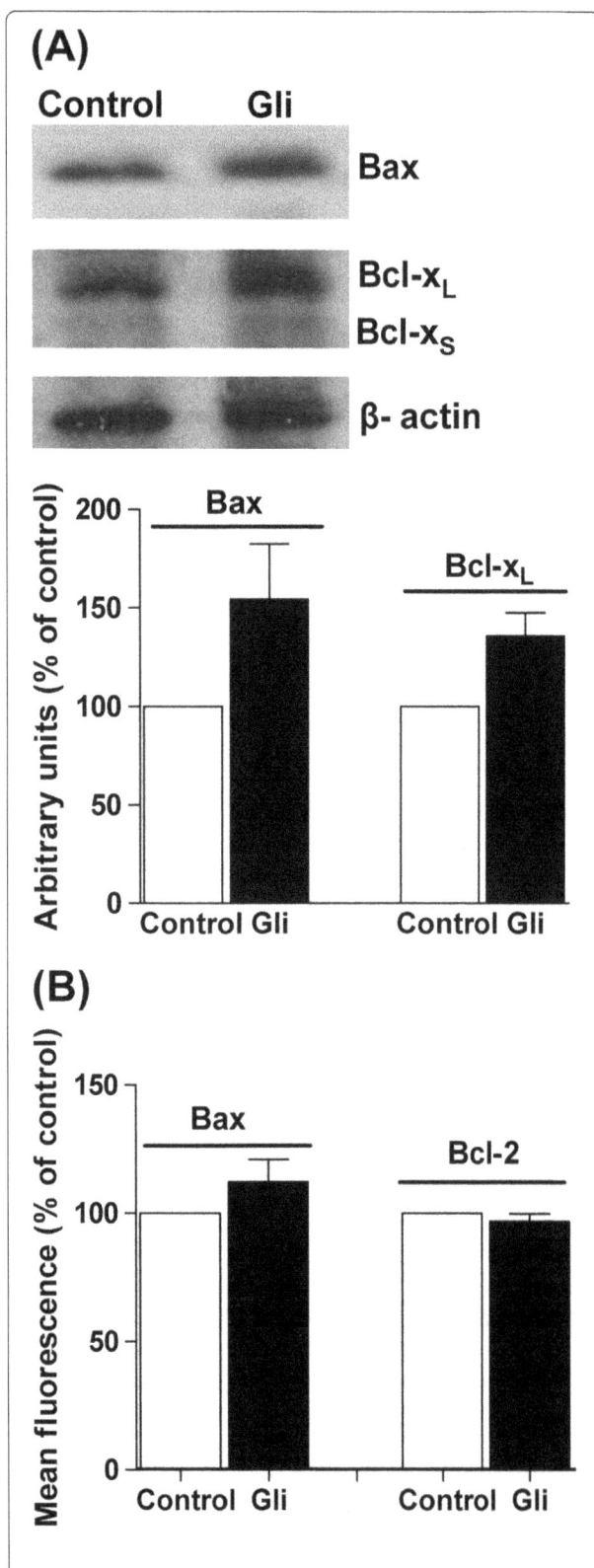

(A)

Figure 4 Expression of proteins involved in apoptosis. Panel **A**: Bax and Bcl-x$_{L/S}$ expression determined by Western Blot employing specific antibodies in MDA-MB-231 cells treated for 72 h with 25 µM Gli (Gli) or vehicle (control) cells. The figure shows a representative Western blot of three independent experiments and the quantification of bands obtained for Bax and Bcl-x$_{L/S}$ protein. Bars represent the mean ± SEM of three independent experiments. p: Non significant (NS), t test. Panel **B**: Expression of Bcl-2 and Bax protein in MDA-MB-231 cells treated by 72 h with 25 µM Gli (Gli) or vehicle, obtained by flow cytometry. Bars represent the mean fluorescence ± SEM obtained by three independent experiments. p: NS, t test.

we demonstrated an increase in MDA-MB-231 cell proliferation in concentrations over 0.05 µM. In addition when different concentrations of minoxidil were combined with 25 µM Gli the increment in proliferation was totally reverted. Taken together, these results suggest that Gli could reduce cell proliferation in MDA-MB-231 cells acting through K$_{ATP}$ channels.

The analysis of cell cycle progression indicated that 25 µM Gli produces an arrest in the G0/G1 phase of cell cycle after 48 h of treatment. After release of serum starvation, the diminution of the proportion of cells in S phase in Gli treated cultures was confirmed by the decrease in BrdU incorporation. The cell division cycle integrates several processes and signal transduction pathways to commit the progression of a cell through or its arrest in a specific cell cycle phase. It is generally accepted that the cell cycle regulators cyclin D1 and cyclin E play an important role in early G1 and late G1 progression. In addition, the progression is tightly regulated by the respective cyclin activated subunits cyclin-dependent kinases (Cdks) and their inhibitors (Cdkis). p27 is a member of the Kip/CIP family of Cdkis known to act in the G1 phase of the cell cycle, preventing G1-S transition [40,41]. The study of proteins involved in the progression through the phases of cell cycle by immunoblot, has evidenced a decrease in cyclin E expression with a raise in cyclin inhibitor p27[Kip1] in Gli treated MDA-MB-231 cells. It is known that the activity of cyclin E in conjunction with its kinase subunit Cdk2, is limiting for the passage of cells through the restriction point needed for the progression of cells from G1 into S-phase [42]. p27[Kip1] binds to the cyclinE/Cdk2 complex and inhibits the kinase thus impeding G1-S passage [43]. Altogether our results suggest that Gli inhibits MDA-MB-231 cell proliferation by hindering G1-S transition. Other authors have also reported that different potassium channels blockers and other agents that cause cell membrane depolarization, produce the arrest of cells in G1 phase with the involvement of different cyclins and inhibitors depending on the cell type [34]. Eto reported that various anticancer agents specifically up-regulate p27[Kip1] expression without affecting expression of the other regulatory proteins of G1-S cell cycle transition in human breast cancer

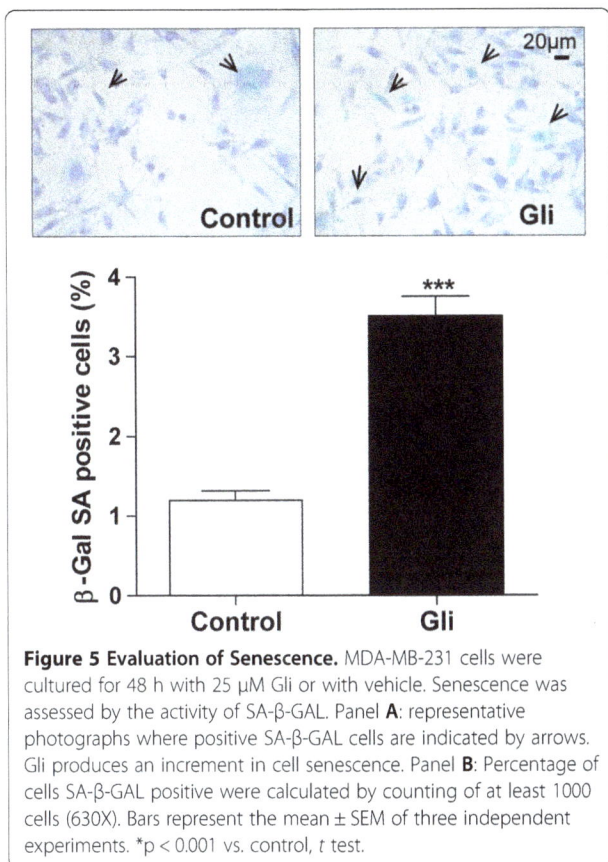

Figure 5 Evaluation of Senescence. MDA-MB-231 cells were cultured for 48 h with 25 µM Gli or with vehicle. Senescence was assessed by the activity of SA-β-GAL. Panel **A**: representative photographs where positive SA-β-GAL cells are indicated by arrows. Gli produces an increment in cell senescence. Panel **B**: Percentage of cells SA-β-GAL positive were calculated by counting of at least 1000 cells (630X). Bars represent the mean ± SEM of three independent experiments. *p < 0.001 vs. control, t test.

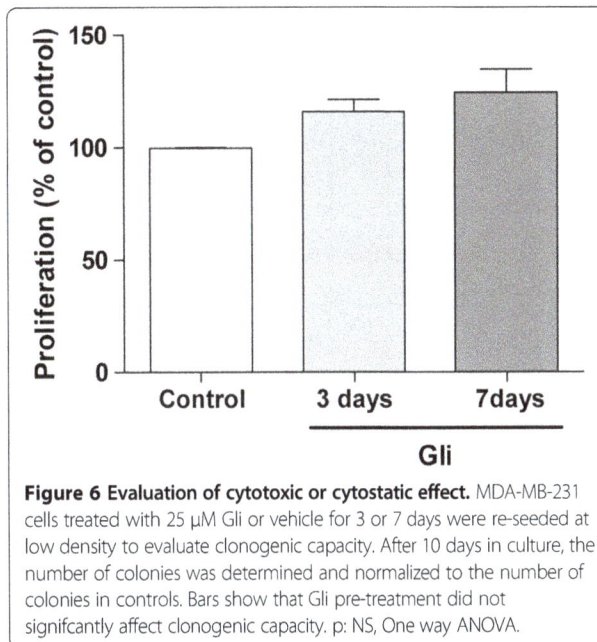

Figure 6 Evaluation of cytotoxic or cytostatic effect. MDA-MB-231 cells treated with 25 µM Gli or vehicle for 3 or 7 days were re-seeded at low density to evaluate clonogenic capacity. After 10 days in culture, the number of colonies was determined and normalized to the number of colonies in controls. Bars show that Gli pre-treatment did not signifcantly affect clonogenic capacity. p: NS, One way ANOVA.

cell lines. Moreover, in concordance with our work, he reported that the up-regulation of p27^{Kip1} expression in these cell lines by anti-cancer agents linearly and positively correlates with the degree of growth inhibition of NMU-induced mammary tumors by the same anti-cancer agent [44].

It has been suggested that chemotherapeutic agents can prevent mammary carcinogenesis and tumor growth through different mechanisms that include apoptosis, differentiation and senescence. Regardless of the mechanism, the evaluation of new antitumoral drugs has as a goal to stop the cell proliferation and produce the death of the tumor cell by apoptotic or non-apoptotic means [45]. Previously, working with NMU-induced mammary

Table 3 Effect of Gli on neutral lipid accumulation

Time (days)	Mean Fluorescence of Nile Red (% of control)	
	Gli	Na Butyrate
2	92.3 ± 4.7	134.3 ± 6.7 ***
3	99.3 ± 1.7	165.7 ± 7.3 ***
7	99.0 ± 10.1	192.7 ± 5.3 ***

Gli: 25 µM glibenclamide. Na Butyrate: 10 mM Sodium butyrate as the positive control. p: NS Gli vs control; *** p < 0.001 butyrate vs control, One way ANOVA and Dunnet test.

tumors in rats, we reported that Gli clearly produced the inhibition of tumor growth through a decrease in cell proliferation and an increase in cell apoptosis and differentiation [31]. It has been reported that Gli produces apoptosis in malignant cell lines such as hepatoblastoma and gastric cancer cells [6,7]. Furthermore, Iwakura and coworkers found that Gli produces a sustained increase in the entrance of Ca^{2+} to the cells inducing their death through apoptosis [46]. On the contrary, we demonstrated that Gli neither produced apoptosis nor triggered the early events of this mechanism of cell death in MDA-MB-231 cells. We also studied the expression of apoptosis related proteins and determined that Gli did not significantly affect the ratio of the expression of Bax/Bcl-2 proteins at any time evaluated. The relation between antiapoptotic and apoptotic proteins of Bcl-2 family is a better determinant of the susceptibility to apoptosis than the expression of each member separately.

In view that some chemotherapeutic agents are able to produce cell senescence as part of their mechanism of action [45], this possible way of action was studied in the MDA-MB-231 cells treated with Gli. Data obtained in our experiments indicate that there is a slight increase in cell senescence after Gli treatment. However, Gli did not result cytotoxic for neoplastic MDA-MB-231 cells so they clearly keep their clonogenic capacity after being exposed to Gli for seven days. Our results are in agreement with the reported by Woodfork et al., showing that Gli induced a cell cycle arrest in G0/G1 phase in MCF-7 cells that could be reverted by the removal of the drug [36].

Mammary tumor cell differentiation is characterized by an arrest in cell proliferation, nuclear and cytoplasmatic

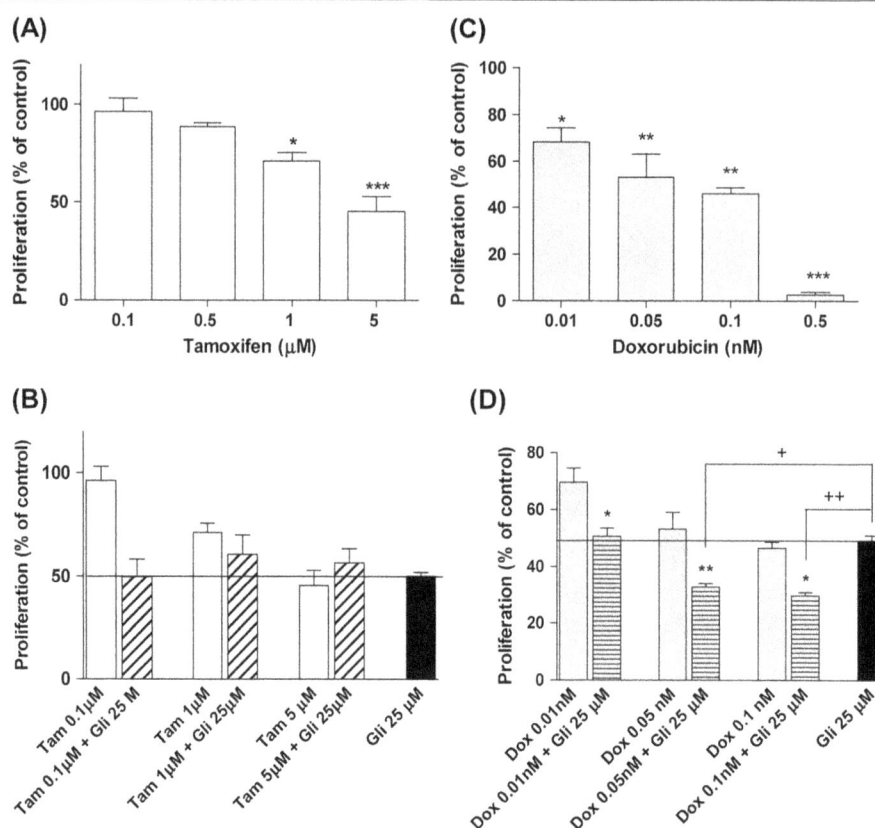

Figure 7 Glibenclamide combination with antineoplasic drugs. MDA-MB-231 cell proliferation was evaluated by counting of colonies with 50 cells or more and expressed as percentage of controls (means ± SEM of three independent experiments). Panel **A**: Results obtained with tamoxifen (Tam) 0.1, 0.5, 1 or 5 μM. Panel **C**: Inhibition of proliferation obtained with doxorubicin (Dox) 0.01, 0.05, 0.1 or 0.5 nM. Panel **B** and **D**: Results obtained for combination of 25 μM Gli plus different concentrations of Tam or Dox. Panel **A** and **C**: *p < 0.05 vs. control; **p < 0.01 vs. control; ***p < 0.001 vs. control, ANOVA and Dunnet post test. Panel **B**: p: NS vs. Gli 25 μM, t test. Panel **D**: *p < 0.05 vs. Dox 0.01 nM, vs. Dox 0.1 nM; **p < 0.001 vs Dox 0.05 nM; ⁺p < 0.05 vs. Dox 0.05 nM + Gli 25 μM; ⁺⁺p < 0.001 vs. Dox 0.1 nM + Gli 25 μM. One way ANOVA and Tuckey post test.

morphological changes and also by the increased expression of the components of milk such as lipids [47,48]. The accumulation of neutral lipid drops in the cell cytoplasm is used as a marker of this process. In our research Gli did not induce differentiation in MDA-MB-231 cells after treatment for seven days.

Antiestrogens such as tamoxifen are widely used for the treatment of ERα (+) breast cancer. Nevertheless, tamoxifen may elicit pro-apoptotic effects in ERα (−) breast cancer cells by the modulation of various cell signaling pathways in an ER-independent manner [49-53]. However, these effects have generally been reported when relatively high concentrations of tamoxifen were used. In the present work we used tamoxifen in combination with Gli as a strategy to enhance its action in ERα (−) breast cancer even if Gli acts as cytostatic in MDA-MB-231 cells. In our experiments tamoxifen inhibited proliferation significantly at quite high concentrations (5 μM) as expected and the combination treatment did not produce a higher inhibitory effect on cell proliferation than each treatment alone. Abdul et al. demonstrated that two nonspecific

potassium channels blockers, amiodarone and dequalinium, potentiated the growth inhibitory effects of tamoxifen on human breast, prostate and colon cancer cell lines [38]. In view of our previous results in NMU-induced mammary tumors [31] it could be suggested that Gli may potentiate tamoxifen action only in breast hormone-dependent cells.

Doxorubicin is extensively used in chemotherapy for patients with metastatic breast cancer. In spite of its excellent anti-tumor activity, the associated acute and chronic toxicities lead to a relatively low therapeutic index [54]. Therefore, combination treatment with a non-toxic drug which can lower the dose would be advantageous. Our results indicate that the combined treatment of Gli and doxorubicin displayed an additive anti-proliferative effect. In this regard, Gli was found to inhibit multidrug resistance protein (MRP1) activity in human lung cancer cells [55]. In addition it has been also demonstrated that the overexpression of the inwardly rectifying K channel Kir2.2 decreased doxorubicin-induced reactive oxygen species accumulation and cell growth inhibition in several cancer cell lines [56]. Further studies are to needed to fully investigate the mechanism involved in the antiproliferative response of MDA-MB-231 cells to the combined treatment glibenclamide with doxorubicin.

Conclusions

Gli, a drug widely used in clinics for the treatment of type 2-diabetes, is atoxic at doses routinely employed and of low cost. Our experimental data clearly demonstrated that it produces a cytostatic effect in MDA-MB-231 cells inhibiting the G1-S phase progression without inducing cell death or differentiation. Nevertheless, in spite of the lack of cytotoxic action, the interesting observation about the effect of the combination of Gli with doxorubicin on proliferation warrants an exhaustive research to elucidate the pathways involved in this interaction, leading to the consideration of a novel role for Gli as an adjuvant in breast cancer treatment.

Competing interests

The authors declare that they have no competing interests.

Authors' contributions

MN is Ph.D and she designed the study, performed the experiments, interpreted the data, and wrote the manuscript. VM, GC, and CC are Ph.D. and carried out clonogenic and flow cytometry assays and participated in data analyses and interpretation. RB and GM are Ph.D. and participated in data analysis and discussion and critically revised the manuscript. MC carried out microscopic observation. ER performed the statistical analysis. All authors have expertise on radiopharmacology and receptors study. VM, CC, GM and RB are members of the National Research Council (CONICET). MN, VM, GC, CC, ER, RB, and GM are professors in the University of Buenos Aires. MC is M. D. and he is specialist in anatomopathology. All authors read and approved the final manuscript.

Acknowledgements

This work was supported by grants from the National Agency of Scientific and Technological Promotion and from Barceló Foundation, Argentina. Vanina Medina, Claudia Cocca, Gabriela Martín and Rosa Bergoc are members of the National Research Council (CONICET).

Author details

[1]Radioisotopes Laboratory, School of Pharmacy and Biochemistry, University of Buenos Aires, Buenos Aires, Argentina. [2]Institute of Immunooncology Dr. EJV Crescenti, Buenos Aires, Argentina. [3]Institute of Health Sciences Barceló, Buenos Aires, Argentina.

References

1. Krentz AJ, Bailey CJ: Oral antidiabetic agents. Current role in type 2 diabetes. *Drugs* 2005, 65:385–411.
2. Lebovitz HE: Treating hyperglycemia in type 2 diabetes: new goals and strategies. *Cleve Clin J Med* 2002, 69:809–820.
3. Lebovitz HE: Oral antidiabetic agents. *Med Clin North Am* 2004, 88:847–863.
4. Shorter K, Farjo NP, Picksley SM, Randall VA: Human hair follicles contain two forms of ATP-sensitive potassium channels, only one of which is sensitive to minoxidil. *FASEB J* 2008, 22:1725–1736.
5. Groop LC: Sulphonylureas in NIDDM. *Diabetes Care* 1992, 15:737–754.
6. Kim JA, Kang YS, Lee SH, Lee EH, Yoo BH, Lee YS: Glibenclamide induces apoptosis through inhibition of cystic fibrosis transmembrane conductance regulator (CFTR) Cl(−) channels and intracellular Ca(2+)

7. Qian X, Li J, Ding J, Wang Z, Duan L, Hu G: Glibenclamide exerts an antitumor activity through reactive oxygen species-c-jun NH2-terminal kinase pathway in human gastric cancer cell line MGC-803. *Biochem Pharmacol* 2008, 76:1705–1715.
8. Wonderlin WF, Strobl JS: Potassium channels, proliferation and G1 progression. *J Membr Biol* 1996, 154:91–107.
9. Pardo LA: Voltage-gated potassium channels in cell proliferation. *Physiology* 2004, 19:285–292.
10. Parkin DM, Bray F, Ferlay J, Pisani P: Global cancer statistics, 2002. *CA Cancer J Clin* 2005, 55:74–108.
11. Al-Dhaheri MH, Shah YM, Basrur V, Pind S, Rowan BG: Identification of novel proteins induced by estradiol, 4-hydroxytamoxifen and acolbifene in T47D breast cancer cells. *Steroid* 2006, 71:966–978.
12. Benson JR, Jatoi I, Keisch M, Esteva FJ, Makris A, Jordan VC: Early breast cancer. *Lancet* 2009, 373:1463–1479.
13. Utsumi T, Kobayashi N, Hanada H: Recent perspectives of endocrine therapy for breast cancer. *Breast Cancer* 2007, 14:194–199.
14. Jordan VC, Brodie AM: Development and evolution of therapies targeted to the estrogen receptor for the treatment and prevention of breast cancer. *Steroids* 2007, 72:7–25.
15. Park BJ, Whichard ZL, Corey SJ: Dasatinib synergizes with both cytotoxic and signal transduction inhibitors in heterogeneous breast cancer cell lines–lessons for design of combination targeted therapy. *Cancer Lett* 2012, 320:104–110.
16. Smith L, Watson MB, O'Kane SL, Drew PJ, Lind MJ, Cawkwell L: The analysis of doxorubicin resistance in human breast cancer cells using antibody microarrays. *Mol Cancer Ther* 2006, 5:2115–2120.
17. Joensuu H, Gligorov J: Adjuvant treatments for triple-negative breast cancers. *Ann Oncol* 2012, 23:vi40–vi45.
18. Soto-Cerrato V, Llagostera E, Montaner B, Scheffer GL, Perez-Tomas R: Mitochondria-mediated apoptosis operating irrespective of multidrug resistance in breast cancer cells by the anticancer agent prodigiosin. *Biochem Pharmacol* 2004, 68:1345–1352.
19. Mody M, Dharker N, Bloomston M, Wang PS, Chou FS, Glickman TS, McCaffrey T, Yang Z, Pumfery A, Lee D, Ringel MD, Pinzone JJ: Rosiglitazone sensitizes MDA-MB-231 breast cancer cells to anti-tumour effects of tumour necrosis factor-alpha, CH11 and CYC202. *Endocr Relat Cancer* 2007, 14:305–315.
20. Jovanović S, Du Q, Mukhopadhyay S, Swingler R, Buckley R, McEachen J, Jovanović A: A patient suffering from hypokalemic periodic paralysis is deficient in skeletal muscle ATP-sensitive K channels. *Clin Transl Sci* 2008, 1:71–74.
21. Bradford MM: A rapid and sensitive method for the quantification of microgram quantities of protein utilizing the principle of protein-dye binding. *Anal Biochem* 1976, 72:248–254.
22. Dimri GP, Lee X, Basile G, Acosta M, Scott G, Roskelley C, Medrano EE, Linskens M, Rubelj I, Pereira-Smith O, et al: A biomarker that identifies senescent human cells in culture and in aging skin in vivo. *Proc Natl Acad Sci USA* 1995, 92:9363–9367.
23. Greespan P, Mayer E, Fowler S: Nile Red: A selective fluorescent stain for intracellular lipid droplets. *J Cell Biol* 1985, 100:965–973.
24. Zhang GJ, Kimijima I, Onda M, Kanno M, Sato H, Watanabe T, Tsuchiya A, Abe R, Takenoshita S: Tamoxifen-induced apoptosis in breast cancer cells relates to down-regulation of bcl-2, but not bax and bcl-x$_{(L)}$, without alteration of p53 protein levels. *Clin Cancer Res* 1999, 5:2971–2977.
25. Mohamad N, Gutiérrez A, Núñez M, Cocca C, Martín G, Cricco G, Medina V, Rivera E, Bergoc R: Mitochondrial apoptotic pathways. *Biocell* 2005, 29:149–161.
26. Schmitt E, Paquet C, Beauchemin M, Bertrand R: DNA-damage response network at the crossroads of cell-cycle checkpoints, cellular senescence and apoptosis. *J Zhejiang Univ Sci B* 2007, 8:377–397.
27. Davis T, Kennedy C, Chiew YE, Clarke CL, De Fazio A: Histone deacetylase inhibitors decrease proliferation and modulate cell cycle gene expression in normal mammary epithelial cells. *Clin Cancer Res* 2000, 6:4334–4342.
28. Felipe A, Vicente R, Villalonga N, Roura-Ferrer M, Martínez-Mármol R, Solé L, Ferreres JC, Condom E: Potassium channels: new targets in cancer therapy. *Cancer Detect Prev* 2006, 30:375–385.

release in HepG2 human hepatoblastoma cells. *Biochem Biophys Res Commun* 1999, 261:682–688.

29. Martin G, Melito G, Rivera E, Levin E, Davio C, Cricco G, Andrade N, Caro R, Bergoc R: Effect of tamoxifen on intraperitoneal N-nitroso-N-methylurea induced tumors. *Cancer Lett* 1996, **100**:227–234.

30. Martin G, Rivera ES, Daivo C, Cricco G, Levin E, Cocca C, Andrade N, Caro R, Bergoc RM: Receptors characterization of intraperitoneally N-nitroso-N-methylurea-induced mammary tumors in rats. *Cancer Lett* 1996, **101**:1–8.

31. Cocca C, Martín G, Núñez M, Gutiérrez A, Cricco G, Mohamad N, Medina V, Croci M, Crescenti E, Rivera E, Bergoc R: Effect of glibenclamide on N-nitroso-methylurea-induced mammary tumors in diabetic and nondiabetic rats. *Oncology Res* 2005, **15**:301–311.

32. Bodenstine TM, Vaidya KS, Ismail A, Beck BH, Diers AR, Edmonds MD, Kirsammer GT, Landar A, Welch DR: Subsets of ATP-sensitive potassium channel (KATP) inhibitors increase gap junctional intercellular communication in metastatic cancer cell lines independent of SUR expression. *FEBS Lett* 2012, **586**:27–31.

33. Du Q, Jovanović S, Sukhodub A, Barratt E, Drew E, Whalley KM, Kay V, McLaughlin M, Telfer EE, Barratt CL, Jovanović A: Human oocytes express ATP-sensitive K(+) channels. *Hum Reprod* 2010, **25**:2774–2782.

34. Ouadid-Ahidouch H, Ahidouch A: K + channel expression in human breast cancer cells: involvement in cell cycle regulation and carcinogenesis. *J Membr Biol* 2008, **221**:1–6.

35. Jang SS, Park J, Hur SW, Hong YH, Hur J, Chae JH, Kim SK, Kim J, Kim HS, Kim SJ: Endothelial progenitor cells functionally express inward rectifier potassium channels. *Am J Physiol Cell Physiol* 2011, **301**:C150–C161.

36. Woodfork KA, Wonderlin WF, Peterson VA, Strobl JS: Inhibition of ATP-sensitive potassium channels causes reversible cell-cycle arrest of human breast cancer cells in tissue culture. *J Cell Physiol* 1995, **162**:163–171.

37. Malhi H, Irani AN, Rajvanshi P, Suadicani SO, Spray DC, McDonald TV, Gupta S: KATP channels regulate mitogenically induced proliferation in primary rat hepatocytes and human liver cell lines. Implications for liver growth control and potential therapeutic targeting. *J Biol Chem* 2000, **275**:26050–26057.

38. Abdul M, Santo A, Hoosein N: Activity of potassium channel-blockers in breast cancer. *Anticancer Res* 2003, **23**:3347–3351.

39. Huang W, Acosta-Martínez M, Levine JE: Ovarian steroids stimulate adenosine triphosphate-sensitive potassium (KATP) channel subunit gene expression and confer responsiveness of the gonadotropin-releasing hormone pulse generator to KATP channel modulation. *Endocrinology* 2008, **149**:2423–2432.

40. Diehl JA: Cycling to cancer with cyclin D1. *Cancer Biol Ther* 2002, **1**:226–231.

41. Gladden AB, Diehl JA: Location, location, location: the role of cyclin D1 nuclear localization in cancer. *J Cell Biochem* 2005, **96**:906–913.

42. Möröy T, Geisen C: Cyclin E. *Int J Biochem Cell Biol* 2004, **36**:1424–1439.

43. Conradie R, Bruggeman FJ, Ciliberto A, Csikász-Nagy A, Novák B, Westerhoff HV, Snoep JL: Restriction point control of the mammalian cell cycle via the cyclin E/Cdk2:p27 complex. *FEBS J* 2010, **277**:357–367.

44. Eto I: Upstream molecular signaling pathways of p27(Kip1) expression in human breast cancer cells in vitro: differential effects of 4-hydroxytamoxifen and deficiency of either D-(+)-glucose or L-leucine. *Cancer Cell Int* 2011, **11**:31.

45. Christov K, Grubbs CJ, Shilkaitis A, Juliana MM, Lubet RA: Short-term modulation of cell proliferation and apoptosis and preventive/therapeutic efficacy of various agents in a mammary cancer model. *Clin Cancer Res* 2007, **13**:5488–5496.

46. Iwakura T, Fujimoto S, Kagimoto S, Inada A, Kubota A, Someya Y, Ihara Y, Yamada Y, Seino Y: Sustained enhancement of Ca(2+) influx by glibenclamide induces apoptosis in RINm5F cells. *Biochem Biophys Res Commun* 2000, **271**:422–428.

47. You H, Yu W, Sanders BG, Kline K: RRR-α-tocopheryl succinate induces MDA-MB-435 and MCF-7 human breast cancer cells to undergo differentiation. *Cell Growth Diff* 2001, **12**:471–480.

48. Münster PN, Srethapakdi M, Moasser MM, Rosen N: Inhibition of heat shock protein 90 function by ansamycins causes the morphological and functional differentiation of breast cancer cells. *Cancer Res* 2001, **61**:2945–2952.

49. Fattman CL, An B, Sussman L, Dou QP: p53-independent dephosphorylation and cleavage of retinoblastoma protein during tamoxifen-induced apoptosis in human breast carcinoma cells. *Cancer Lett* 1998, **130**:103–113.

50. Ferlini C, Scambia G, Marone M, Distefano M, Gaggini C, Ferrandina G, Fattorossi A, Isola G, Benedetti Panici P, Mancuso S: Tamoxifen induces oxidative stress and apoptosis in oestrogen receptor-negative human cancer cell lines. *Br J Cancer* 1999, **79**:257–263.

51. Mandlekar S, Yu R, Tan TH, Kong AN: Activation of caspase-3 and c-Jun NH2-terminal kinase-1 signaling pathways in tamoxifen-induced apoptosis of human breast cancer cells. *Cancer Res* 2000, **60**:5995–6000.

52. Scandlyn MJ, Stuart EC, Somers-Edgar TJ, Menzies AR, Rosengren RJ: A new role for tamoxifen in oestrogen receptor-negative breast cancer when it is combined with epigallocatechin gallate. *Br J Cancer* 2008, **99**:1056–1063.

53. Zhang X, Ding L, Kang L, Wang ZY: Estrogen receptor-alpha 36 mediates mitogenic antiestrogen signaling in ER-negative breast cancer cells. *PLoS One* 2012, **7**:e30174.

54. Chen JH, Ling R, Yao Q, Li Y, Chen T, Wang Z, Li KZ: Effect of small-sized liposomal Adriamycin administered by various routes on a metastatic breast cancer model. *Endocr Relat Cancer* 2005, **12**:93–100.

55. Payen L, Delugin L, Courtois A, Trinquart Y, Guillouzo A, Fardel O: The sulphonylurea glibenclamide inhibits multidrug resistance protein (MRP1) activity in human lung cancer cells. *Br J Pharmacol* 2001, **132**(3):778–784.

56. Lee I, Park C, Kang WK: Knockdown of inwardly rectifying potassium channel Kir2.2 suppresses tumorigenesis by inducing reactive oxygen species-mediated cellular senescence. *Mol Cancer Ther* 2010, **9**(11):2951–2959.

9

The prognostic value of blood pH and lactate and metformin concentrations in severe metformin-associated lactic acidosis

Farshad Kajbaf[1] and Jean-Daniel Lalau[1,2]*

Abstract

Aims: Analysis of the prognostic values of blood pH and lactate and plasma metformin concentrations in severe metformin-associated lactic acidosis may help to resolve the following paradox: metformin provides impressive, beneficial effects but is also associated with life-threatening adverse effects.

Research design and methods: On the basis of 869 pharmacovigilance reports on MALA with available data on arterial pH and lactate concentration, plasma metformin concentration and outcome, we selected cases with a pH < 7.0 and a lactate concentration >10 mmol/L. Outcomes were compared with those described for severe metformin-independent lactic acidosis.

Results: Fifty-six patients met the above-mentioned criteria. The mean arterial pH and lactate values were 6.75 ± 0.17 and 23.07 ± 6.94 mmol/L, respectively. The survival rate was 53%, even with pH values as low as 6.5 and lactate and metformin concentrations as high as 35.3 mmol/L and 160 mg/L (normal < 1 mg/L), respectively. Survivors and non-survivors did not differ significantly in terms of the mean arterial pH and lactate concentration. The mean metformin concentration was higher in patients who subsequently died but this difference was due to a very high value (188 mg/L) in one patient in this group, in whom several triggering factors were combined. Sepsis, multidrug overdoses and the presence of at least two triggering factors for lactic acidosis were observed significantly more frequently in non-survivors ($p = 0.007$, 0.04, and 0.005, respectively). This contrasts with a study of metformin-independent lactic acidosis in which there were no survivors, despite less severe acidosis on average (mean pH: 6.86).

Conclusions: In 56 cases of severe metformin-associated lactic acidosis, blood pH and lactate did not have prognostic value. One can reasonably rule out the extent of metformin accumulation as a prognostic factor. Ultimately, the determinants of metformin-associated lactic acidosis appear to be the nature and number of triggering factors. Strikingly, most patients survived - despite a mean pH that is incompatible with a favorable outcome under other circumstances.

Keywords: Type 2 diabetes, Lactate, Lactic acidosis, Metformin, Prognosis

Background

We have previously shown that neither blood lactate concentration nor plasma metformin concentration was of prognostic value with respect to mortality in so-called metformin-associated lactic acidosis (MALA) [1,2]. However, given that arterial pH and blood lactate concentration may vary (from ≤ 7.34 to 6.4 and from > 5 mmol/L to 35.5 mmol/L, respectively, in our experience [2]), a focus on severe MALA is needed in order to try to better understand the paradox whereby metformin provides impressive, beneficial effects but is also associated with life-threatening adverse effects.

Methods

Merck Serono provided us with access to its pharmacovigilance database on metformin. We systematically searched for and studied cases recorded as "metformin-

---

* Correspondence: lalau.jean-daniel@chu-amiens.fr
[1]Service d'Endocrinologie-Nutrition, Hôpital Sud, Amiens cedex 1 F-80054, France
[2]Université de Picardie Jules Verne, Amiens, France

associated lactic acidosis" between January 1995 and August 2010.

The database is a compilation of all cases worldwide brought to Merck Serono's attention during the study period. Most entries are indirect, i.e. cases for which information is transmitted to Merck Serono by local or national health authorities. Other cases are documented through spontaneous declarations (from physicians, pharmacists, patients, etc.) or via the medical literature.

On the basis of these cases, the criteria for study selection were the presence of severe lactic acidosis at admission (defined as an arterial pH < 7.0 and a blood lactate concentration >10 mmol/L) and the availability of data on the plasma metformin concentration (regardless of the assay used) and survival (defined as discharge from the intensive care unit).

Comparisons between survivors and non-survivors were made using Student's unpaired t-test for quantitative, demographic variables and a chi-2 test for qualitative variables. Test results with p-values ≤0.05 were considered to be statistically significant.

Outcomes were compared with those in Friesecke et al. recent study [3], in which cases of severe MALA were compared with cases of similarly severe metformin-independent lactic acidosis.

The present study was approved by the local investigational review board (Commission d'Evaluation Ethique des Recherches Non Interventionnelles, avis n° 101, Espace Ethique Hospitalier Amiens Picardie, Amiens, France).

Results

Fifty-six patients (17 males and 39 females) met the selection criteria (out of a series of 869 case reports of MALA from 32 countries. Most cases (74.7%) came from Europe.

The population's main characteristics are summarized in Table 1. The mean ± SD (range) age was 62.9 ± 12.1 (39–83) and the mean serum creatinine level was 587 ± 279 μmol/L (57–1000). The mean arterial pH was 6.75 ± 0.17 (6.28-6.99), the mean lactate concentration was 23.07 ± 6.94 mmol/L (10.9-55.7) and the mean plasma metformin concentration was 50.64 ± 42.19 mg/L

(0.8-188 mg/L). The latter value may well be the highest ever reported.

Only 2 patients (3.5%) had a plasma metformin concentration within the therapeutic range (based on the upper limit of 2.5 mg/L recently proposed [4]). The majority of patients (73%) displayed marked metformin accumulation, with a value over 25 mg/L.

The overall survival rate in these patients was 53.6% (30 out of 56). This rate did not depend on the date during the study period (data not shown). In other words, the outcome was not more favorable because of more recent observations in survivors. Some patients survived even with pH values as low as 6.5 and lactate and metformin concentrations as high as 35.3 mmol/L and 160 mg/L (N < 1 mg/L), respectively.

Survivors and non-survivors did not differ significantly in terms of the mean arterial pH and lactate concentration. Individual patient data for these two parameters are shown in Figure 1. The mean metformin concentration was higher in non-survivors.

The main presumed triggering factors for lactic acidosis are presented in Table 2 and are grouped into four categories: kidney failure, other organ failures, overdose and other conditions. Sepsis and multi-drug intoxication rates were significantly higher in non-survivors than in survivors (p = 0.007 and 0.04, respectively).

We also analyzed the number of presumed triggering factors per patient as a function of the outcome (Table 3). The presence of only one factor was more frequent in survivors (p = 0.01) than in non-survivors; conversely, the presence of two or more combined factors appeared to be significantly more frequent in non-survivors than survivors (p = 0.005).

A comparison of our study results with those of Friesecke et al. [4] shows the same proportion of MALA survivors (around 50%) and the same mean pH (pH 6.75 in both studies). In contrast, Friesecke et al. did not report on any survivors in metformin-independent lactic acidosis, despite the presence of less severe acidosis (mean pH: 6.86).

Discussion

To the best of our knowledge, this is the largest series of metformin-treated patients with severe lactic acidosis yet

Table 1 Characteristics of the study population (mean ± SD) [range]

	All patients (n = 56)	Survivors (n = 30)	Non-survivors (n = 26)	p-value for the survivor/non-survivor comparison
Age	62.9 ± 12.1 [39–83]	61.7 ± 11.1 [40–81]	64.2 ± 13.1 [39–83]	0.44
Creatinine, μmol/L	587 ± 270 [57–1000]	672 ± 265 [133–1000]	508 ± 310 [57–929]	0.09
pH	6.75 ± 0.17 [6.28-6.99]	6.73 ± 0.17 [6.30-6.98]	6.79 ± 0.17 [6.28-6.99]	0.16
Lactate, mmol/L	23.07 ± 6.94 [10.9-55.7]	22.24 ± 4.72 [14–35.3]	24.0 ± 8.9 [10.9-55.7]	0.26
Plasma metformin level, mg/L	48.3 ± 39.6 [0.8-188]	39.66 ± 34.22 [0.8-160]	63.3 ± 47.4 [1.01-188]	0.04

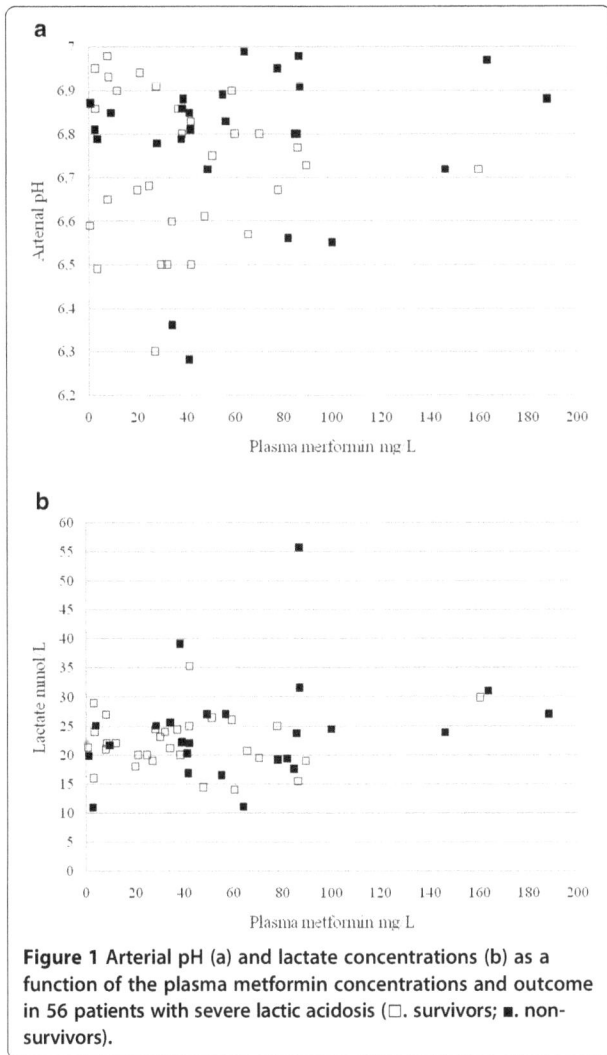

Figure 1 Arterial pH (a) and lactate concentrations (b) as a function of the plasma metformin concentrations and outcome in 56 patients with severe lactic acidosis (□. survivors; ■. non-survivors).

reported. The first striking feature is that the majority of patients (53%) survived, despite a mean arterial pH of 6.73 and a mean lactate concentration of over 20 mmol/L (22.24 mmol/L). In comparison, the mean arterial pH in our previous series of unselected MALA patients was much higher, at 7.04 (arterial lactate concentration: 15.1 mmol/L) [2].

Even though most of the patients survived (independently of age), it is important to know whether survival was related to the severity of lactic acidosis, the extent of metformin accumulation and/or the nature and number of triggering factors. A link with lactic acidosis *per se* can be ruled out, since mean pH and lactate values were similar in survivors and non-survivors. Even though the mean metformin concentration was higher in non-survivors, metformin responsibility can also be ruled out with a good degree of confidence because this concentration difference was due to a very high value (188 mg/L, N < 1 mg/L) in only one non-survivor having combined triggering factors.

Indeed, outcomes appeared to be strongly correlated with (i) the nature of the triggering factors, since some conditions were significantly more frequent in non-survivors (i.e. sepsis and multidrug intoxication, with p values of 0.007 and 0.04, respectively) and (ii) the number of triggering factors, since the presence of just one factor was more frequent in survivors and two or more factors were more frequently observed in non-survivors.

The fact that metformin concentrations may widely vary in MALA complicates analysis of outcomes. Indeed, metformin-treated patients do not necessarily develop lactic acidosis - even in the presence of marked metformin accumulation [5]. It is nevertheless possible to distinguish patients according to their metformin level: (i) undetectable or low, (ii) normal, (iii) slight to moderate elevation or (iv) marked elevation [6]. In our previous report, we noted that 6 of the 49 patients (12.2%) had a plasma metformin concentration at or below the upper limit of the therapeutic range [2]. The homogeneous distribution of metformin concentrations in the present series enabled us to better test for an association between metformin accumulation and outcome. Indeed, only 3.5% of the patients had a low value, whereas the great majority (almost 80%) had marked accumulation, >10 mg/L.

Lastly, we are keen to reconcile the impressively beneficial metabolic and vascular effects of metformin on one hand with the drug's widely assumed, potentially lethal toxicity in MALA on the other – as summed up by a sentence like "metformin-associated lactic acidosis is rare but is still associated with a high mortality rate".

Indeed, our report on a rather large series of patients with severe MALA and a death rate of almost 50% highlights how severe the complication really is. However, the problem is much more complex than that, since MALA is not a clearly defined clinical entity [7]. One way to circumvent this difficulty is thus to compare the outcome in MALA with that in metformin-independent lactic acidosis. The data from Friesecke et al. recent study (in which MALA was compared with similarly severe lactic acidosis due to other causes) showed the same proportion of survivors (around 50%) and the same mean pH (6.75) for MALA as in our (much larger) series but, strikingly, did not feature any survivors in metformin-independent lactic acidosis (despite less severe acidosis (mean pH: 6.86)) [4]. There are two possible explanations for this striking difference in survival when comparing MALA and metformin-independent lactic acidosis: (i) the presence of less severe, acidosis-triggering co-morbidities in MALA patients (because metformin accumulation is responsible for a proportion of cases of observed acidosis) and/or (ii) a protective effect of metformin (due to its vascular properties [8] and its action on the respiratory-chain complex [9]).

Table 2 Prognosis according to the presumed main triggering medical conditions (one condition per patient or more)

Associated condition	Total n	Survivors n (%)	Non-survivors n (%)	p-value for survivor/ non-survivor comparison
Kidney failure				
Total	34	19 (55.9)	15 (44.1)	0.87
Acute failure	21	11	10	0.89
Chronic failure	7	5	2	0.43
Duration unspecified	6	3	3	1.00
Other organ failures				
Total	10	6	4	0.74
Liver	4	2	2	1.00
Cardiovascular system	3	3	0	0.24
Lung	3	1	2	0.59
Overdose				
Total	8	3	5	0.45
Metformin (alone)	4	3	1	0.61
Multidrug (including metformin)	4	0	4	0.04
Other conditions				
Total	13	3	10	0.02
Sepsis	6	0	6	0.007
Alcohol abuse	3	2	1	1.00
Cancer	1	0	1	0.46
Pancreatitis	1	1	0	1.00
Neurological disorder	1	0	1	0.46
Acute denutrition	1	0	1	0.46
Indetermined	3	2	1	1.00

Whatever the underlying reason, the present report's most remarkable finding is the unexpectedly high proportion of MALA survivors - despite an arterial pH as low as 6.5 (in 5 patients) and a lactate concentration as high as 35.3 mmol/L. However, this observation is coherent with the growing body of preclinical and clinical evidence demonstrating unexpectedly rapid recovery and survival in massive metformin accumulation and/or very severe MALA [8-13].

Conclusions

In comparison with common forms of lactic acidosis, severe MALA is particular in that the majority of patients survive – despite a mean pH that is usually thought to be fatal. For this type of MALA patients, the outcome was related to the nature and number of triggering factors, rather than the severity of lactic acidosis or the extent of metformin accumulation.

Key messages

- Analysis of the outcomes in severe metformin-associated lactic acidosis may help to resolve the following paradox: metformin provides beneficial effects but is also associated with life-threatening adverse effects.
- In 56 cases of severe metformin-associated lactic acidosis (pH < 7.0 and a lactate concentration >10 mmol/L), blood pH and lactate did not have prognostic value.
- The extent of metformin accumulation cannot not be considered as a prognostic factor.

Table 3 Prognosis according to the number of presumed triggering medical conditions

Number of medical conditions	Total n	Survivors n (%)	Non-survivors n (%)	p-value for the survivor/non-survivor comparison
No identified conditions or scarce information	3	2	1	1.00
1	38	25 (65.8)	13 (34.2)	0.01
2 or more	15	3 (20)	12 (80)	0.005

- The determinants of metformin-associated lactic acidosis appeared to be the nature and number of triggering factors.
- Most patients survived despite a mean pH that is incompatible with favorable outcomes under other circumstances. Such an unexpectedly favorable outcome prompted to form a challenging hypothesis whereby metformin may be protective in severe lactic acidosis that occurs for other reasons in patients taking this drug.

Abbreviation

MALA: Metformin-associated lactic acidosis.

Competing interests

The authors declare that they have no competing interests.

Authors' contributions

FK and JDL both contributed to conception, design, acquisition of data or analysis and interpretation of data; J.D.L. was involved in drafting and revising the manuscript. Both authors read and approved the final manuscript.

References

1. Lalau JD, Lacroix C, Compagnon P, *et al*: Role of metformin accumulation in metformin-associated lactic acidosis. *Diabetes Care* 1995, **18**:779–784.
2. Lalau JD, Race J: Lactic acidosis in metformin-treated patients. Prognostic value of arterial lactate levels and plasma metformin concentrations. *Drug Saf* 1999, **20**:377–384.
3. Friesecke S, Abel P, Roser M, *et al*: Outcome of severe lactic acidosis associated with metformin accumulation. *Crit Care* 2010, **14**:R226.
4. Graham GG, Punt J, Arora M, *et al*: Clinical pharmacokinetics of metformin. *Clin Pharmacokinet* 2011, **50**:81–98.
5. Lalau JD, Lemaire-Hurtel A, Lacroix C: Establishment of a database of metformin plasma concentrations and erythrocyte levels in normal and emergency situations. *Clin Drug Investig* 2011, **31**:425–438.
6. Lalau J, Race J: Metformin and lactic acidosis in diabetic humans. *Diabetes Obes Metab* 2000, **2**:131–137.
7. Lalau JD: Lactic acidosis induced by metformin. *Drug Saf* 2010, **33**:727–740.
8. Bouskela E, Wiensperger N: Effects of metformin on hemorrhagic shock, concentration volume and ischemia/reperfusion on nondiabetic hamsters. *J Vasc Med Biol* 1993, **4**:41–46.
9. Batandier C, Guigas B, Detaille D, *et al*: The ROS production induced by a reverse-electron flux at respiratory complex 1 is hampered by metformin. *J Bioenerg Biomembr* 2006, **38**:33–42.
10. Gjedde S, Christiansen A, Pedersen S, *et al*: Survival following a metformin overdose of 63 g: a case report. *Pharmacol Toxicol* 2003, **93**:98–99.
11. Lalau JD, Masmoudi K: Unexpected recovery from prolonged hypoglycaemic coma: a protective role of metformin? *Intensive Care Med* 2005, **3**:493.
12. Nyirenda MJ, Sandeep T, Grant I, *et al*: Severe acidosis in patients taking metformin - rapid reversal and survival despite high APACHE score. *Diabet Med* 2006, **23**:432–435.
13. Seidowsky A, Nseir S, Houdret N, *et al*: Metformin-associated lactic acidosis: a prognosis and therapeutic study. *Crit Care Med* 2009, **37**:2191–2196.

10

A cost effectiveness analysis of the preferred antidotes for acute paracetamol poisoning patients in Sri Lanka

S M D K Ganga Senarathna[1,2,3*], Shalini Sri Ranganathan[1], Nick Buckley[2,4] and Rohini Fernandopulle[1]

Abstract

Background: Acute paracetamol poisoning is a rapidly increasing problem in Sri Lanka. The antidotes are expensive and yet no health economic evaluation has been done on the therapy for acute paracetamol poisoning in the developing world. The aim of this study is to determine the cost effectiveness of using N-acetylcysteine over methionine in the management of acute paracetamol poisoning in Sri Lanka.

Methods: Economic analysis was applied using public healthcare system payer perspective.
Costs were obtained from a series of patients admitted to the National Hospital of Sri Lanka with a history of acute paracetamol overdose. Evidence on effectiveness was obtained from a systematic review of the literature. Death due to hepatotoxicity was used as the primary outcome of interest. Analysis and development of decision tree models was done using Tree Age Pro 2008.

Results: An affordable treatment threshold of Sri Lankan rupees 1,537,120/death prevented was set from the expected years of productive life gained and the average contribution to GDP. A cost-minimisation analysis was appropriate for patients presenting within 10 hours and methionine was the least costly antidote. For patients presenting 10-24 hours after poisoning, n-acetylcysteine was more effective and the incremental cost effectiveness ratio of Sri Lankan rupees 316,182/life saved was well under the threshold. One-way and multi-way sensitivity analysis also supported methionine for patients treated within 10 hours and n-acetylcysteine for patients treated within 10-24 hours as preferred antidotes.

Conclusions: Post ingestion time is an important determinant of preferred antidotal therapy for acute paracetamol poisoning patients in Sri Lanka. Using n-acetylcysteine in all patients is not cost effective. On economic grounds, methionine should become the preferred antidote for Sri Lankan patients treated within 10 hours of the acute ingestion and n-acetylcysteine should continue to be given to patients treated within 10-24 hours.

Background

Paracetamol is the most common cause of drug poisoning in the world [1] and the single most commonly taken drug in overdoses that lead to hospital presentation and admission [2].

Poisoning with paracetamol is an emerging problem in Sri Lanka with rapidly increasing admissions to the National Hospital of Sri Lanka (NHSL): from only 35 cases in 2003 to 515 cases in 2005 [3]. Paracetamol poisoning is one of the most expensive poisonings

management in Sri Lanka [4,5]. The average cost of managing a patient with acute paracetamol poisoning was even higher than the average cost of managing a organophosphate poisoning patient; the most costly poisoning management at the Anuradhapura General Hospital in Sri Lanka [4,5]. However it is important to note that eighty percent of the current total cost of management of acute paracetamol poisoning is due to cost of antidotes unlike in organophosphate poisoning [5].

Even though paracetamol poisoning has been researched far more than other pharmaceutical poisonings, there is limited literature on the pharmaco-economics of treatment. So far no full economic evaluation on interventions on paracetamol poisoning has been

* Correspondence: ganga136@yahoo.com
[1]Department of Pharmacology, Faculty of Medicine, University of Colombo, Colombo, Sri Lanka
Full list of author information is available at the end of the article

carried out [6]. Two antidotes, N-acetylcysteine (NAC) and methionine, are available in Sri Lanka. NAC is the most expensive and also the most commonly used antidote. The evidence on effectiveness of antidotes used in acute paracetamol poisoning is weak [7]. However, on the basis of the current best available evidence NAC is considered to be more effective than methionine in the management of patients with acute paracetamol poisoning [7]. Considering that NAC is also more costly than providing methionine, it should be useful to determine the comparative cost effectiveness of the two treatments, and whether the additional benefit of NAC over methionine is worth the extra cost. Cost effectiveness analysis is based on the premise that it is the wider community interest which is paramount; therefore extra lives saved from use of a more expensive antidote have to be balanced against the extra costs involved in doing so. It is easy to make the management decision; if an intervention is dominant (i.e. the new intervention is less costly and yields higher benefit). But in situations where an intervention is not dominant, we have to find out the point at which the intervention is cost effective. The question of an intervention is cost-effective depends upon whether the relevant decision maker is willing and able to pay the additional costs to achieve the additional benefits that can be achieved by introducing the alternative program. The magnitude of this value will be controversial. In this analysis it was considered that the program is cost effective if it can gain a year of healthy life for less than a country's national income per person per capita gross national income [8].

The objective of the present cost effectiveness analysis is to determine the incremental cost effectiveness of NAC over methionine in the management of acute paracetamol poisoning patients (with suicidal intent) in Sri Lanka.

Methods
Structure of the decision tree model
The evidence on effectiveness of both antidotes; NAC and methionine depends on the post ingestion time. According to the best available evidence, all antidotes are much more effective if given within 10 hours of the acute ingestion [7].

Therefore we constructed two decision tree models: for patients treated within 10 hours, and for patients treated within10 to 24 hours after acute ingestion of paracetamol (Figure 1). Both models compared use of methionine and NAC in patients where the risk was assessed using plasma paracetamol levels according to the Rumack-Matthew nomogram.

Acute paracetamol poisoning can result in fulminant hepatic failure which can lead to death. The most frequently applied definition for significant paracetamol

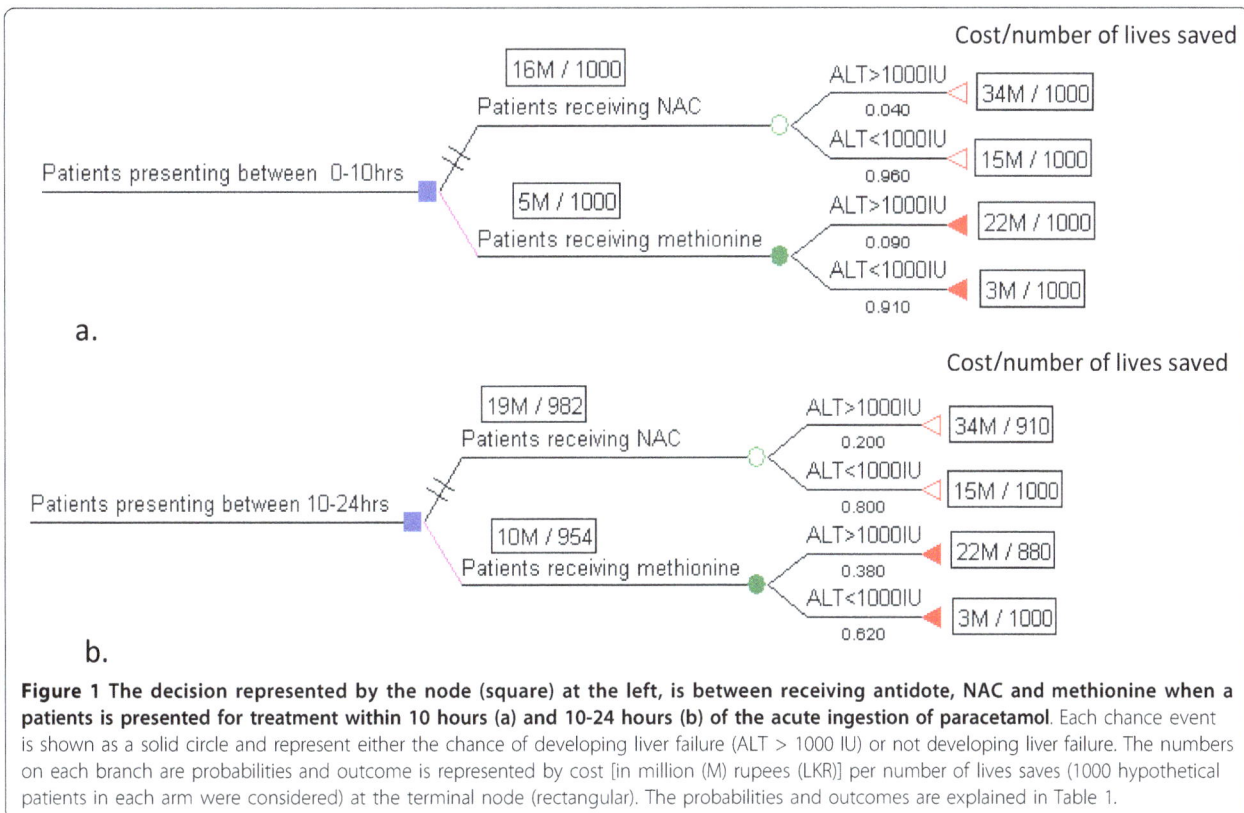

Figure 1 The decision represented by the node (square) at the left, is between receiving antidote, NAC and methionine when a patients is presented for treatment within 10 hours (a) and 10-24 hours (b) of the acute ingestion of paracetamol. Each chance event is shown as a solid circle and represent either the chance of developing liver failure (ALT > 1000 IU) or not developing liver failure. The numbers on each branch are probabilities and outcome is represented by cost [in million (M) rupees (LKR)] per number of lives saves (1000 hypothetical patients in each arm were considered) at the terminal node (rectangular). The probabilities and outcomes are explained in Table 1.

hepatotoxicity is having liver transaminases (ALT or AST) > 1000 U/L at any time [9,10].

Therefore the decision tree model adopted death following hepatotoxicity (ALT or AST > 1000 U/L) as the final outcome measure (Figure 1).

Population considered

The analysis was applied to patients admitted to the National Hospital of Sri Lanka (NHSL). The ethics approval was obtained from ethical review boards of the NHSL and the Faculty of Medicine, Colombo. In Sri Lanka healthcare is free at the point of delivery. Therefore the analysis was done from the public healthcare system payers' perspective. The time horizon was 2006 and the analysis was performed with reference to 1000 hypothetical patients in each arm.

Data and assumptions on costs and effectiveness of antidotes

Costs

The direct costs linked to the treatment options were measured as the total cost of drug treatment and hospitalisation. The total cost of drug treatment includes the cost of NAC/methionine (obtained from the medical supplies division of Sri Lanka), cost of hospital stay (obtained from accounts branch of the NHSL and follow up of case series) and cost of person hours (obtained from accounts branch of the NHSL and follow up of case series). The cost of antidotal therapy was based on the usual NAC (IV NAC 300 mg/kg over 20.25 hours) and methionine regimen(2.5 g every four hours for four doses) used in Sri Lanka. The costs in LKR (Sri Lankan rupees) (100 LKR = 1 US dollar) of items included in the analysis are given in Additional file 1: annexure1.

Effectiveness data

Antidotal effectiveness data was obtained from the systematic review and meta-analysis on the interventions for paracetamol poisoning by Brok et al. 2002 and 2006 [6,7]. The meta analysis included randomised controlled trials (RCTs), quasi-RCTs, RCTs with volunteers and observational studies. According to the review, no RCTs were of high quality. Further, no RCT compared NAC with methionine or no treatment for the relevant time frame (within24 hours of the acute ingestion) for this analysis. The review provided an exploratory analysis on antidotes and gave pooled probabilities for developing hepatotoxicity and death following acute paracetamol poisoning in patients with plasma paracetamol levels above possible or probable risk line of the nomogram [10,11]. Summary of the studies included in the exploratory analysis are given in Additional file 2: annexure 2 [9-21].

Incremental cost effectiveness

The total costs and outcomes for each treatment arm were presented. The expected value of each

management alternatives identified at the root. The incremental cost effectiveness ratio (ICER) for two alternative treatments was calculated (incremental analysis produces a summary measure of relative efficiency) by dividing the cost difference by the outcome difference.

$$ICER = (Cost\ of\ NAC - cost\ of\ methionine) / (Outcome\ for\ NAC - outcome\ for\ methionine)$$

When there was no difference in outcome between management alternatives, cost minimisation analysis was done and the least costly management alternative was chosen.

Development of decision tree models and the analysis were done using Tree Age Pro Excel healthcare 2008 software, Serial number GXT2J-2B6KK-3D3DV-G.

Discounting and sensitivity analysis

Acute paracetamol poisoning is an acute condition and costs and outcomes occur during a short span of time: two to ten days. Therefore costs or outcomes were not discounted to adjust for elapsed time between expenditure and outcome when ICERs are calculated. When treatment threshold value was calculated, future income of the study patients were considered and therefore it was discounted at the rate of 3.5% to bring it to the present value [22],

One-way-sensitivity analysis was done by increasing and decreasing costs and mortality by 50% and also by taking the upper and lower confidence interval of the probability on the systematic review estimates of mortality and hepatotoxicity with each antidote. Multi- ways sensitivity analysis was done to examine the worst combination of the single factors for both NAC and methionine in both time periods.

Results
Medical care cost

When a 60 kg patient is treated with NAC and does not develop hepatotoxicity, the cost to the healthcare system was 15,038 rupees. However if the patient develops hepatotoxicity, the cost rises to 34,329 rupees due to infusion of additional NAC and supportive care. The total cost for the methionine option was 2,839 rupees when patients do not develop hepatotoxicity and 22,481 when the patient develops hepatotoxicity. The breakdown on direct medical care costs are given in Additional file 1: annexure 1.

Outcome data

The exploratory analysis of the systematic review pooled studies together and gave pooled probabilities as shown in Table 1[7]. The probability for death following the use of both antidotes was zero for patients treated within 10 hours of the acute ingestion. However, the 95% CI of the case-fatality had an upper CI of 0.5% for NAC and 2.4% for methionine.

Table 1 Probability for hepatotoxicity and death, when antidotes are administered within 0-10 and 10-24 hours from the acute ingestion

	Probability for AST/ALT > 1000 IU/l (n/N) [6,7]	Probability for death (n/N)	Note
IV NAC 300 mg/kg over 20.25 hours			
Within 10 hours	4% (13/315)	0[†](0/13)	*
	(95% CI 2.5 to 7.0)	(95% CI 0 to 24)	
Within 10-24 hours	20% (67/322)	9%[‡] (6/67)	*
	(95% CI 17 to 26)	(95% CI 3.8 to 18)	
Methionine 1 g 4 hourly 4 doses			
Within 10 hours	9% (13/143)	0[†]	#
	(95% CI 4.5 to 15)	(95% CI 0 to 24)	
Within 10-24 hours	38%(17/41)	12%[II](2/17)	#
	(95% CI 26.3 to 57.9)	(95% CI 2 to 36)	

* Probabilities were derived by pooling results of Prescott et al. 1979, Smilkstein et al. 1988, Burkhart et al. 1995, Buckley et al. 1999, Parker et al. 1990, Smilkstein et al. 1991, Woo et al. 2000, Ayonrinde et al. 2005 and Kerr et al. 2005 [9-17]. # Probabilities were derived by pooling results of Prescott et al. 1979, Crome et al. 1976, Hamlyn et al. 1981, Prescott et al. 1976 and Vale et al. 1981 [9,18-21]. † No patient treated (NAC/methionine) within 10 hours died due to hepatototoxicity, therefore the probability of death due to hepatototoxicity was zero

Threshold value

The mean per capita income for a Sri Lankan in 2006 was LKR 6,463/month [23]. The average age for the case series of patients was 20 years and the average number of working years for a Sri Lankan is 55 years which is the retirement age. When patients poisoned with paracetamol dies at the age of 20, the society will lose average earning at the rate of percapita income per month up to the retirement age. Therefore the discounted present value of a life saved at the age of 20 would be LKR 1,537,120

(Discounted present value = $\sum^{35-1} 77556_n (1-0.035)^n$) and this value was used as the treatment threshold value to prevent a death due to acute paracetamol poisoning in Sri Lanka. Therefore the study considered that it is cost effective to prevent an additional death by NAC at a cost of ≤ LKR 1,537,120.

Baseline results

The decision tree models with expected outcomes for patients presenting within 10 and 10-24 hours is given in Figure 1.

The incremental cost effectiveness ratios reveal how much it would cost to prevent an extra death by shifting to the more costly antidote (NAC) from the cheaper alternative antidote (methionine). When treated within 10 hours of the acute ingestion, the incremental cost for treatment with NAC over methionine came to LKR 11,588,680, but outcome resulted from alternative interventions were similar. Therefore base line ICER was not calculated for this group and cost minimisation analysis was done (Table 2).

Cost effectiveness analysis was done for patients treated within 10 to 24 hours, the ICER for this group of patients

was LKR 316,182 per life saved (below the threshold value) where the incremental cost was LKR 8,726,620 and additional lives saved by NAC was 28 (Table 2).

Sensitivity analysis
One way sensitivity analysis
Incremental cost effectiveness ratios for one way sensitivity analysis, taking mortality as outcome measure are given in Table 2.
Multi-way-sensitivity analysis
According to the base-case analysis, methionine was the lease costly antidote for patients treated within 10 hours and NAC had an ICER below the threshold value for patients treated within 10 to 24 hours after ingestion. The robustness of this decision was further tested by assessing the worse case for methionine when given within 10 hours and the worse case for NAC when given 10-24 hours in a multi-way sensitivity analysis.

Worse case analysis for methionine within 10 hours gave an ICER of LKR 2,718,784 for NAC. Worse case analysis for NAC given within 10-24 hours showed dominance for methionine where methionine saved 42 more lives at a lower cost.

Discussion

The most important factor influencing total cost in the management of acute paracetamol poisoning in Sri Lanka is the antidotal therapy. This cost pattern would also be observed in other developing country settings where hospital stay and human resources are cheaper. Economic modeling should inform the most cost effective way of using these two antidotes which can reduce the total cost of management in developing country settings.

Table 2 Incremental cost per life saved for baseline data and following one way sensitivity analysis (Number of lives saved as the final outcome measure)

| | Incremental cost per life saved(LKR/Life saved) | |
	0-10 hrs	10-24 hrs
Baseline results	Not applicable[‡]	316,182
One way sensitivity analysis results		
Increasing by 50%		
NAC deaths	Not applicable[‡]	469,173
NAC cost	Not applicable[‡]	565,805
Methionine deaths	Not applicable[‡]	173,147
Methionine cost	Not applicable[‡]	265,107
Decreasing by 50%		
NAC deaths	Not applicable[‡]	238,432
NAC cost	Not applicable[‡]	55,312
Methionine deaths	Not applicable[‡]	1,818,046
Methionine cost	Not applicable[‡]	366,486
Upper confidence interval(CI)		
NAC deaths	Dominance for methionine [†]	909,023
NAC hepatotoxicity	Not applicable[‡]	445,229
Methionine deaths	5,365,130	73,456
Methionine hepatotoxicity	Not applicable[‡]	94,349
Lower confidence interval(CI)		
NAC deaths	Not applicable[‡]	229,648
NAC hepatotoxicity	Not applicable[‡]	268,907
Methionine deaths	Not applicable[‡]	Dominance for methionine [†]
Methionine hepatotoxicity	Not applicable	836,480

[‡] The outcome resulted from alternative interventions were similar therefore cost effectiveness ratios were not calculated.

[†] Methionine shows strong dominance for a decision as the incremental effectiveness was lower while the incremental cost is higher for NAC (methionine saves more lives at a lower cost)

The most suitable economic analysis for patients treated within 10 hours of the acute ingestion is the cost minimization analysis, as the evidence suggests the probability of death is zero for patients treated with either antidote. With this premise, methionine is clearly the least costly alternative for this group of patients. One-way sensitivity analysis and multi-way sensitivity analysis calculated ICERs (on instances where there is an outcome difference) were above our pre-defined threshold for an acceptable cost per life saved by NAC. Therefore, methionine is the antidote of choice for patients treated within 10 hours.

The ICER for NAC for patients presenting within 10-24 hours was LKR 316,182 for a death prevented. This is a value much lower than the treatment threshold value and suggests the use of NAC in preference to methionine is very cost-effective. One way sensitivity analysis in all instances had ICERs lower than the threshold value except when the lower confidence interval for death following methionine was considered where it showed dominance for methionine.

Worse case analysis for NAC also indicated dominance for methionine. Therefore the conclusion ranged from dominance for methionine to NAC being cost effective. However in most of the sensitivity analysis and in the base case analysis the ICER for NAC was much lower than the threshold value. Therefore use of NAC for patients presenting within 10-24 hours of the acute ingestion appears to be a cost effective option in Sri Lanka.

The effectiveness data for the decision tree was based on the systematic review and meta analysis by Brok et al. 2006. The meta-analysis referred to 10 studies to produce estimates of effectiveness in respect to these two antidotes; five studies for NAC, four studies for methionine and one study on both antidotes. According to the levels of evidence and grade of recommendation proposed by Cook et al. 1992 [24], studies used for methionine were in grade B(1), grade C(1) and grade D (2), studies used for effectiveness of NAC were in grade B(1), Grade D(2)and grade E(2) and the study on both NAC and methionine was grade D quality.

The meta-analysis did not use any studies which provided grade A recommendations and eight out of 10 studies were in grade D or worse. An RCT directly comparing these two antidotes would provide much better effectiveness data. Such a trial might be worthwhile and should be strongly supported. The trial could not easily be blinded due to the different routes of administration. However, the outcome measures are largely objective and there is a low likelihood of bias.

Conclusions

Post ingestion time is an important determinant of preferred antidotal therapy for acute paracetamol poisoning patients in Sri Lanka. Using N-acetylcysteine in all patients is not cost effective.

If policy makers are wishing to utilise economic evaluations to improve decision making, the findings from this study suggest that, within the first 10 hours, the use of methionine may be more cost-effective than NAC for paracetamol poisoning in Sri Lanka. This would potentially more than halve the total expenditure on this increasingly common poisoning. N-acetylcysteine should continue to be given to patients treated within 10-24 hours.

Limitations

The study recommends the use of methionine for patients treated within 10 hours of the acute ingestion. There is some literature suggestive of methionine induce adverse effects such as nausea and vomiting. However our prospective case series didn't identify such incidences even though 55 patients received methionine compared 68 of IV NAC. Two patients received both antidotes owing to unavailability of IV NAC at the time of patient admission [3].

Additional material

Additional file 1: Annexure 1. Cost per patient (body weight: 60 kg) for different treatment alternatives.
Additional file 2: Annexure 2. Summary of the studies included in the exploratory analysis of the systematic review [9-21].

Abbreviations
GDP: Gross domestic product; NHSL: National Hospital of Sri Lanka; NAC: N-acetylcysteine; ALT: Serum alanine aminotransferase; AST: Serum aspartate aminotransferase; LKR: Sri Lankan rupees; RCTs: Randomised controlled trials; ICER: Incremental cost effectiveness ratio.

Acknowledgements
The authors are grateful to director and the consultant physicians of the NHSL for providing facility to carry out the study in the hospital. We are also thankful to medical, nursing and other staff of medical wards and staff of record room, accounts, salaries, and transport divisions of NHSL for providing assistance to do the data collection. We are also thankful to Professor Andrew Dawson and South Asian Clinical Toxicology Research Collaboration for funding.

Author details
[1]Department of Pharmacology, Faculty of Medicine, University of Colombo, Colombo, Sri Lanka. [2]South Asian Clinical Toxicology Research Collaboration, Kandy, Sri Lanka. [3]Pharmacy Program, Department of Medical Education and Health Sciences, Faculty of Medical Sciences, University of Sri Jayewardenepura, Nugegoda , Sri Lanka. [4]Faculty of Medicine, University of New South Wales, Sydney, Australia.

Authors' contributions
SMDKGS participated in the design and planning of the study, drafted the study proposal, collected patient information, conducted the economic evaluation and interpreted results, wrote the first draft and took part in revising the paper and finalizing the paper. SSR participated in the design and planning of the study, edited and revised the study proposal, edited the paper and took part in revising the paper and approved the final version. NB participated in the design and planning of the study, edited and revised the study proposal, edited the paper and took part in revising the paper and approved the final version. RF participated in the design and planning of the study, edited and revised the study proposal, edited the paper and took part in revising the paper and approved the final version. All authors read and approved the final manuscript.
Study design
Cost effectiveness analysis based on exploratory analysis of a systematic review

Competing interests
The authors declare that they have no competing interests.

References
1. Sanaei-Zadeh H, Tagghaddosinejad F, Jalali N, Kariman H: **Adverse effects of intravenous N-acetylcysteine.** *Clin Drug Investig* 2003, **23(2)**:129-133.
2. Buckley N, Eddleston M: **Paracetamol (acetaminophen) poisoning.** *Clin Evid* 2005, **14**:1738-1744.
3. Senarathna SMDKG, Sri Ranganathan S, Dawson AH, Buckley N, Fernandopulle BMR: **Management of acute paracetamol poisoning patients in a tertiary care hospital.** *Ceylon Med J* 2008, **53(3)**:89-92.
4. Wickramasinghe K, Steele P, Dawson A, Dharmaratne D, Gunawardena A, Senarathna L, *et al*: **Cost to government health-care services of treating acute self-poisonings in a rural district in Sri Lanka.** *Bull World Health Organ* 2009, **87**:180-185.
5. Senarathna SMDKG, Sri Ranganathan S, Fernandopulle BMR: **Cost-outcome description of management of patients with acute paracetamol poisoning [Abstract].** *Ceylon Med J* 2008, **53(Suppl 1)**:53.
6. Brok J, Buckley N, Gluud C: **Interventions for paracetamol (acetaminophen) overdoses.** *Cochrane Database Syst Rev* 2002, **3,**
7. Brok J, Buckley N, Gluud C: **Interventions for paracetamol (acetaminophen) overdoses (Review).** *Cochrane Database Systemic Review* 2006, **2,**
8. Investing in Health: *World Development Report* Oxford: Oxford. University Press; 1993, 213-25, Ref Type: Report.
9. Prescott LF, Illingworth RN, Critchely JA, Stewart MJA, Proud foot AT: **Intravenous Nacetylcysteine: the treatment of choice for paracetamol poisoning.** *Br Med J* 1979, **2(6198)**:1097-1100.
10. Smilkstein MJ, Knapp GI, Kulig KW, Rumack BH: **Efficacy of oral Nacetylcysteine in the treatment of acetaminophen overdose. Analysis of a national multi centre study (1976-1985).** *N Engl J Med* 1988, **319(24)**:1557-1562.
11. Burkhart KK, Janco N, Kulig KW, Rumack BH: **Cimetidine as adjunctive treatment for acetaminophen overdose.** *Hum Exp Toxicol* 1995, **14(3)**:299-304.
12. Buckley NA, Whyte IM, O'Connell DL, Dawson AH: **Oral or intravenous Nacetylcysteine: which is the treatment of choice for acetaminophen (paracetamol) poisoning.** *J Toxicol Clin Toxicol* 1999, **37(6)**:759-767.
13. Parker D, White P, Paton D, Routledge A: **Safety of late acetylcysteine treatment in paracetamol poisoning.** *Hum Exp Toxicol* 1990, **9**:25-27.
14. Smilkstein MJ, Bronskin AC, Linden C, Augenstein WL, Kulig KW, Rumack BH: **Acetaminophen overdose: A 48-h intravenous N-acetylcysteine treatment protocol.** *Ann Emerg Med* 1991, **20**:1058-1063.
15. Woo OF, Mueller PD, Olson KR, Anderson IB, Kim SY: **Shorter duration of oral N-acetylcysteine therapy for acute acetaminophen overdose.** *Ann Emerg Med* 2000, **35(4)**:363-368.

16. Ayonrinde OT, Phelps GJ, Hurley JC, Ayonrinde OA: **Paracetamol overdose and hepatotoxicity at a regional Australian hospital: a 4 year experience.** *Intern Med J* 2005, **35**:655-660.

17. Kerr F, Dawson A, Whyte IM, Buckley N, Murray L, Graudins A, *et al*: **The Australian clinical toxicology Investigators collaboration, Randomised Trails of Different loading infusion rates of Nacetylcysteine.** *Ann Emerg Med* 2005, **45(4)**:402-408.

18. Crome P, Valem JA, Volans GN, Widdop B, Goulding R: **Oral methionine in the treatment of severe paracetamol (Acetaminophen) overdose.** *Lancet* 1976, **2(7990)**:829-830.

19. Hamlyn AN, Lesna M, Record CO, Smith PA, Path FRC, Watson AJ: **Methionine and cysteamine in paracetamol overdose, prospective controlled trial of early therapy.** *J Int Med Res* 1981, **9**:226-231.

20. Prescott LF, Park J, Sutherland GR, Smith IJ: **Cysteamine, methionine, and penicillamine in the treatment of paracetamol poisoning.** *Lancet* 1976, **2**:109-113.

21. Vale JA, Meredith TJ, Goulding R: **Treatment of acetaminophen poisoning. The use of oral methionine.** *Arch Intern Med* 1981, **141(3)**:394-396.

22. National Institute for Clinical Excellence (NICE): *Guide to the methods of technology appraisal London* London: NICE; 2004.

23. Census and statistics Sri Lanka: **Household income and expenditure survey 2006/07 summary findings. [On line].** *Department of Census and statistics Sri Lanka* 2007, Available at: http://www.statistics.gov.lk/HIES/ HIES2006_07Website/Publications/SummaryFfindingsHIES2006_07.pdf [Accessed on 1st April 2008].

24. Cook DJ, Guyatt GH, Laupacis A, Sackett DL: **Rules of evidence and clinical recommendations on the use of antithrombitic agents.** *Chest* 1992, **102**:305s-311s.

11

Comparison of renal effects of ibuprofen versus indomethacin during treatment of patent ductus arteriosus in contiguous historical cohorts

Alla Kushnir[1,2†] and Joaquim MB Pinheiro[1*†]

Abstract

Background: Ibuprofen treatment of patent ductus arteriosus (PDA) has been shown to be as effective as indomethacin in small randomized controlled trials, with possibly fewer adverse effects. However, adverse renal effects of ibuprofen have been noted in some trials and suspected in our practice.
The purpose of this study was to examine whether ibuprofen and indomethacin treatment of PDA have comparable effects on renal function as evidenced by urine output and serum creatinine.

Methods: Retrospective chart review of 350 patients. Serum creatinine and urine output were recorded prior to start of treatment, during each course and after the last course of treatment. Pre-treatment mean creatinine and urine output values were compared to treatment and post treatment means using 2-factor repeated measures ANOVA.

Results: 165 patients were treated with indomethacin (2005-2006) and 185 received ibuprofen (2007-2008). There was no difference between treatment groups in demographics or baseline renal function. For both groups, the number of treatment courses was inversely correlated with birth weight and gestational age. Analysis of the first course including all patients, revealed significant increase in creatinine and decrease in urine output with both drugs, with a more pronounced effect of indomethacin on creatinine. In the subgroup of 219 patients who received only one treatment course, there was a significant increase in creatinine after indomethacin, but not after ibuprofen. In the 131 who received 2 or more courses, the decrease in urine output and increase in creatinine were not different between drugs. There were significant decreases in urine output observed in the second and third courses of ibuprofen treatment (both by 0.9 mL/kg/hr).

Conclusion: Both drugs have a similar short-term effect on renal function. Indomethacin had a more prominent initial effect, while ibuprofen decreased renal function during the second and third courses similarly to indomethacin. The changes in renal function seen with ibuprofen treatment should be considered in fluid and electrolyte management, especially if treatment beyond one course is required.

Background

Patent ductus arteriosus (PDA) is a common occurrence in very low birth weight (VLBW, ≤1500 g) infants, which often causes significant morbidities. Left-to-right shunting through the ductus may increase the risk of intraventricular hemorrhage [1,2], necrotizing enterocolitis [3], bronchopulmonary dysplasia, and death [4,5].

Successful pharmacological closure of PDA with indomethacin was first reported in 1976, with subsequent reports that indomethacin reduced neonatal morbidity [6,7]. However, indomethacin may lead to complications such as transient or permanent renal dysfunction [8,9], necrotizing enterocolitis, and reduced cerebral oxygenation [10]. These indomethacin-related complications have prompted researchers to seek safer pharmacological treatment for closure of PDA.

In recent years another cyclooxygenase inhibitor, ibuprofen, has been proposed for the treatment of PDA, and several randomized controlled trials have shown it

* Correspondence: pinheij@mail.amc.edu
† Contributed equally
[1]Division of Neonatology, Department of Pediatrics; Albany Medical Center 43 New Scotland Avenue, Albany, NY 12208 USA
Full list of author information is available at the end of the article

to be as efficacious as indomethacin, with possibly fewer adverse effects [11]. It is thought that ibuprofen is better tolerated due to less effects on renal function, renal and mesenteric blood flow [12-14], and cerebral blood flow [15]. Adverse effects of ibuprofen have been noted in some trials [16] and suspected in our practice. This difference might be due to the fact that the infants in the previous trials were more mature (gestational age ~28 weeks) than the age of the infants at greatest risk for PDA (younger than 26 weeks); thus, it is difficult to extrapolate the clinical effects observed in those trials to the younger and unselected population typically treated in the clinical care context. Our primary objective was to ascertain whether ibuprofen and indomethacin treatment of PDA have comparable effects on renal function as evidenced by urine output and serum creatinine, during routine clinical usage.

Methods
Study design
This was a retrospective cohort study with a hypothesis that ibuprofen and indomethacin treatment of PDA have comparable effects on renal function as evidenced by urine output and serum creatinine. In October 2006 Neonatology staff switched from indomethacin to ibuprofen as the drug of choice for medical treatment of PDA. The cohort of neonates treated with indomethacin from January 2005 to October 2006 was compared to those treated with ibuprofen from October 2006 through December 2008. The study was approved by the Institutional Review Board of the Albany Medical Center, and exempted from requiring informed consent.

Patient population
Records were reviewed for inborn or outborn preterm neonates born at any gestation and birth weight, admitted to the NICU of Albany Medical Center Hospital (New York State-designated Level IV Regional Perinatal Center) and requiring treatment for PDA, from January 2005 through December 2008. The clinical approach to the PDA was unchanged throughout the study period and it is summarized here. Prophylactic indomethacin was not used in our institution. Cardiology consultation was requested if a symptomatic PDA was suspected (extremely low birth weight neonate, widened pulse pressures, murmur, bounding pulses, or significant respiratory disease) and an echocardiogram was performed. The size of the PDA was described qualitatively by the cardiologists (as absent, small, mild, moderate, large, or synonymous terms), along with blood flow direction. Attending neonatologists generally initiated medical treatment if predominant left-to-right shunting was noted through a PDA larger than "small", while also considering the patient's clinical status,

expected course given postnatal age, and potential contraindications. The day after the last treatment dose was administered, a follow-up echo was performed, and another course of either ibuprofen or indomethacin was given based on the same criteria used for the initial course. The decision to use further courses of medical treatment or resort to surgical ligation was made jointly by the attending neonatologist, cardiologist and cardiothoracic surgeon. A mildly restrictive fluid therapy regimen was used, beginning with a weight-based guideline, and then tailored to each infant's condition and postnatal age. The fluid regimen was further restricted (by approximately 20 mL/kg/day below the individualized daily target) as cyclooxygenase inhibitor therapy was initiated.

Indomethacin was dosed at 0.2 mg/kg/dose once, then 0.1 mg/kg/dose IV daily for 2 more doses for neonates <750 g; 0.2 mg/kg/dose daily for 3 doses for neonates 750 g to 1 kg; and 0.2 mg/kg/dose every 12 hours for those over 1 kg. Ibuprofen was dosed at 10 mg/kg/dose once and then 5 mg/kg/dose daily for 2 more doses.

Data collected
Demographic data were recorded into an Excel spreadsheet and de-identified. These data included gender, date of birth and date of discharge, birth weight, and gestational age. PDA-related data recorded included: date indomethacin or ibuprofen started, number of courses of medical treatment given, whether PDA was closed after the last treatment and whether surgical ligation of the PDA was performed.

Renal function prior to, during and after medical treatment of PDA was assessed by recording urine output and serum creatinine. Serum creatinine on the morning prior to administration of the first dose of ibuprofen or indomethacin was used as the baseline level. If no creatinine value was available from that day, the one from the prior day was used. During each treatment course, the last available serum creatinine was recorded. Resolution of the drug effect on renal function was assessed by evaluation of creatinine on the third to fifth day after the last drug dose.

Evaluation of urine output was done on the same schedule as creatinine, for 24 hours previous to, during treatment, and three to five days after the last dose of ibuprofen or indomethacin. Urine output was calculated as mL/kg/hour.

Secondary outcomes noted were necrotizing enterocolitis (NEC), bronchopulmonary dysplasia (BPD), and retinopathy of prematurity (ROP). NEC (defined using Bell's criteria [17]), spontaneous intestinal perforation (defined using Vermont Oxford Network criteria [18]), NEC-like illness, and whether NEC required surgical intervention were recorded. NEC-like illness was defined by the presence of clinical symptoms and radiographic appearance of bowel ischemia without pneumatosis or portal gas on abdominal radiograph. BPD was defined as oxygen requirement at 36 weeks post-menstrual age. ROP exam and the stage of retinopathy were also evaluated [19]. Presence of IVH and periventricular leukomalacia (PVL) were recorded, as well as the stage of IVH [20].

Sample size and statistical analysis

An a-priori power analysis setting the α error at 0.05 and ß error at 0.20 revealed that a minimum of 50 patients in each group was required to detect a 20% difference in urine output - well within the expected size of the cohorts. SPSS for Windows (SPSS version 12.0.1, Chicago, IL), as well as Minitab (Minitab version 15.0, State College, PA) and Stata (Stata version 8, College Station, TX) were used to conduct statistical data analyses. Pre-treatment mean creatinine and urine output values were compared to treatment and post treatment means using 2-factor repeated measures ANOVA (generalized linear model, including terms for treatment, time, treatment-by-time interaction, and with patients nested within treatment group). Dunnett's post-hoc test was used to compare within-group changes in mean creatinine and urine output from baseline to each treatment course. A p value of < 0.05 was considered significant.

Chi-square analysis was performed to compare the proportion of patients experiencing the secondary outcomes of PDA closure, BPD, ROP, and NEC between treatment groups.

In order to assess whether there is a difference in the rate of PDA closure, number of doses of medical treatment required, or changes in renal function depending on gestational age or birth weight, these variables were evaluated in subgroup analyses. Gestational age categories were divided into: <25 weeks, 25 0/7-27 6/7 weeks, 28 0/7 - 29 6/7 weeks, and ≥ 30 0/7 weeks. Birth weight categories were divided into: ≤ 750 grams, 751 -1000 grams, 1001 - 1500 grams, and >1500 grams.

Results

Of the 350 patients, 165 were treated with indomethacin and 185 received ibuprofen. The 7 cases where both drugs were used were excluded from the analyses of outcomes subsequent to the first course of treatment [Table 1].

The overall efficacy was the same for ibuprofen (71%) and indomethacin (68%) [Table 2]. The rate of ligation overall was the same after treatment with indomethacin and ibuprofen, with the exception of the neonates that required 2 courses of treatment for PDA closure. More babies required PDA ligation after receiving 2 courses of

Table 1 Baseline Population Characteristics

	Indomethacin	Ibuprofen
Birth Weight, grams (mean)	1048	1083
Birth Weight Categories, n (%)		
≤ 750 grams	54 (33)	56 (30)
751 - 1000 grams	38 (23)	41 (22)
1001 - 1500 grams	51 (31)	54 (29)
> 1500 grams	22 (13)	35 (19)
Gestational Age, weeks (mean)	27.7	27.8
Gestational Age Categories, n (%)		
< 25 weeks	33 (20)	34 (18)
25 - 27 6/7 weeks	61 (37)	68 (37)
28 - 29 6/7 weeks	35 (21)	37 (20)
≥ 30 weeks	36 (22)	47 (25)
Gender		
Male	82 (50)	108 (58) *
Female	83 (50)	78 (42)
Number of courses, n (%)	165	185
1	101 (61)	118 (63)
2	41 (25)	28 (15)
3	19 (12)	37 (20)
4	4 (2)	2 (1)
Baseline urine output, mL/kg/h mean (SD)	3.9 (1.4)	4.2 (1.6)
Baseline creatinine, mg/dL mean (SD)	0.96 (0.2)	0.93 (0.2)

PDA, patent ductus arteriosus
* denotes statistically significant difference between treatments, p < 0.05

indomethacin (53.7%) compared to ibuprofen (28.6%) (p < 0.05) [Table 3].

Date of birth was considered as day of life one. There was no difference in the initial treatment day between indomethacin and ibuprofen [Table 4]. Second and third treatment courses started at a median of one day after conclusion of the previous course. There was, also, no statistical difference in the intervals between first and second (p = 0.2) or second and third treatment courses (p = 0.4) [Table 4]. There was no difference between drug treatment groups in gestational age, birth weight, or baseline creatinine or urine output. We found a significantly larger proportion of male infants in the ibuprofen group (58% males; p = 0.04) [Table 1]. However, ANOVA with gender as a covariate revealed no significant gender effect on baseline urine output or creatinine values, nor in their response to each treatment; crosstabulations revealed no statistically significant differences between genders in the number of treatment courses, PDA closure or ligation rates in the ibuprofen group (data not shown). The number of treatment courses had a significant (p = 0.0001) inverse relation with both birth weight and gestational age, in chi-square analyses.

When all patients were included in the analysis of the first treatment course, there was a statistically significant

Table 2 Secondary Outcomes According to Treatment Group

	Indomethacin	Ibuprofen	
	(N = 161)	(N = 182)	p value
Day of Life at Start of Treatment (mean, SD)	3.3 ± 2.3	3.5 ± 2.7	NS
PDA Closed, n (%)	109 (68)	129 (71)	0.4
PDA Ligation, n (%)	45 (28)	38 (21)	0.1
BPD, n (%)	72 (45)	90 (49)	0.2
NEC-related conditions, any, n (%)	27 (17)	32 (18)	0.8
NEC, n (%)	6 (4)	15 (8)	0.08
NEC-Like Illness (%)	13 (8)	5 (3)	0.03*
Spontaneous Intestinal Perforations, n (%)	8 (5)	12 (7)	0.5
ROP, n (%)	65 (52)	41 (30)	<0.001*
Severe ROP: Grades III-V	15 (12)	15 (11)	0.8
IVH, any, n (%)	58 (36)	57 (31)	0.4
Severe IVH: Grade III/IV	12 (8)	12 (9)	0.6
PVL	4 (2.4)	3 (1.6)	0.4
Death, n (%)	12 (7)	16 (9)	0.4

PDA, patent ductus arteriosus; BPD, bronchopulmonary dysplasia; NEC, necrotizing enterocolitis; ROP, retinopathy of prematurity; IVH, intraventricular hemorrhage; PVL, periventricular leukomalacia.

The denominator for the percent (%) for each secondary outcome reflects the number of patients with evaluation of that outcome - for ROP in particular, 82 infants did not have a retinal exam.

* denotes statistically significant difference between treatments, p < 0.05

increase in creatinine (by 0.1 mg/dL) and decrease in urine output (by 0.3 mL/kg/hr) from baseline, after indomethacin [Figure 1][Table 5]. With ibuprofen treatment, only the increase in creatinine was significant. The ANOVA revealed that the increase in creatinine was significantly greater with indomethacin than with ibuprofen (p < 0.05 for both the treatment effect and the treatment-time interaction) [Table 5 and Figure 1]. However, there was no statistically significant difference in the effect of both drugs on urine output.

In the subgroup of 219 patients who received only one course of therapy, there was a significant increase in creatinine (by 0.1 mg/dL, p = 0.001) after indomethacin, but not after ibuprofen [Figure 2], with a significant drug-by-time interaction (p = 0.029). Regarding urine output, ANOVA revealed no significant differences between drugs, although post-hoc tests showed a significant decrease in urine output only in the indomethacin group [Figure 2]. For the 131 neonates who received 2 or more total courses of treatment, there were significant decreases in urine output and increases in

creatinine from baseline values, which were not significantly different between drugs [Figure 2]. Post hoc analyses revealed significant decreases in urine output from baseline observed during the last course of ibuprofen treatment (both by 0.9 mL/kg/hr, p < 0.05), in the subgroups receiving 2 or 3 courses [Figure 2]. Creatinine and urine output post-treatment returned to baseline values in both groups, regardless of the number of courses. Fluid intake was similar in both groups (data not shown).

There was no difference in secondary outcomes between the two drugs, except for ROP and NEC-like illness. There was a significantly higher rate of ROP in the indomethacin group [Table 2]. However, there was no difference in the rate of severe ROP between the groups. There was a significantly higher rate of NEC-like illness in the indomethacin group (8% vs. 3% for ibuprofen, p = 0.03); conversely, there was a trend towards more frequent diagnosis of NEC in the ibuprofen group (8% vs. 4% for indomethacin, p = 0.08) [Table 2], but no difference in the rate of spontaneous

Table 3 Treatment Efficacy by Number of Treatment Courses

	Indomethacin			Ibuprofen		
Number of Courses Used	1	2	3	1	2	3
Total N	101	41	19	118	28	37
PDA Closed, n (%)	89 (88.1)	18 (43.9)	3 (15.8)	108 (92.3)	15 (53.6)	7 (18.9)
PDA Ligations	8 (7.9)	22 (53.7)*	15 (78.9)	3 (2.6)	8 (28.6)*	26 (70.3)

PDA, patent ductus arteriosus.

Not all patients whose PDA remained open needed to have a surgical ligation.

* denotes statistically significant difference between treatments, p < 0.05.

Table 4 Treatment Start Day

	Indomethacin	Ibuprofen
Initial Day of Treatment		
Median	3	3
Mean	3.3	3.5
Minimum	1	1
Maximum	18	22
Interquartile range	2	2
Days between 1st and 2nd courses		
Median	1	1
Mean	4.1	2.7
Minimum	1	1
Maximum	32	18
Interquartile range	2	0
Days between 2nd and 3rd courses		
Median	1	1
Mean	1.9	2.6
Minimum	1	1
Maximum	9	13
Interquartile range	0	2

intestinal perforations between the two treatment groups [Table 2].

Discussion

The purpose of this study was to examine whether ibuprofen and indomethacin treatment of PDA have comparable effects on renal function as typically used in a NICU, where it is common for ELBW neonates to receive more than one course of cyclooxygenase inhibitor therapy in order to close the PDA. In addition to the renal effects, our observations on less common potential adverse effects of cyclooxygenase inhibitors add substantially to the available information on safety of these therapies, as this is the largest comparison study conducted in the US examining efficacy and side effects.

Van Overmeire et al. studied the efficacy of indomethacin and ibuprofen given to larger premature infants (≤32 weeks) at the age of 2-4 days. They reported that the closure rate was similar (66% and 70%, respectively) after the first course and that there was no significant difference in side effects, although ibuprofen was associated with significantly less impairment of renal function [5]. The study showed that infants of lower gestational age (<28 weeks) had a lower pharmacological closure rate and underwent surgical ligation more frequently. This and several other studies [11,13,21-23] found that there was similar efficacy in PDA closure when using indomethacin or ibuprofen. Most of these reports found that ibuprofen had fewer side effects than indomethacin. However, these studies enrolled small numbers of neonates, that were more mature (mean gestational age >28 weeks) than those in our study. Van Overmeire described 40 preterm infants

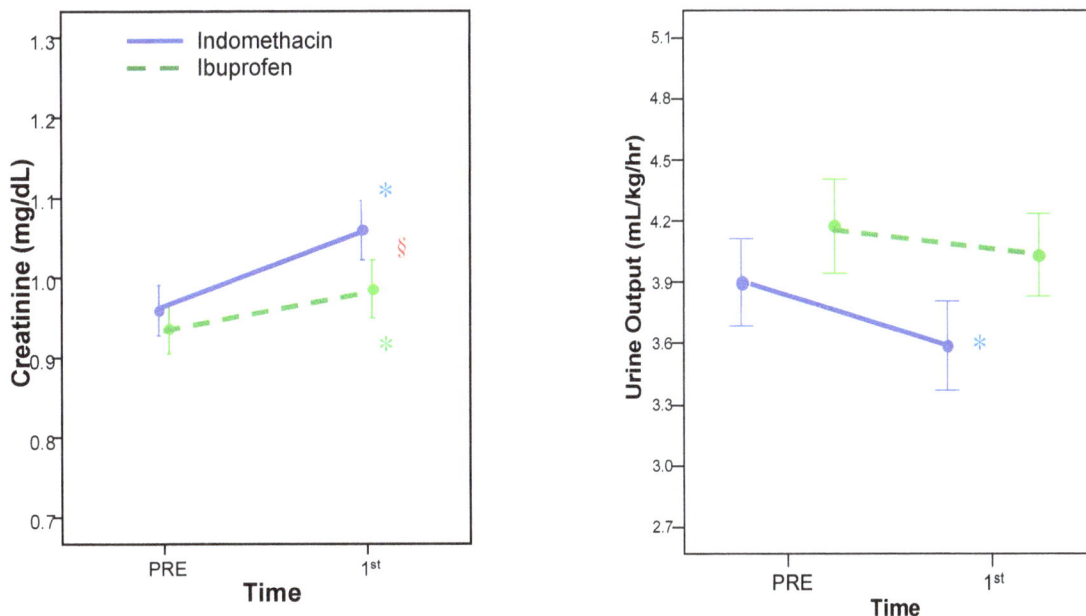

Figure 1 Mean urine output and creatinine values for all patients by drug. Comparison of mean urine output and creatinine values for all patients during the first course of therapy, by treatment drug. Indomethacin group (solid line) and Ibuprofen group (dashed line). PRE - pretreatment baseline; 1st - end of first course of treatment. * denotes statistically significant (p < 0.05) change from treatment baseline; § denotes statistically significant (p < 0.05) difference in change from baseline between treatment groups.

Table 5 Effect of Each Initial Treatment Course on Renal Function

	Indomethacin			Ibuprofen			Comparison between treatments on changes from baseline (ANOVA)	
	Baseline	1st course	p value for change with indomethacin (t-test)	Baseline	1st course	p value for change with ibuprofen (t-test)	p value for main treatment effect	p value for treatment - time interaction
Urine output (mL/kg/hr; mean ± SD)	3.9 ± 1.4	3.6 ± 1.4	0.033 *	4.2 ± 1.6	4.0 ± 1.4	0.24	0.51	0.50
Serum Creatinine (mg/dL; mean + SD)	0.96 ± 0.21	1.06 ± 0.24	<0.001*	0.93 ± 0.2	0.98 ± 0.24	0.005 *	0.039*	0.047 *

Supplemental analyses of the effect of each initial treatment course on renal function.

* denotes statistically significant (p < 0.05) change from baseline within a treatment group

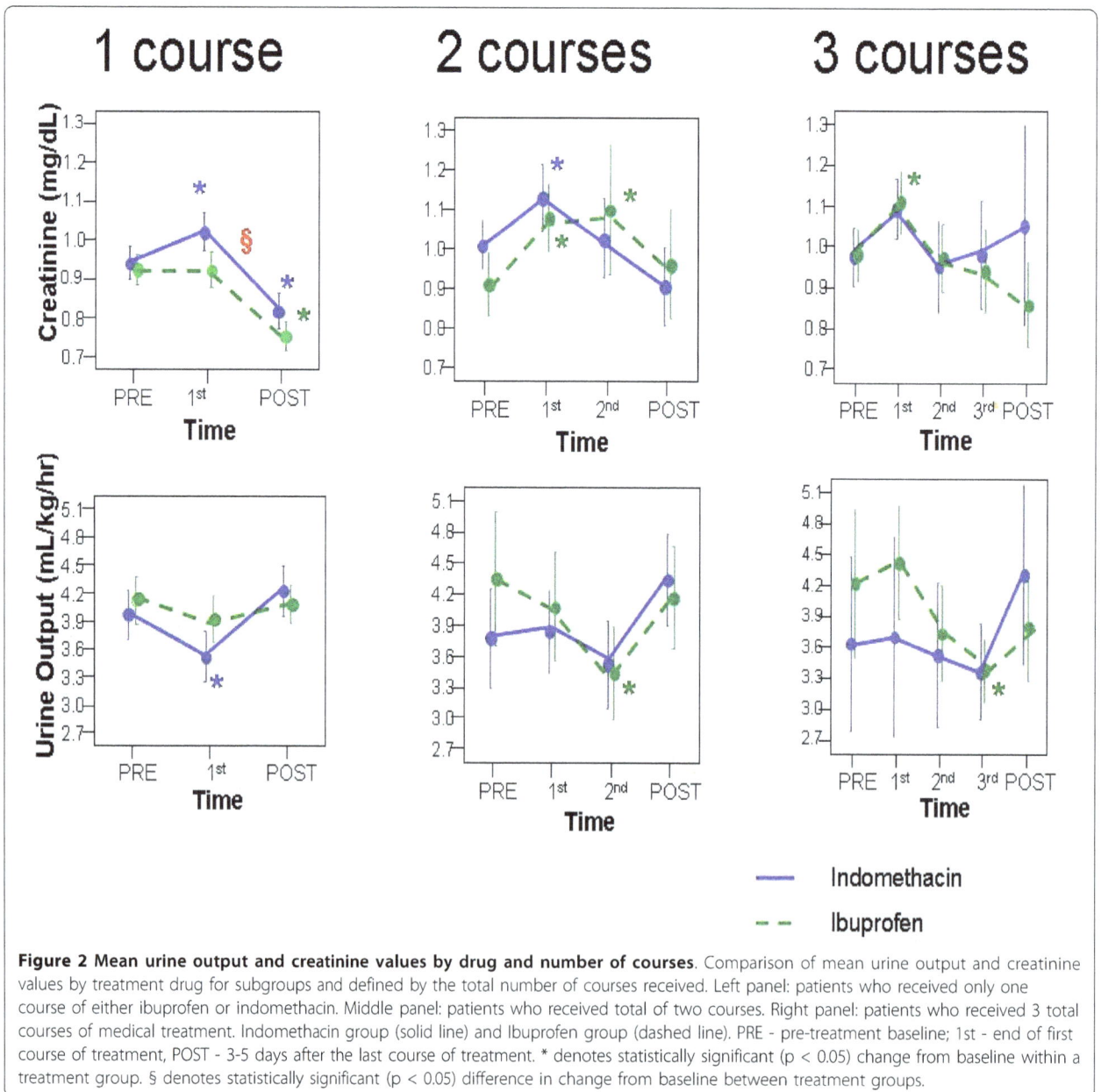

Figure 2 Mean urine output and creatinine values by drug and number of courses. Comparison of mean urine output and creatinine values by treatment drug for subgroups and defined by the total number of courses received. Left panel: patients who received only one course of either ibuprofen or indomethacin. Middle panel: patients who received total of two courses. Right panel: patients who received 3 total courses of medical treatment. Indomethacin group (solid line) and Ibuprofen group (dashed line). PRE - pre-treatment baseline; 1st - end of first course of treatment, POST - 3-5 days after the last course of treatment. * denotes statistically significant (p < 0.05) change from baseline within a treatment group. § denotes statistically significant (p < 0.05) difference in change from baseline between treatment groups.

most of whom required a single course of medical treatment; only 7 required a repeat course [23]. Su *et al.* compared efficacy and side effects of ibuprofen and indomethacin in neonates ($\leq$ 28 weeks) with echographically present PDA. They found both efficacy and side effect profile to be the same in both groups, except for a greater tendency toward oliguria after one course of indomethacin compared to ibuprofen [16]. Because surgical ligation was performed if the PDA was still present after one course, that study does not elucidate effects on renal function with further medical treatment.

The findings of our study confirm that indomethacin has a more prominent initial effect on measures of renal function than ibuprofen. However, ibuprofen had a detrimental effect on renal function in the second and third courses equal to that of indomethacin. Both drugs had a similar overall detrimental effect on renal function, with repeated courses.

Other recent studies support the notion that ibuprofen therapy is not devoid of renal effects in neonates [24-26]. Gournay *et al.* noted an increase in creatinine in the prophylactic ibuprofen group and in those who received a second course of ibuprofen, which resolved in the second week of life. They also noted a decrease in urine output with ibuprofen as compared with placebo that returned to baseline after the first course. Ticker and Yildirim described temporary oliguria and/or renal dysfunction after treatment with one course of ibuprofen that is similar to that seen with indomethacin. Vieux *et al.* found a significant decrease in glomerular filtration and tubular function impairment in the ibuprofen group that was not seen in the patients who did not receive ibuprofen [25]. Richards *et al.* reported that the effectiveness of ibuprofen in closing a PDA decreased with a second course, and that creatinine was significantly higher in neonates receiving a second course as compared to controls [27].

Our study also adds information pertaining to the safety of cyclooxygenase inhibitor treatment. There was no difference in morbidities potentially associated with cyclooxygenase inhibitor therapy between patients receiving ibuprofen or indomethacin, except for the incidence of ROP and NEC-like disease. These findings may be incidental to secondary analyses, or they may hint at clinically significant relationships. The higher rate of ROP in the indomethacin group was related primarily to higher incidence of stages 1 and 2 diseases, not of severe ROP. This has not been seen in previous studies [23,28,29]. It is possible that the difference in ROP rates is related to the more stringent oxygen saturation targets implemented in 2006 [30].

In the ibuprofen group there was a trend towards a higher frequency of NEC, but not of spontaneous intestinal perforations [Table 2]; NEC-like disease was significantly less frequent. There was no increase in the incidence of NEC seen in other studies of ibuprofen [5] and this finding is unexpected since ibuprofen does not significantly reduce mesenteric blood-flow velocity [13]. Diagnostic drift is unlikely since neither neonatology nor radiology staff physicians changed during the study period; furthermore, diagnostic criteria in the database remained constant. However, over the last decade there has been an increase in the incidence of NEC in a nationally representative sample of NICUs, and our observation may reflect this background trend [31].

Since this study compares two historical cohorts, it is possible that unmeasured confounders may have changed over time, and affected the primary or secondary study outcomes. However, in our NICU, indomethacin and ibuprofen were used for treatment of PDA during two immediately contiguous eras. Because the switch in management occurred through mutual agreement of all neonatologists, indomethacin was exclusively used before October 2006 and ibuprofen thereafter. In our analysis we excluded the few patients who received both indomethacin and ibuprofen. The study comprises only a 4 year time span, so the effects of therapeutic drift should be minimal; furthermore, there were no other planned or perceived changes in clinical management related to PDA.

The larger number of patients evaluated in this study increased our ability to detect important differences in adverse events between the two drugs. Most of the previous studies, both retrospective and prospective, had lower numbers of patients enrolled [5,11,14,16,23,29]. The retrospective nature of the study facilitated observation of the effects of both indomethacin and ibuprofen during unrestricted clinical usage. In particular, we demonstrated the consequences of repeated courses of cyclooxygenase inhibitor treatment in a large cohort of ELBW neonates.

This study confirms the findings or prior trials, revealing comparable effectiveness of indomethacin and ibuprofen in closing a PDA [11,13,21-23]. It also adds substantial weight to the notion that the likelihood of successful medical closure of the PDA diminishes with each subsequent course [27].

A limitation of our study is that it was retrospective. This allowed for some variability in treatment approaches by attending neonatologists; however, all clinicians used the same dosage regimen of PDA therapy and had similar approaches to PDA diagnosis. There was a wide range in the gestational age as well as acuity level of the neonates, which allows the results of this study to be more broadly generalizable. The larger proportion of males in the ibuprofen era is likely a chance finding, since review of our data on more than 1900 VLBW newborns over 14 years did not reveal a gender predilection of significant (treatable) PDAs or of PDA ligations. Furthermore, the gender difference between our study groups is unlikely to influence the results, since we found no gender-related differences in indices of renal function at baseline or in changes in urine output or creatinine during treatment courses.

Conclusion

In summary, our data indicated that both indomethacin and ibuprofen appear to have a similar overall effect on renal function, particularly with repeated courses of therapy. This effect may be clinically apparent with decreased urine output and potential fluid overload, and it is more prominent during the first course of indomethacin. Whereas a decrease in urine output of nearly 10 mL/kg/day may be anticipated during the first course of indomethacin therapy for PDA, both indomethacin and ibuprofen will produce a decrease in urine output of about 20 mL/kg/day during subsequent courses. These changes in renal function should be considered and reflected in fluid and electrolyte management by prospectively decreasing fluid intake by approximately 20 mL/kg/day, especially if treatment is required beyond one course.

List of abbreviations
PDA: patent ductus arteriosus; BPD: bronchopulmonary dysplasia; ROP: retinopathy of prematurity; NEC: necrotizing enterocolitis; IVH: intraventricular hemorrhage; PVL: periventricular leukomalacia; VLBW: very low birth weight

Acknowledgements
I would like to acknowledge Dr. Angel Rios, Dr. Michael Horgan, and Dr. Rubia Khalak for the time they gave being on A.K.'s Scholarship Oversight Committee and overseeing the progress of this study.

Author details
[1]Division of Neonatology, Department of Pediatrics; Albany Medical Center 43 New Scotland Avenue, Albany, NY 12208 USA. [2]Division of Neonatology, Department of Pediatrics; Cooper Hospital 1 Cooper Plaza, Camden, NJ 08103 USA.

Authors' contributions
JMBP participated in the design of the study, performed the statistical analysis, and helped draft the manuscript. AK conceived of the study, participated in its design and data acquisition, performed statistical analysis, and drafted the manuscript. All authors read and approved the final manuscript.

Competing interests
Research support provided by an educational grant from Ovation Pharmaceuticals (Lundbeck, Inc.)

References
1. Evans N, Kluckow M: Early ductal shunting and intraventricular haemorrhage in ventilated preterm infants. *Arch Dis Child Fetal Neonatal Ed* 1996, **75**(3):F183-F186.
2. Martin CG, Snider AR, Katz SM, Peabody JL, Brady JP: Abnormal cerebral blood flow patterns in preterm infants with a large patent ductus arteriosus. *J Pediatr* 1982, **101**(4):587-93.
3. Wong SN, Lo RN, Hui PW: Abnormal renal and splanchnic arterial Doppler pattern in premature babies with symptomatic patent ductus arteriosus. *J Ultrasound Med* 1990, **9**(3):125-30.
4. Cotton RB, Stahlman MT, Kovar I, Catterton WZ: Medical management of small preterm infants with symptomatic patent ductus arteriosus. *J Pediatr* 1978, **92**(3):467-73.
5. Van Overmeire B, Smets K, Lecoutere D, Van de Broek H, Weyler J, Degroote K, Langhendries JP: A comparison of ibuprofen and indomethacin for closure of patent ductus arteriosus. *N Engl J Med* 2000, **343**(10):674-81.
6. Friedman WF, Hirschklau MJ, Printz MP, Pitlick PT, Kirkpatrick SE: Pharmacologic closure of patent ductus arteriosus in the premature infant. *N Engl J Med* 1976, **295**(10):526-9.
7. Heymann MA, Rudolph AM, Silverman NH: Closure of the ductus arteriosus in premature infants by inhibition of prostaglandin synthesis. *N Engl J Med* 1976, **295**(10):530-3.
8. Betkerur MV, Yeh TF, Miller K, Glasser RJ, Pildes RS: Indomethacin and its effect on renal function and urinary kallikrein excretion in premature infants with patent ductus arteriosus. *Pediatrics* 1981, **68**(1):99-102.
9. van Bel F, Guit GL, Schipper J, van de Bor M, Baan J: Indomethacin-induced changes in renal blood flow velocity waveform in premature infants investigated with color Doppler imaging. *J Pediatr* 1991, **118**(4 (Pt 1)):621-6.
10. Edwards AD, Wyatt JS, Richardson C, Potter A, Cope M, Delpy DT, Reynolds EO: Effects of indomethacin on cerebral haemodynamics in very preterm infants. *Lancet* 1990, **335**(8704):1491-5.
11. Varvarigou A, Bardin CL, Beharry K, Chemtob S, Papageorgiou A, Aranda JV: Early ibuprofen administration to prevent patent ductus arteriosus in premature newborn infants. *JAMA* 1996, **275**(7):539-44.
12. Romagnoli C, De Carolis MP, Papacci P, Polimeni V, Luciano R, Piersigilli F, Delogu AB, Tortorolo G: Effects of prophylactic ibuprofen on cerebral and renal hemodynamics in very preterm neonates. *Clin Pharmacol Ther* 2000, **67**(6):676-83.
13. Pezzati M, Vangi V, Biagiotti R, Bertini G, Cianciulli D, Rubaltelli FF: Effects of indomethacin and ibuprofen on mesenteric and renal blood flow in preterm infants with patent ductus arteriosus. *J Pediatr* 1999, **135**(6):733-8.
14. Lago P, Bettiol T, Salvadori S, Pitassi I, Vianello A, Chiandetti L, Saia OS: Safety and efficacy of ibuprofen versus indomethacin in preterm infants treated for patent ductus arteriosus: a randomised controlled trial. *Eur J Pediatr* 2002, **161**(4):202-7.
15. Mosca F, Bray M, Lattanzio M, Fumagalli M, Tosetto C: Comparative evaluation of the effects of indomethacin and ibuprofen on cerebral perfusion and oxygenation in preterm infants with patent ductus arteriosus. *J Pediatr* 1997, **131**(4):549-54.
16. Su BH, Lin HC, Chiu HY, Hsieh HY, Chen HH, Tsai YC: Comparison of ibuprofen and indometacin for early-targeted treatment of patent ductus arteriosus in extremely premature infants: a randomised controlled trial. *Arch Dis Child Fetal Neonatal Ed* 2008, **93**(2):F94-F99.
17. Bell MJ, Ternberg JL, Feigin RD, Keating JP, Marshall R, Barton L, Brotherton T: Neonatal necrotizing enterocolitis. Therapeutic decisions based upon clinical staging. *Ann Surg* 1978, **187**(1):1-7.
18. Vermont Oxford Network Database: Manual of Operations. Burlington, VT: Vermont Oxford Network; 2007, Release 12.0.
19. International Committee for the Classification of Retinopathy of Prematurity: The International Classification of Retinopathy of Prematurity Revisited., 123 2005, 991-9.
20. Papile LA, Burstein J, Burstein R, Koffler H: Incidence and evolution of subependymal and intraventricular hemorrhage: a study of infants with birth weights less than 1,500 gm. *J Pediatr* 1978, **92**(4):529-34.
21. Clyman RI: Ibuprofen and patent ductus arteriosus. *N Engl J Med* 2000, **343**(10):728-30.
22. Patel J, Roberts I, Azzopardi D, Hamilton P, Edwards AD: Randomized double-blind controlled trial comparing the effects of ibuprofen with indomethacin on cerebral hemodynamics in preterm infants with patent ductus arteriosus. *Pediatr Res* 2000, **47**(1):36-42.
23. Van Overmeire B, Follens I, Hartmann S, Creten WL, Van Acker KJ: Treatment of patent ductus arteriosus with ibuprofen. *Arch Dis Child Fetal Neonatal Ed* 1997, **76**(3):F179-F184.

24. Tiker F, Yildirim SV: **Acute renal impairment after oral ibuprofen for medical closure of patent ductus arteriosus.** *Indian Pediatr* 2007, **44(1)**:54-5.

25. Vieux R, Desandes R, Boubred F, Semama D, Guillemin F, Buchweiller MC, Fresson J, Hascoet JM: **Ibuprofen in very preterm infants impairs renal function for the first month of life.** *Pediatr Nephrol* 2010, **25(2)**:267-74.

26. Gournay V, Roze JC, Kuster A, Daoud P, Cambonie G, Hascoet JM, Chamboux C, Blanc T, Fichtner C, Savagner C, Gouyon JB, Flurin V, Thiriez G: **Prophylactic ibuprofen versus placebo in very premature infants: a randomised, double-blind, placebo-controlled trial.** *Lancet* 2004, **364(9449)**:1939-44.

27. Richards J, Johnson A, Fox G, Campbell M: **A second course of ibuprofen is effective in the closure of a clinically significant PDA in ELBW infants.** *Pediatrics* 2009, **124(2)**:e287-e293.

28. Aranda JV, Clyman R, Cox B, Van Overmeire B, Wozniak P, Sosenko I, Carlo WA, Ward RM, Shalwitz R, Baggs G, Seth A, Darko L: **A randomized, double-blind, placebo-controlled trial on intravenous ibuprofen L-lysine for the early closure of nonsymptomatic patent ductus arteriosus within 72 hours of birth in extremely low-birth-weight infants.** *Am J Perinatol* 2009, **26(3)**:235-45.

29. Cotton RB, Stahlman MT, Bender HW, Graham TP, Catterton WZ, Kovar I: **Randomized trial of early closure of symptomatic patent ductus arteriosus in small preterm infants.** *J Pediatr* 1978, **93(4)**:647-51.

30. SUPPORT Study Group of the Eunice Kennedy Shriver NICHDNeonatal Research Network: **Target Ranges of Oxygen Saturation in Extremely Preterm Infants.** *N Engl J Med* 2010, **362(21)**:1959-69.

31. Vermont Oxford Network: **Vermont Oxford Network Database: 2009 Annual NICU Quality Management Report.** Burlington, VT, Vermont Oxford Network; 2010.

12

Safety, pharmacokinetics and pharmacodynamics of remogliflozin etabonate, a novel SGLT2 inhibitor, and metformin when co-administered in subjects with type 2 diabetes mellitus

Elizabeth K Hussey[1], Anita Kapur[1*], Robin O'Connor-Semmes[1], Wenli Tao[1], Bryan Rafferty[1^], Joseph W Polli[1], Charles D James Jr[2] and Robert L Dobbins[1]

Abstract

Background: The sodium-dependent glucose co-transporter-2 (SGLT2) is expressed in absorptive epithelia of the renal tubules. Remogliflozin etabonate (RE) is the prodrug of remogliflozin, the active entity that inhibits SGLT2. An inhibitor of this pathway would enhance urinary glucose excretion (UGE), and potentially improve plasma glucose concentrations in diabetic patients. RE is intended for use for the treatment of type 2 diabetes mellitus (T2DM) as monotherapy and in combination with existing therapies. Metformin, a dimethylbiguanide, is an effective oral antihyperglycemic agent widely used for the treatment of T2DM.

Methods: This was a randomized, open-label, repeat-dose, two-sequence, cross-over study in 13 subjects with T2DM. Subjects were randomized to one of two treatment sequences in which they received either metformin alone, RE alone, or both over three, 3-day treatment periods separated by two non-treatment intervals of variable duration. On the evening before each treatment period, subjects were admitted and confined to the clinical site for the duration of the 3-day treatment period. Pharmacokinetic, pharmacodynamic (urine glucose and fasting plasma glucose), and safety (adverse events, vital signs, ECG, clinical laboratory parameters including lactic acid) assessments were performed at check-in and throughout the treatment periods. Pharmacokinetic sampling occurred on Day 3 of each treatment period.

Results: This study demonstrated the lack of effect of RE on steady state metformin pharmacokinetics. Metformin did not affect the AUC of RE, remogliflozin, or its active metabolite, GSK279782, although C_{max} values were slightly lower for remogliflozin and its metabolite after co-administration with metformin compared with administration of RE alone. Metformin did not alter the pharmacodynamic effects (UGE) of RE. Concomitant administration of metformin and RE was well tolerated with minimal hypoglycemia, no serious adverse events, and no increase in lactic acid.

Conclusions: Coadministration of metformin and RE was well tolerated in this study. The results support continued development of RE as a treatment for T2DM.

Trial registration: ClinicalTrials.gov, NCT00376038

Keywords: Remogliflozin etabonate, SGLT2 inhibitor, Metformin, Pharmacokinetics, Type 2 diabetes mellitus

* Correspondence: anita.x.kapur@gsk.com
^Deceased
[1]GlaxoSmithKline, 5 Moore Drive, Research Triangle Park, NC 27709, USA
Full list of author information is available at the end of the article

Background

Type 2 diabetes mellitus (T2DM) is a chronic disease characterized by deteriorating glycemic control and an associated risk of complications. Evidence from controlled clinical trials suggests that improving glycemic control can substantially reduce the long-term microvascular complications of diabetes [1-5]. Current guidelines recommend that T2DM patients should be initially managed with diet and exercise followed by pharmacological treatment with metformin as the preferred step 1 agent, unless there are contraindications to metformin use. When glycemic goals are not achieved, the dose of metformin is increased or a second agent is added [6,7]. In this treatment algorithm, suitability for combination with metformin becomes a critical concern in developing new antidiabetic agents.

Metformin is a dimethylbiguanide that reduces elevated blood glucose levels primarily through its effects on reducing hepatic glucose production and improving peripheral tissue sensitivity to insulin. Metformin is typically administered with meals and has an oral bioavailability of approximately 40 to 60% [8]. It undergoes extensive renal excretion 3 times the glomerular filtration rate [9] and has a mean plasma elimination half-life between 4.0 and 8.7 hours. There are no clinically relevant metabolic interactions reported with metformin, and it is neither metabolized nor inhibits the metabolism of other drugs [10]. However, there are several transporter related drug interactions, in particular with cationic drugs that have been reported [9]; these typically don't require a dose adjustment. The main adverse event of clinical concern with metformin is lactic acidosis, a potentially life-threatening side effect that may be associated with high plasma concentrations of metformin and renal insufficiency [11-13].

The low-affinity, high-capacity sodium-dependent glucose co-transporter-2 (SGLT2), which is expressed specifically in the renal proximal tubule [14,15], plays a major role in the reabsorption of glucose by the kidney. SGLT2 has recently gained recognition as a potential therapeutic target for reducing hyperglycemia in T2DM, and several selective SGLT2 inhibitors are being evaluated in the clinic [16-22]. In diabetic animal models, pharmacological inhibition of SGLT2 leads to glucosuria followed by normalization of plasma glucose levels and consequent improvement in insulin resistance [23-25]. This mechanism may provide improvements in both fasting and postprandial hyperglycemia without causing weight gain or other dose-limiting side effects observed with other oral antidiabetic approaches [26].

Remogliflozin etabonate is the prodrug of the highly selective and potent SGLT2 inhibitor, remogliflozin. Administration of remogliflozin etabonate has been shown to increase urinary glucose excretion in a dose-dependent manner in mice and rats and to exhibit antidiabetic efficacy in several diabetic rodent models [27]. Remogliflozin is further metabolized to GSK279782, which is an equally potent inhibitor of SGLT2 [28] but circulates at approximately 20% of the plasma concentrations of remogliflozin; thus GSK279682 is expected to contribute to some of the observed SGLT-2 inhibitor pharmacology. Single oral doses of remogliflozin etabonate up to 1000 mg in healthy subjects and repeated dosing in subjects with T2DM (up to 1000 mg BID for 2 weeks) have been safe and well tolerated [29,30]. Remogliflozin etabonate is intended for use in the treatment of T2DM as monotherapy. Given its mechanism of action, it would be a candidate for combination with metformin and other antidiabetic therapies as well. The osmotic diuresis associated with increased urine glucose excretion provides a potential mechanism for pharmacokinetic drug–drug interactions due to the extensive renal clearance of metformin, although treatment with the diuretic hydrochlorothiazide for 2 weeks had no significant effect on the clearance of metformin in subjects with T2DM [31].

This study was designed to evaluate the effect of remogliflozin etabonate on metformin exposure in T2DM subjects. Secondarily, the effect of metformin on steady state plasma concentrations of remogliflozin etabonate, remogliflozin (active entity) and the active metabolite, GSK279782 was evaluated. Three days of dosing (total of 5 doses) was considered adequate to achieve steady-state conditions for both metformin and remogliflozin. Safety problems that might be related to a pharmacokinetic drug–drug interaction were also monitored.

Methods

This single-center, Phase 1 study was conducted at Medica Sur Hospital and Clinical Foundation Pharma Unit (CIF-BIOTEC), Mexico. This study was approved by the investigational center ethics committee (Hospital Medical Sur Ethics Committee) and was conducted in accordance with Good Clinical Practice and the principles of the Declaration of Helsinki. All subjects provided their written informed consent before study participation. The study was registered at http://clinicaltrials.gov with the identifier NCT00376038.

Subjects

Male and female subjects (post-menopausal women or pre-menopausal women with documented hysterectomy or tubal ligation) with documented T2DM (≥3 months), ranging in age from 30 to 64 years and with a body mass index of 22 to 35 kg/m^2, were eligible for the study. Enough subjects were to be enrolled to ensure completion of at least 12 evaluable subjects. Pre-study screening included a medical history, physical examination, medical and laboratory evaluations, including 12-lead ECG, and a urinary drug screen. Subjects were required to be free of clinically significant medical and laboratory abnormalities, to have glycosylated hemoglobin (HbA1c) <10%, and fasting plasma glucose (FPG) <280 mg/dL, and to be controlled by diet alone or metformin. Standard exclusion criteria concerning blood donation, alcohol and drug use, caffeine intake, and participation in other recent investigational drug studies were applied. In addition, subjects were excluded from participation in the study if they required insulin, had received insulin within the past 3 months, or if they had significant renal disease (as manifested by one or more of the following: creatinine clearance <60 mL/min/1.73 m^2, urine albumin concentration ≥300 µg/mg of creatinine, or a spot urine sample with a urine protein/creatinine ratio >2.5 mg/mg (a ratio that approximates the common cut off of 3 g of protein in urine per 24 hours to exclude subjects with nephrotic range proteinuria [32]).

Study design

The study was a randomized, open-label, repeat-dose, two-sequence, cross-over study in subjects with T2DM who were taking metformin or who were drug naive. Before randomization, eligible subjects were stratified on the basis of their pre-entry treatment regimen: metformin or drug naive. Subjects were randomized to receive one of two treatment sequences depicted in Table 1. Each treatment sequence included three treatment regimens [A = metformin 500 mg every 12 hours (MET BID), B = remogliflozin etabonate 500 mg every 12 hours (RE BID), and C = metformin 500 mg + remogliflozin etabonate 500 mg every 12 hours (MET + RE)] administered over three 3-day dosing periods that were separated by two non-treatment intervals of variable duration (minimum of 2 days up to a maximum of 15 days). The last dose of drug for each study period was before breakfast on day 3. Metformin was administered as Glucophage® (Bristol-Myers Squibb, New York, NY) and subjects were allowed to continue taking metformin during the non-treatment interval between the first and second treatment periods. On the evening before each treatment period, subjects were admitted and confined to the clinical site for the duration of the 3-day treatment period. Pharmacokinetic (PK), pharmacodynamic (PD; urine glucose and FPG), and safety (adverse events, vital signs, ECG, clinical laboratory parameters including lactic acid) assessments were performed at check-in and throughout the treatment periods. For each treatment period, the PK sampling occurred on Day 3.

Subjects were asked to refrain from drinking grapefruit juice or eating grapefruit for at least 3 days before the first dose until collection of the final PK sample for each treatment period. Subjects were to abstain from alcohol or caffeine- or xanthine-containing products from up to 24 hours prior to admission until collection of the final blood/urine sample. Subjects who smoked had to be able to abstain from use of tobacco products for the 12-hour PK sampling interval. On days 1–3 of each treatment regimen, while in-house, subjects were fed breakfast, lunch, and dinner as standard meals with identical meals provided on the PK sampling days. Subjects were given 1700 kcal per day, with calories distributed as 55% carbohydrate, 25% fat, and 20% protein. Breakfast was served at approximately 7am and dinner at approximately 7 pm. Subjects were instructed to complete these meals within 30 minutes. Within 15 minutes of completing the meal, the study medications were administered with 240 mL of water per the randomization schedule. Use of the following concomitant medications was allowed if the dosing regimen had been stable for at least 3 months prior to study enrollment: 3-hydroxy-3-methyl-glutaryl-CoA reductase inhibitors, ACE inhibitors, angiotensin receptor blockers, hydrochlorothiazide (dose of ≤25 mg/day), calcium channel blockers, alpha or beta blockers, thyroid hormone (only if TSH in normal range), hormone replacement therapy, inhaled and intranasal corticosteroids, antidepressants (SSRIs only) and multivitamins. Low-dose acetaminophen or ibuprofen (≤1.2 g/day), and any medications prescribed for treatment of adverse events occurring during the study were also allowed. Concomitant medications were not permitted within 4 hours of study drug administration.

Clinical and laboratory monitoring for safety

For each treatment period, subjects were admitted to the clinical facility on the evening of Day −1 to undergo check-in procedures including a physical examination, 12-lead ECG, vital signs, clinical laboratory tests (chemistry, hematology and urinalysis), lactic acid measurement, fasting blood glucose measurement, alcohol screen, drugs of abuse screen and pregnancy test (if applicable). On each study day morning, a fasting blood sugar measurement was determined by glucose monitor. On Days 1 and 2, vital signs and a 12-lead ECG were recorded. Samples for clinical laboratory measure were also taken on Days 1 and 3.

Table 1 Treatment sequence regimens

Treatment sequence	Period 1	Interval between dosing	Period 2	Interval between dosing	Period 3
	3 Days	2 to 15 days	3 days	2 to 15 days	3 days
1	A	Continue metformin only	C	Stop all trial medications	B
2	C	Continue metformin only	A	Stop all trial medications	B

Treatment A (MET BID): Metformin IR 500 mg every 12 hours. Treatment B (RE BID): Remogliflozin etabonate 500 mg every 12 hours. Treatment C (MET + RE BID): Metformin IR 500 mg every 12 hours + remogliflozin etabonate 500 mg every 12 hours. Metformin was administered starting from the morning of Day 1 of Period 1 and stopped after the morning dose on Day 3 of Period 2. For any Treatment Period when remogliflozin etabonate was administered, remogliflozin etabonate dosing was stopped after the morning dose was given on Day 3.

Subjects returned to the clinic 7–10 days following the last dosing day for a follow-up physical examination and laboratory evaluation. During the between-treatment intervals, subjects were provided with glucose monitors to measure fasting blood glucose concentrations; subjects were instructed as to how to recognize and treat symptoms of hypoglycemia. Adverse events were monitored throughout the entire study (randomization to follow-up visit). Any adverse events reported during the study were assessed by the investigator for intensity (mild, moderate, severe) and relationship to the study drug (causality). Where possible, all adverse events were followed until stabilization, resolution, or until the event was otherwise explained.

Pharmacokinetic assessment
Blood sampling
Serial blood (two 2 mL samples for metformin and for remogliflozin etabonate and metabolites) were collected predose, 0.25, 0.5, 0.75, 1, 1.5, 2, 3, 4, 6, 8, and 12 hours post-dose for determination of plasma metformin, remogliflozin etabonate (prodrug), remogliflozin (active entity) and GSK279782 (metabolite) concentrations. All sample times are relative to the time of the administration of the first dose of study medication on Day 3 of each period. Blood samples for metformin were collected into tubes containing EDTA and immediately placed on ice and centrifuged at approximately 3000 rpm for 10 minutes at approximately 4°C. The harvested plasma was separated, frozen and stored at −20°C or lower until analysis for metformin concentrations. Blood samples for remogliflozin etabonate, remogliflozin and GSK279782 were collected into tubes containing potassium-oxalate/ sodium fluoride, placed on ice and centrifuged at approximately 3000 rpm for 10 minutes at approximately 4°C. The harvested plasma was frozen at −70°C until analysis for remogliflozin etabonate, remogliflozin and GSK279782 concentrations.

Drug assays
The concentrations of remogliflozin etabonate, remogliflozin, and GSK279782 in deproteinized plasma samples and standards were determined by high-performance liquid chromatography (HPLC) with tandem mass spectrometry (MS/MS) using isotopically labelled internal standards ($[^2H_7]$-remogliflozin etabonate, $[^2H_7]$- remogliflozin and $[^2H_7]$-GSK279782 as previously described [28].

The concentrations of metformin in plasma were determined by HPLC-MS/MS using a $[^2H_6]$-metformin isotopically labelled internal standard. Plasma proteins from a 50 mL plasma aliquot were precipitated using acetonitrile containing the internal standard (200 ng mL-1). Samples were vortex mixed then centrifuged. The resulting supernatant was transferred and mixed with 200 mL of HFBA buffer (water containing 10 mM ammonium acetate and 0.26% (v/v) of heptofluorobutyric acid) prior to injection.

HPLC was performed on a Shimadzu LC-10A HPLC system. Chromatography was performed on a MAC-MOD Ace 3 C18, 4.6 × 50 mm column at a flow rate of 1.0 mL min-1. An isocratic mobile phase elution with 82:18 (v/v) HFBA buffer : Acetonitrile was used. Samples were analysed in positive ion mode by Turbo Ionspray LC/MS/MS with a PE/Sciex API 3000. The calibration range was 20 to 5000 ng mL-1. Performance of the method was assessed during a 3 day validation study using quality control samples at 5 concentrations 20, 80, 500, 4000 and 5000 ng mL-1. The average within-run precision [coefficient of variation (CV %)] was <9.6% and the between-run precision CV% was < 4.7%. Similar assay performance was observed during study sample analyses.

Pharmacokinetic calculations
PK analyses of plasma concentration–time data of each analyte (i.e., metformin, remogliflozin etabonate, remogliflozin, and GSK279782) were conducted using the noncompartmental Model 200 (for extravascular administration) of WinNonlin Professional Edition version 4.1 (Pharsight Corporation, Mountain View, CA, USA). Actual elapsed time from dosing was used to estimate all individual plasma PK parameters. Values for the following PK parameters were estimated for each analyte, as appropriate, following administration of 3 days dosing of metformin, remogliflozin etabonate, or both.

- C_{max} and t_{max} were the actual observed values.
- $AUC_{(0-12)}$ or $AUC_{(0-last)}$ was calculated by a combination of linear and logarithmic trapezoidal methods. The linear trapezoidal method was used for all incremental trapezoids arising from increasing concentrations and the logarithmic trapezoidal method was used for those arising from decreasing concentrations.

Pharmacodynamic assessment
Plasma PD
FPG concentrations were collected on Day −1, 1, 2 and 3. Changes in plasma glucose from baseline (Day 1) to Day 2 and 3 were calculated.

Urine PD
Urine was collected on Days 1 to 3 of each treatment period, and urine glucose concentrations were analyzed for the following intervals: 0–4 hours, 4–8 hours, 8–12 hours and 12–24 hours. The quantity of glucose and creatinine excreted in urine was determined by multiplying the urine glucose or creatinine concentration for each time interval by the volume of urine for the corresponding collection interval. The total 24-hour quantity of glucose excreted in urine on Day 2 was calculated by adding the amounts collected during each interval. Urine glucose and creatinine

amounts were summarized for each collected interval and for the total 24-hour collection period.

Creatinine clearance (CLcr) was calculated on Day 2 and used to determine the percent of filtered glucose load excreted in urine. By using the urine collections on Day 2, CLcr was calculated as follows:

$$\text{Clcr} = \text{total amount of urine creatinine } 0 - xxh \text{ interval}$$
$$/\text{nearest associated serum creatinine}$$
$$= ((\text{urine creatinine(mg/xx hours)}$$
$$/\text{serum creatinine(mg/dL))*100 mL/dL)}$$
$$/(xx*60)(\text{minutes/xx hours}),$$

where urine creatinine (mg/xx hours) is the amount of urine excreted in a xx-hour period. Urine creatinine was calculated by multiplying the urine creatinine concentration by the urine volume (mL) for a 0-xxh time interval as follows:

$$\text{urine creatinine (mg/xx hours)}$$
$$= (\text{urine creatinine concentration(mg/dL)*}$$
$$(\text{interval volume(mL)}/100(\text{mL/dL}).$$

CLcr was reported in mL/minutes on Day 2 for collection intervals 0–4 hours, 4–8 hours, 8-12 hours, 12–24 hours, and the total daily interval of 0–24 hours.

The serum creatinine concentration used for the above calculations was the pre-dose value for the same day as the urine collection or the one closest to the day of urine collection if no serum creatinine was collected on that day.

Percent of filtered glucose excreted in the urine

Percent of filtered glucose excreted in the urine was estimated for all collection intervals on Day 2 as follows:

$$(\text{Glucose Amount Excreted})/(\text{Clcr*PG*Time Interval}) \text{ or}$$
$$[\text{Urine glucose (mg/dL)*Serum Creatinine (mg/dL)}]/$$
$$[\text{urine creatinine (mg/dL)*PG(mg/dL)}]$$

where glucose amount excreted is the amount of glucose excreted during the xx-hour period, and CLcr is calculated for the xx-hour time interval. PG is the plasma glucose concentration reported closest to the midpoint of the time interval. Because only pre-dose PG was collected in this study, the pre-dose PG on Day 2 was used. Time interval is the number of minutes of urine collection for that interval.

Total fluid intake, urine volume, and fluid balance (intake minus output) were summarized over the 0–24-hour interval of Day 1 and Day 2 and the 0–12-hour interval of Day 3 of each treatment period.

Statistical analysis

The sample size was based on the primary endpoint, metformin $\text{AUCs}_{(0-12)}$ and assumed a within-subject standard deviation of 0.15 [33,34] for natural log-transformed AUC. Using the two one-sided t-test [35] at type I error $\alpha=0.05$ under a crossover design, 12 subjects should provide at least 90% power to demonstrate lack of an interaction if the ratio of test to reference is truly 1 and the equivalence criteria for the 90% confidence interval (CI) is 0.8–1.25.

Safety and PD parameters were summarized using descriptive statistics. Analyses of steady-state plasma metformin $\text{AUC}_{(0-12)}$ and C_{max} were conducted with metformin alone as the reference treatment. A mixed effect model with $\ln(\text{AUC}(0-12))$ as the dependent variable; treatment, period and sequence as fixed effects; and subject-within-sequence as a random effect was used to estimate the treatment difference and its associated 90% CI on the log scale. The PROC MIXED from SAS (Version 8.2, Cary, NC, USA) was used to fit the model. The estimates and the 90% CI were exponentiated in order to obtain the ratio of geometric means and its CI. The assumptions underlying the model were assessed by visual inspection of residual plots.

Similar analyses were performed for the secondary PK endpoints for remogliflozin etabonate, remogliflozin and its metabolite, with and without metformin. T_{max} was analysed non-parametrically using Hodges–Lehmann method [36,37].

Results

Thirteen subjects (7 females [54%] and 6 males [46%]) were randomized and completed the study. Of these 13 subjects, 10 subjects were being treated with metformin before study entry and three subjects were drug naive before study entry. The median age was 54 years (range 38 to 62 years); the median BMI was 29 kg/m^2 (range 22.5 to 34.3 kg/m^2); mean fasting plasma glucose at baseline was 7.21 mmol/L (SD 1.77; range 4.8 to 10.9 mmol/L). All subjects were Hispanic or Latino.

Pharmacokinetics

The summary data of PK parameters for metformin, remogliflozin etabonate, remogliflozin and GSK279782 are presented in Table 2. The primary PK objective was to demonstrate a lack of effect of remogliflozin etabonate on the PK parameters of metformin. Results from the primary comparison, are summarized in Table 3 and mean concentration vs time profiles are shown in Figure 1. There was no effect of remogliflozin etabonate on metformin PK parameters.

One of the secondary objectives included a comparison of PK parameters for remogliflozin etabonate, remogliflozin and GSK279782 after treatment with remogliflozin etabonate alone and with MET + RE. A summary of these

Table 2 Summary of plasma metformin, remogliflozin etabonate, remogliflozin, and GSK279782 PK parameters

Metformin PK parameter	MET BID	MET + RE BID
	N = 13	N = 13
$AUC_{(0-12)}$ (h.ng/mL)	7141.3 (24)	7520.8 (27)
C_{max} (ng/mL)	1018.2 (26)	1025.3 (25)
t_{max} (h)	4.0 (1.0 - 6.0)	4.0 (1.0–6.0)
Remogliflozin etabonate (prodrug) PK Parameter	**RE BID**	**MET + RE BID**
	N = 12-13[a]	N = 12-13[a]
$AUC_{(0-last)}$ (h.ng/mL)	98.9 (69)	102.1 (49)
C_{max} (ng/mL)	79.5 (107)	67.7 (77)
t_{max} (h)	3.0 (1.0–4.0)	3.0 (1.0–6.0)
Remogliflozin (active entity) PK Parameter	**RE BID**	**MET + RE BID**
	N = 13	N = 13
$AUC_{(0-12)}$ (h.ng/mL)	6814.3 (33)	6425.9 (33)
C_{max} (ng/mL)	2688.6 (52)	2124.6 (63)
t_{max} (h)	3.0 (1.0–4.0)	3.0 (1.0 - 6.0)
GSK279782 (active metabolite) PK Parameter	**RE BID**	**MET + RE BID**
	N = 13	N = 13
$AUC_{(0-12)}$ (h.ng/mL)	1527.9 (37)	1472.9 (36)
C_{max} (ng/mL)	462.8 (39)	361.9 (38)
t_{max} (h)	4.0 (1.0–4.0)	4.0 (1.0–8.0)

Values are geometric mean (%CVb) for each parameter, except for t_{max} which is median (range). PK, pharmacokinetic; MET BID, metformin 500 mg every 12 hours; MET + RE BID, metformin 500 mg + remogliflozin etabonate 500 mg every 12 hours; RE BID, remogliflozin etabonate 500 mg every 12 hours.
[a] AUC not evaluable for one subject.

results is presented in Table 3 and concentration vs. time profiles are provided in Figures 2, 3, 4. There were no effects of metformin on the AUC of remogliflozin etabonate, remogliflozin, or its metabolite, GSK279782. However, C_{max} was lower with the combination. For C_{max}, on average, there was a decrease of 21% in remogliflozin and a decrease of 22% in GSK279782 with MET + RE compared to remogliflozin etabonate alone. The 90% CI indicates that the true difference lies between a decrease of 40% and an increase of 5% for remogliflozin and between a decrease of 33% and 9% for GSK279782.

Pharmacodynamics

Fasting plasma glucose

A summary of the FPG concentration data by treatment period and study day is presented in Figure 5. When the changes in fasting plasma glucose concentrations from baseline (pre-dose on Day 1) to Day 2 and Day 3 were considered for the three treatment periods, it appeared that the fasting glucose concentrations remained relatively stable during the MET BID period, whereas small decreases were observed during both the RE BID and MET + RE BID treatment periods.

Table 3 Statistical comparisons of PK parameters of metformin, remogliflozin etabonate, remogliflozin, and GSK279782 with and without remogliflozin etabonate

Compound	PK parameter	Treatment comparison	Point estimate (GLSM Ratio)	90% CI
Metformin	AUC(0–12) [1]	MET + RE / MET	1.05	(0.98, 1.12)
	Cmax	MET + RE / MET	1.01	(0.92, 1.10)
Remogliflozin etabonate (prodrug)	$AUC_{(0-last)}$	MET + RE / RE	1.00	(0.77, 1.29)
	C_{max}	MET + RE / RE	0.85	(0.54, 1.35)
Remogliflozin (active entity)	$AUC_{(0-12)}$	MET + RE / RE	0.94	(0.86, 1.04)
	C_{max}	MET + RE / RE	0.79	(0.60, 1.05)
GSK279782 (active metabolite)	$AUC_{(0-12)}$	MET + RE / RE	0.96	(0.92, 1.01)
	C_{max}	MET + RE / RE	0.78	(0.67, 0.91)

[1] primary comparison; MET + RE, metformin 500 mg + remogliflozin etabonate 500 mg every 12 hours; GLSM : Geometric least-squares mean.

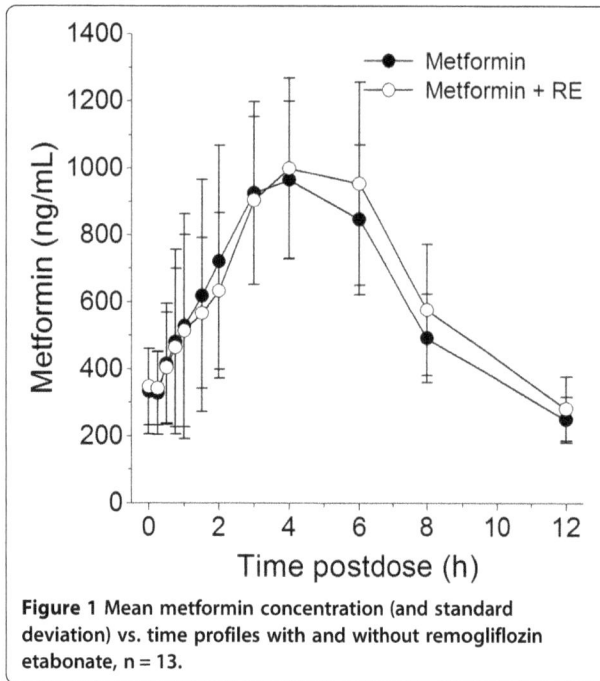

Figure 1 Mean metformin concentration (and standard deviation) vs. time profiles with and without remogliflozin etabonate, n = 13.

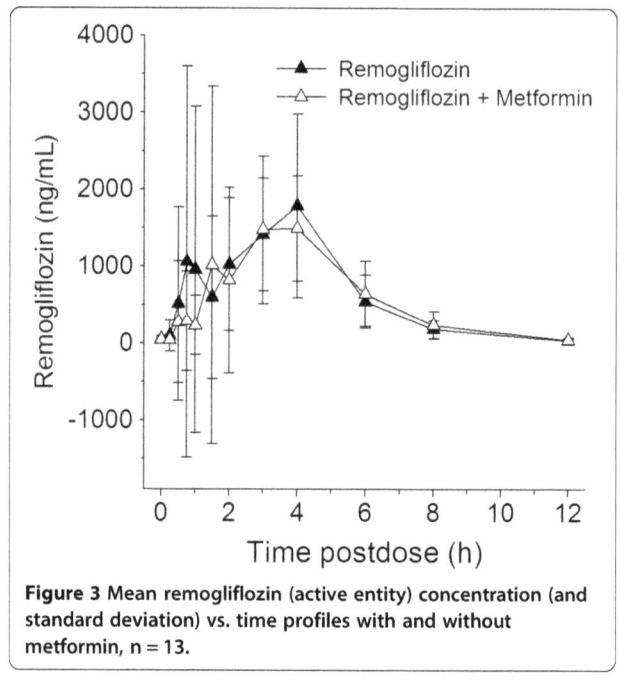

Figure 3 Mean remogliflozin (active entity) concentration (and standard deviation) vs. time profiles with and without metformin, n = 13.

Urinary glucose excretion and percent of filtered glucose excreted

Mean cumulative 24-hour urinary glucose excretion was approximately 500 mmol following treatment with RE BID or MET + RE BID (Day 2), whereas MET BID had relatively no effect on urine glucose output (Table 4).

The effect of remogliflozin etabonate on urine glucose excretion was not diminished by co-administration with metformin. The greatest increase in urine glucose excretion was evident within the first 4 hours of dosing following both remogliflozin etabonate regimens. The 24-hour creatinine clearance on Day 2 was comparable across the three treatment periods and was approximately 110 mL/min. During the RE BID and MET + RE BID periods, mean and median values for the percent

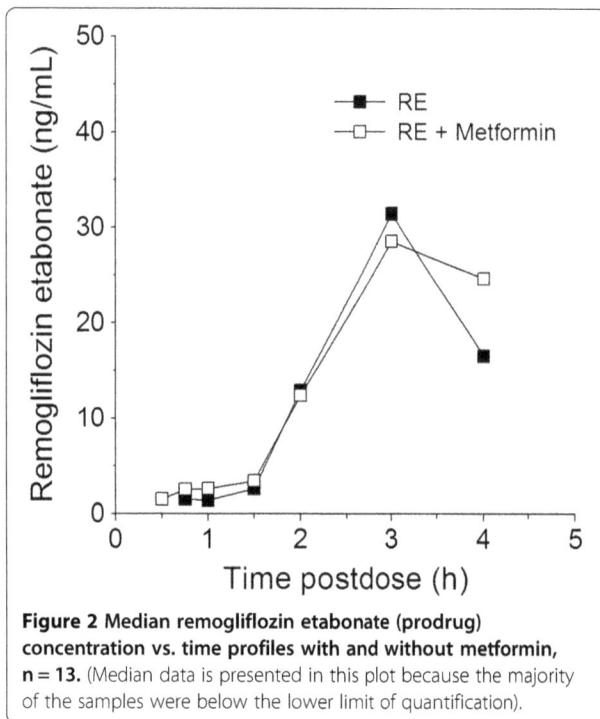

Figure 2 Median remogliflozin etabonate (prodrug) concentration vs. time profiles with and without metformin, n = 13. (Median data is presented in this plot because the majority of the samples were below the lower limit of quantification).

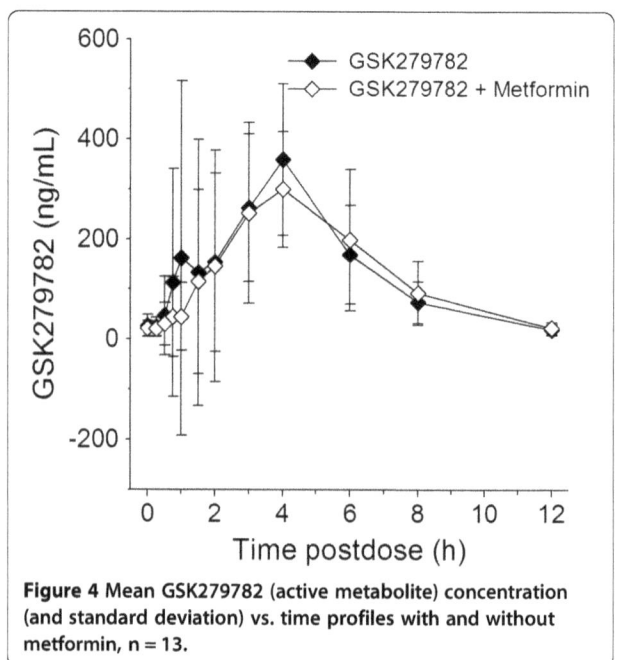

Figure 4 Mean GSK279782 (active metabolite) concentration (and standard deviation) vs. time profiles with and without metformin, n = 13.

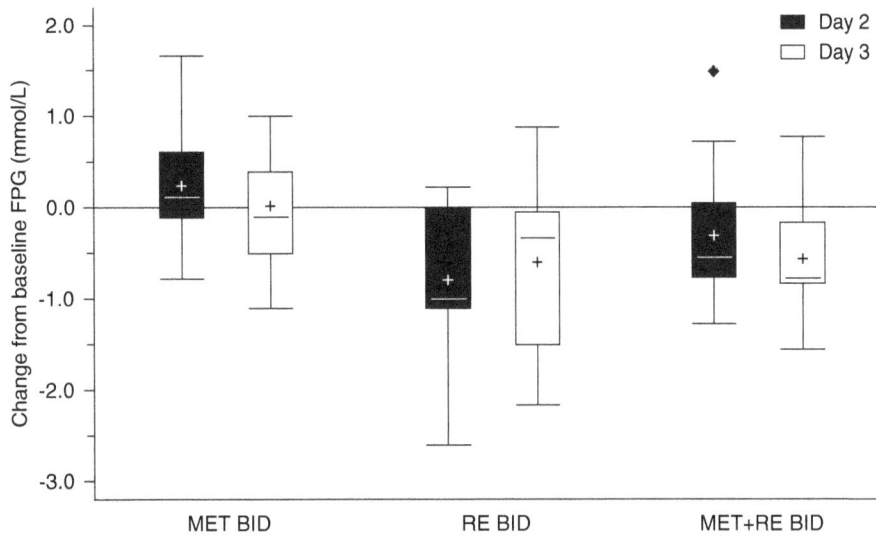

Figure 5 Fasting plasma glucose concentration (FPG; mmol/L) – Change from baseline (pre- dose on Day 1 of each treatment period).
MET BID, metformin 500 mg every 12 hours; RE BID, remogliflozin etabonate 500 mg every 12 hours; MET + RE BID, metformin 500 mg + remogliflozin etabonate 500 mg every 12 hours. Mean (and standard deviation) baseline FPG values for each treatment period: MET BID: 6.72 (1.88); RE BID, 6.98 (2.06); MET + RE BID, 6.42 (1.15).

of filtered glucose excreted in the urine ranged from 43% up to 68% during the individual collection intervals, with a mean of approximately 50% for the combined 24 hour collection for both remogliflozin etabonate containing regimens compared to 1.4% with metformin alone (Table 5).

Fluid balance
Total fluid intake, total urine volume, and fluid balance data for the 24-hour collection intervals on Days 1 and 2 and the initial 12-hour collection interval on Day 3 were compared by treatment. On Days 1 and 2, mean total 24-hour fluid intake ranged from approximately 2500 mL to 3000 mL across the three treatment periods. During the 12-hour collection period on Day 3, mean fluid intake ranged from approximately 1800 to 2200 mL for any one treatment period. Because fluid intake was less than total urine volume throughout all treatment periods, mean fluid balance values were considered negative during most intervals. On Day 1, fluid balance (median, range) appeared more negative on RE BID (-1145 mL, -1630 to +335 mL)

and MET + RE BID (−1200 mL, -2395 to −90 mL) compared to MET BID (−775 mL, -2280 to +400 mL). Fluid balance neutrality seemed to be reached on Day 3 for all drug regimens.

Safety and tolerability
There were no serious adverse events reported. The only adverse event considered related to study drug was hypoglycemic symptoms reported by 2 subjects, one event with metformin alone and one with MET + RE. However, plasma glucose measurements were unfortunately not performed to confirm hypoglycemia. In both cases, the symptoms of hypoglycemia were considered mild in intensity. The events were reported in the time before scheduled meals; the symptoms resolved with provision of food, and did not require a change in study drug. Back pain and headache were the only events reported by more than one subject during any treatment period (reported during MET BID by 2 different subjects). All adverse events are summarized in Table 6.

Table 4 Summary of 24-hour urine glucose (mmol) on day 2 by treatment

	Met BID N = 13	RE BID N = 13	Met + RE BID N = 13
Mean (SD)	13.6 (13.4)	528 (130)	458 (98)
Median	10.9	497	485
Min, Max	1.1, 43.9	384, 796	242, 573

Table 5 Summary of percent filtered glucose excreted in urine on day 2 by treatment

	Met BID N = 13	RE BID N = 13	Met + RE BID N = 13
Mean (SD)	1.41 (1.52)	51.3 (7.02)	48.7 (9.87)
Median	0.95	51.8	49.3
Min, Max	0.10, 4.71	38.4, 61.3	35.7, 67.9

Table 6 Summary of adverse events by treatment

Preferred term	MET BID	RE BID	MET + RE BID
	N = 13	N = 13	N = 13
	n (%)	n (%)	n (%)
Any Event	5 (38%)	2 (15%)	7 (54%)
Headache	2 (15%)	0	1 (8%)
Back pain	2 (15%)	0	0
Muscle spasms	1 (8%)	1 (8%)	0
Hypoglycemia	1 (8%)	0	1 (8%)
Neck pain	1 (8%)	0	0
Osteoarthritis	0	0	1 (8%)
Abdominal pain upper	0	1 (8%)	0
Dyspepsia	0	0	1 (8%)
Toothache	1 (8%)	0	0
Dizziness	1 (8%)	0	0
Fatigue	1 (8%)	0	0
Nasopharyngitis	0	0	1 (8%)
Wound	0	0	1 (8%)
Rash	0	0	1 (8%)

No clinically significant changes in laboratory parameters or vital signs were reported for any treatment regimen. As an increased exposure to metformin can result in lactic acidosis, lactic acid levels were measured. While there were no instances of lactic acidosis, a trend toward increasing lactic acid was observed with metformin monotherapy relative to regimens including remogliflozin (Figure 6).

Discussion

Despite the availability of multiple classes and combinations of antihyperglycemic agents, the clinical management of T2DM is currently suboptimal, with the majority of patients failing to achieve and maintain target glycemic levels in practice [38]. Consequently, there is a continued need for novel therapeutic approaches, particularly those with complementary modes of action that will enable further improvement of glycemic control.

Remogliflozin etabonate, by inhibiting glucose reabsorption, offers a potential treatment for T2DM as monotherapy and in combination with existing therapies. Remogliflozin etabonate is being developed for use for the treatment of T2DM as monotherapy, and in combination with existing therapies including metformin. In this study, no effect of remogliflozin etabonate on metformin PK parameters was observed. The findings from this study are consistent with the reported lack of inhibition by remogliflozin etabonate, remogliflozin, and GSK279782 on a panel of metabolic enzymes and transporters, including organic cation transporters involved with metformin renal secretion [39].

This study was not adequately powered to test the effect of metformin on remogliflozin etabonate PK parameters. Metformin did not appear to affect the AUC of remogliflozin etabonate, remogliflozin and its metabolite; however, C_{max} was lower after the co-administration of remogliflozin etabonate and metformin than with remogliflozin etabonate alone. Under the conditions of this study, the peak plasma concentration of remogliflozin considerably exceeded the concentration required for full

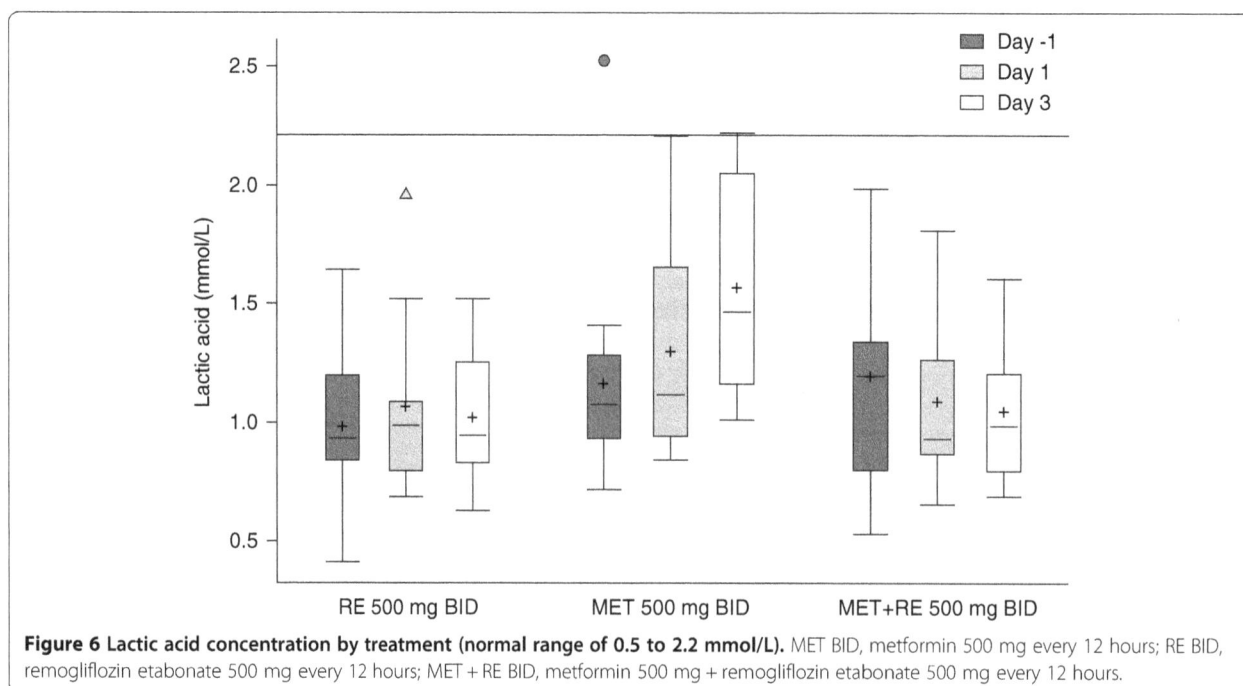

Figure 6 Lactic acid concentration by treatment (normal range of 0.5 to 2.2 mmol/L). MET BID, metformin 500 mg every 12 hours; RE BID, remogliflozin etabonate 500 mg every 12 hours; MET + RE BID, metformin 500 mg + remogliflozin etabonate 500 mg every 12 hours.

inhibition of the SGLT2 transporter. However, it is possible that a clinically significant decrease would be observed when administering the combination if low doses of remogliflozin etabonate or considerably higher doses of metformin were given.

As expected on the basis of its pharmacological properties, the administration of remogliflozin etabonate with or without metformin greatly increased urine glucose excretion and the percent of filtered glucose excreted in the urine. The evidence of pharmacological effect was seen within the first 4 hours of dosing with remogliflozin etabonate and sustained while on treatment. Co-administration of metformin with remogliflozin etabonate did not diminish the glucosuric effect of remogliflozin etabonate. Only small changes in fasting glucose concentration were observed during both the RE BID and MET + RE BID treatment periods for this cohort of subjects with good glucose control. Mean fasting glucose concentrations were <7 mmol/L on Day −1 of each treatment period, leaving little room for substantial improvement.

Concomitant administration of remogliflozin etabonate with metformin for 3 days was well tolerated in subjects with T2DM. Hypoglycemia was the only adverse event that was considered related to study drug (and occurred with metformin alone, as well as with the combination). However, neither case was confirmed with plasma glucose concentrations. Antidiabetic treatments that increase urine glucose may increase risk of urinary tract infections (UTIs); however, no documented UTIs were observed over the limited duration of remogliflozin etabonate treatment in this study. Mean lactate concentrations showed an increase or increasing trend during the three day MET BID treatment period. In contrast, mean lactate concentrations are unchanged or decreased slightly during RE BID and MET + RE BID periods. Potential mechanisms to explain the decreased lactate concentrations include reduced glucose concentrations with less production from glycolysis, enhanced extraction of lactic acid by the liver for gluconeogenesis or increased clearance of lactic acid by the kidney. No symptoms suggestive of lactic acidosis occurred during the study.

Conclusions

In summary, the findings of this study do not indicate a safety concern when multiple oral doses of remogliflozin etabonate 500 mg are administered with metformin 500 mg BID in the intended patient population. Because remogliflozin etabonate does not affect the PK profile of metformin, there is a low risk for adverse events resulting from a PK drug interaction and increased metformin exposure. The approximate 20% decline in remogliflozin Cmax under conditions of coadministration is likely a reflection of the 15% decline in the Cmax of the prodrug

(RE) when given with metformin (Table 3). It appears that metformin reduces the Cmax of RE without an effect on RE AUC, suggesting a change in the shape of the 12-hour, steady state, concentration-time profile. Even though the confidence interval is wide for the prodrug Cmax point estimate (0.54, 1.35) and contains 1.0, it is plausible that coadministration of metformin altered GI motility enough to affect the absorption or hydrolysis of RE resulting in a lower Cmax of RE. The lower Cmax values for remogliflozin and GKS279782 following dosing with metformin collectively support this conclusion since they are downstream metabolites of RE.

Although administration with metformin resulted in a 21% reduction in C_{max}, the PD properties of remogliflozin etabonate were not altered when administered with metformin. There was an indication that remogliflozin etabonate alone improves plasma blood glucose by increasing the excretion of urine glucose, and this effect by remogliflozin etabonate was not impaired by the co-administration of metformin. Future studies in a larger patient population are warranted to definitively test the safety and efficacy of remogliflozin etabonate in combination with metformin in patients with T2DM who have not achieved the desired glycemic target.

Competing interests
At the time of study, EKH, AK, ROCS, WT, BR, JWP, CJ, and RLD are employees of GlaxoSmithKline.

Authors' contributions
EKH, AK, ROCS, WT, BR, JWP, CJ, and RLD participated in the design of the study, its co-ordination and performed the statistical analysis. All authors were involved in critically revising the drafts of the manuscript, and read and approved the final manuscript.

Acknowledgements
The authors would like to acknowledge Drs. Jorge Poo and Esteban Rios, clinical investigators (Medica Sur Hospital and Clinical Foundation, CIF-BIOTEC, Mexico City, Mexico) for their efforts in conduct of this clinical study. Editorial assistance in the preparation of this manuscript was provided by Katie Green, International Medical Press, funded by GlaxoSmithKline.

Author details
[1]GlaxoSmithKline, 5 Moore Drive, Research Triangle Park, NC 27709, USA.
[2]Tandem Labs, Durham, NC, USA.

References
1.   DCCT Research Group: The relationship of glycemic exposure (HbA1c) to the risk of development and progression of retinopathy in the Diabetes Control and Complications Trial. *Diabetes* 1995, **44**:968–983.
2.   Ohkubo Y, Kishikawa H, Araki E, Miyata T, Isami S, Motoyoshi S, Kojima Y, Furuyoshi N, Shichiri M: Intensive insulin therapy prevents the progression of diabetic microvascular complications in Japanese patients with non-insulin-dependent diabetes mellitus: a randomized prospective 6-year study. *Diabetes Res Clin Pract* 1995, **28**:103–117.
3.   Stratton IM, Adler AI, Neil HA, Matthews DR, Manley SE, Cull CA, Hadden D, Turner RC, Holman RR: Association of glycaemia with macrovascular and microvascular complications of type 2 diabetes (UKPDS 35): prospective observational study. *Br Med J* 2000, **321**:405–412.

4. UK Prospective Diabetes Study (UKPDS) Group: **Effect of intensive blood-glucose control with metformin on complications in overweight patients with type 2 diabetes (UKPDS 34).** *Lancet* 1998, **352:**854–865.

5. UK Prospective Diabetes Study (UKPDS) Group: **Intensive blood-glucose control with sulphonylureas or insulin compared with conventional treatment and risk of complications in patients with type 2 diabetes (UKPDS 33).** *Lancet* 1998, **352:**837–853.

6. American Diabetes Association: **Standards of medical care in diabetes.** In *PhD Thesis*; 2007.

7. Nathan D, Buse J, Davidson M, Heine R, Holman R, Sherwin R, Zinman B: **Management of hyperglycaemia in type 2 diabetes: a consensus algorithm for the initiation and adjustment of therapy.** *Diabetologia* 2006, **49:**1711–1721.

8. Scheen AJ: **Clinical pharmacokinetics of metformin.** *Clin Pharmacokinet* 1996, **30:**359–371.

9. Graham GG, Punt J, Arora M, Day R, Doogue MP, Duopng JK, Furlong TJ, Greenfield JR, Greenup LC, Kirkpatrick CM, Ray JE, Timmins P, Williams KM: **Clinical pharmacokinetics of metformin.** *Clin Pharmacokinet* 2011, **50:**81–98.

10. Scheen AJ: **Drug interactions of clinical importance with antihyperglycaemic agents: an update.** *Drug Saf* 2005, **28:**601–631.

11. Bodmer M, Meier C, Krahenbuhl S, Jick SS, Meier CR: **Metformin, sulfonylureas, or other antidiabetes drugs and the risk of lactic acidosis or hypoglycemia: a nested case–control analysis.** *Diabetes Care* 2008, **31:**2086–2091.

12. Davis TM, Jackson D, Davis WA, Bruce DG, Chubb P: **The relationship between metformin therapy and the fasting plasma lactate in type 2 diabetes: the fremantle diabetes study.** *Br J Clin Pharmacol* 2001, **52:**137–144.

13. Salpeter SR, Greyber E, Pasternak GA, Salpeter EE: **Risk of fatal and nonfatal lactic acidosis with metformin use in type 2 diabetes mellitus: systematic review and meta-analysis.** *Arch Intern Med* 2003, **163:**2594–2602.

14. Kanai Y, Lee WS, You G, Brown D, Hediger MA: **The human kidney low affinity Na+/glucose cotransporter SGLT2. Delineation of the major renal reabsorptive mechanism for D-glucose.** *J Clin Invest* 1994, **93:**397–404.

15. Wright EM, Hirayama BA, Loo DF: **Active sugar transport in health and disease.** *J Intern Med* 2007, **261:**32–43.

16. Handlon AL: **Sodium glucose co-transporter 2 (SGLT2) inhibitors as potential antidiabetic agents.** *Expert Opin Ther Pat* 2005, **13:**1531–1540.

17. Hussey E, Clark R, Amin D, Kipnes M, O'Connor-Semmes R, O'Driscoll E, Leong J, Murray S, Dobbins R, Layko D, *et al:* **The single-dose pharmacokinetics and pharmacodynamics of sergliflozin etabonate, a novel inhibitor of glucose reabsorption, in healthy volunteers and subjects with type 2 diabetes mellitus.** *J Clin Pharmacol* 2010, **50:**623–635.

18. Hussey EK, Dobbins RL, Stoltz RR, Stockman NL, O'Connor-Semmes RL, Kapur A, Murray SC, Layko D, Nunez DJR: **Multiple-dose pharmacokinetics and pharmacodynamics of sergliflozin etabonate, a novel inhibitor of glucose reabsorption, in healthy overweight and obese subjects: a randomized double-blind study.** *J Clin Pharmacol* 2010, **50:**636–646.

19. Idris I, Donnelly R: **Sodium-glucose co-transporter-2 inhibitors: an emerging new class of oral antidiabetic drug.** *Diabetes Obes Metab* 2009, **11:**79–88.

20. Isaji M: **Sodium-glucose cotransporter inhibitors for diabetes.** *Curr Opin Investig Drugs* 2007, **8:**285–292.

21. Komoroski B, Vachharajani N, Feng Y, Li L, Kornhauser D, Pfister M: **Dapagliflozin, a novel, selective SGLT2 inhibitor, improved glycemic control over 2 weeks in patients with type 2 diabetes mellitus.** *Clin Pharmacol Ther* 2009, **85:**513–519.

22. Komoroski B, Vachharajani N, Boulton D, Kornhauser D, Geraldes M, Li L, Pfister M: **Dapagliflozin, a novel SGLT2 inhibitor, induces dose-dependent glucosuria in healthy subjects.** *Clin Pharmacol Ther* 2009, **85:**520–526.

23. Asano T, Ogihara T, Katagiri H, Sakoda H, Ono H, Fujishiro M, Anai M, Kurihara H, Uchijima Y: **Glucose transporter and Na+/glucose cotransporter as molecular targets of anti-diabetic drugs.** *Curr Med Chem* 2004, **11:**2717–2724.

24. Ehrenkranz JR, Lewis NG, Kahn CR, Roth J: **Phlorizin: a review.** *Diabetes Metab Res Rev* 2005, **21:**31–38.

25. Katsuno K, Fujimori Y, Takemura Y, Hiratochi M, Itoh F, Komatsu Y, Fujikura H, Isaji M: **Sergliflozin, a novel selective inhibitor of low-affinity sodium glucose cotransporter (SGLT2), validates the critical role of SGLT2 in renal glucose reabsorption and modulates plasma glucose level.** *J Pharmacol Exp Ther* 2007, **320:**323–330.

26. Jabbour SA, Goldstein BJ: **Sodium glucose co-transporter 2 inhibitors: blocking renal tubular reabsorption of glucose to improve glycaemic control in patients with diabetes.** *Int J Clin Pract* 2008, **62:**1279–1284.

27. Fujimori Y, Katsuno K, Nakashima I, Ishikawa-Takemura Y, Fujikura H, Isaji M: **Remogliflozin etabonate, in a novel category of selective low-affinity sodium glucose cotransporter (SGLT2) inhibitors, exhibits antidiabetic efficacy in rodent models.** *J Pharmacol Exp Ther* 2008, **327:**268–276.

28. Sigafoos J, Bowers G, Castellino S, Culp AG, Wagner DS, Reese JM, Humphreys JE, Hussey EK, O'Connor-Semmes RL, Kapur A, Tao W, Dobbins RL, Polli JW: **Assessment of the drug interaction risk for remogliflozin etabonate, a sodium-dependent glucose cotransporter-2 inhibitor: evidence from in vitro, human mass balance, and ketoconazole interaction studies.** *Drug Metab Dispos* 2012, **40:**2090–2101.

29. Dobbins R, Kapur A, Kapitza C, O'Connor-Semmes R, Tao W, Hussey E: **Remogliflozin etabonate, a selective inhibitor of the sodium-glucose transporter 2 (SCLT2) reduces serum glucose in type 2 diabetes mellitus (T2DM) patients.** *Diabetes* 2009, **58:**1573-P.

30. Kapur A, O'Connor-Semmes R, Hussey E, Dobbins R, Tao W, Hompesch M, Nunez D: **First human dose escalation study with remogliflozin etabonate (RE) in healthy subjects and in subjects with type 2 diabetes mellitus (T2DM).** *Diabetes* 2009, **58:**509-P.

31. Sung EY, Moore MP, Lunt H, Doogue M, Zhang M, Begg EJ: **Do thiazide diuretics alter the pharmacokinetics of metformin in patients with type 2 diabetes already established on metformin?** *Br J Clin Pharmacol* 2009, **67:**130–131.

32. Thurman J, Wiseman A: **The patient with glomerulonephritis or vasculitis.** In *Manual of Nephrology*. 7th edition. Edited by Schrier RW. Philadelphia: Lippincott Williams & Wilkins; 2009:140–153.

33. Saffar F, Aiache JM, Andre P: **Influence of food on the disposition of the antidiabetic drug metformin in diabetic patients at steady-state.** *Methods Find Exp Clin Pharmacol* 1995, **17:**483–487.

34. Timmins P, Donahue S, Meeker J, Marathe P: **Steady-state pharmacokinetics of a novel extended-release metformin formulation.** *Clin Pharmacokinet* 2005, **44:**721–729.

35. Schuirmann DJ: **A comparison of the two one-sided tests procedure and the power approach for assessing the equivalence of average bioavailability.** *J Pharmacokinet Biopharm* 1987, **15:**657–680.

36. Hauschke D, Steinijans VW, Diletti E: **A distribution-free procedure for the statistical analysis of bioequivalence studies.** *Int J Clin Pharmacol Ther Toxicol* 1990, **28:**72–78.

37. Hollander M, Wolfe DA: *Nonparametric Statistical Methods*. New York: Wiley; 1973.

38. Del Prato S, Felton A-M, Munro N, Nesto R, Zimmet P, Zinman B, on behalf of the Global Partnership for Effective Diabetes Management: **Improving glucose management: ten steps to get more patients with type 2 diabetes to goal. Recommendations from the Global Partnership for Effective Diabetes Management.** *Int J Clin Pract* 2005, **59:**1345–1355.

39. Polli JW, Humphreys JE, Harmon KA, Webster LO, Reese MJ, MacLauchlin CC: **Assessment of remogliflozin etabonate, a sodium-dependent glucose co-transporter-2 inhibitor, as a perpetrator of clinical drug interactions: a study on drug transporters and metabolic enzymes.** *J Diabetes Metab* 2012, **3:**5. http://dx.doi.org/10.4172/2155-6156.1000200.

13

Adherence to medication for the treatment of psychosis: rates and risk factors in an Ethiopian population

Menna Alene[1], Michael D Wiese[2], Mulugeta T Angamo[3], Beata V Bajorek[4], Elias A Yesuf[1] and Nasir Tajure Wabe[3*]

Abstract

Background: Medication-taking behavior, specifically non-adherence, is significantly associated with treatment outcome and is a major cause of relapse in the treatment of psychotic disorders. Non-adherence can be multifactorial; however, the rates and associated risk factors in an Ethiopian population have not yet been elucidated. The principal aim of this study was to evaluate adherence rates to antipsychotic medications, and secondarily to identify potential factors associated with non-adherence, among psychotic patients at tertiary care teaching hospital in Southwest Ethiopia.

Methods: A cross-sectional study was conducted over a 2-month period in 2009 (January 15th to March 20th) at the Jimma University Specialized Hospital. Adherence was computed using both a compliant fill rate method and self-reporting via a structured patient interview (focusing on how often regular medication doses were missed altogether, and whether they missed taking their doses on time). Data were analyzed using SPSS for windows version 16.0, and chi-square and Pearsons r tests were used to determine the statistical significance of the association of variables with adherence.

Result: Three hundred thirty six patients were included in the study. A total of 75.6% were diagnosed with schizophrenia, while the others were diagnosed with other psychotic disorders. Most (88.1%) patients were taking only antipsychotics, while the remainder took more than one medication. Based upon the compliant fill rate, 57.5% of prescription fills were considered compliant, but only 19.6% of participants had compliant fills for all of their prescriptions. In contrast, on the basis of patients self-report, 52.1% of patients reported that they had *never* missed a medication dose, 32.0% *sometimes* missed their daily doses, 22.0% only missed taking their dose at the specific scheduled time, and 5.9% missed *both* taking their dose at the specific scheduled time and *sometimes* missed their daily doses. The most common reasons provided for missing medication doses were: forgetfulness (36.2%); being busy (21.0%); and a lack of sufficient information about the medication (10.0%). Pill burden, medication side-effects, social drug use, and duration of maintenance therapy each had a statistically significant association with medication adherence (P ≤ 0.05).

Conclusion: The observed rate of antipsychotic medication adherence in this study was low, and depending upon the definition used to determine adherence, it is either consistent or low compared to previous reports, which highlights its pervasive and problematic nature. Adherence must therefore be considered when planning treatment strategies with antipsychotic medications, particularly in countries such as Ethiopia.

Keywords: Medication adherence, Antipsychotic, Compliant fill rate, Jimma

* Correspondence: nasir.wabe@ju.edu.et
3Clinical Pharmacy Unit, Pharmacy Department, College of Public Health and Medical Science, Jimma University, Jimma, Ethiopia
Full list of author information is available at the end of the article

Background

Medication adherence relates to a patient's medication-taking behavior, and specifically refers to the extent to which a patient follows the mutually agreed treatment plan. Non-adherence to medication is known to be associated with poorer treatment outcomes, particularly in the management of chronic disease, yet numerous clinical studies have reported an average adherence rate of only 43.1% to 78.0% among patients receiving treatment for various conditions.

In the treatment and management of psychotic disorders, non-adherence to medication is particularly problematic. Antipsychotic medications are effective in treating psychiatric problems, including schizophrenia; however, the maximum benefit that a patient derives from these medications is highly dependent on their adherence to treatment [1]. The favorable rates of relapse prevention reported in controlled trials cannot usually be applied to everyday practice, due to poorer adherence in the 'real world' setting; as highlighted by Cramer and Rosenheck [2], outside of clinical trial settings, the average rate of adherence to antipsychotic regimens is only 58%.

Although non-adherence is a ubiquitous problem in medicine [3], the nature of schizophrenia and other psychotic disorders makes it especially difficult for patients to adhere to treatment [4]. First, schizophrenia is an illness in which insight into the condition, and therefore need for treatment, is more likely to be impaired compared to other illnesses [5]; this lack of insight has been shown to be associated with non-adherence to medications [6-8] and other psychosocial treatment [9]. Second, disorganization and cognitive impairment are additional symptoms of schizophrenia that interfere with medication management [10-12], particularly over the long-term given the chronic nature of the illness. In general, the more prolonged the medication treatment period, the lower the rates of adherence, and this has been reported in other chronic diseases [13]. Furthermore, the greater the exposure to treatment the more likely the patient is to experience side-effects, increasing the patient's reluctance to adhere to treatment; unfortunately, the advent of atypical antipsychotics has not significantly reduced the potential for adverse drug events [14,15]. Finally, schizophrenia and its treatment (antipsychotics) are subject to stigma [16].

The impact of medication non-adherence on clinical outcomes in the treatment of schizophrenia is significant, as studies have shown that deviation from maintenance antipsychotic treatment leads to disease relapse, increased clinic and emergency room visits, and re-hospitalization [17,18]. Furthermore, mortality in persons with schizophrenia is two to four times greater than that in the general population [19,20], which is in part

due to the out-right increased risk of suicide, but also to non-adherence to treatment for both the psychosis as well as other underlying physical illnesses [21]. Subsequently, this compromises the individual's quality of life and function, and increases the economic burden to the health-system [22].

In Ethiopia, due to the under-resourced health-care system, medication non-adherence rates are potentially much higher, thereby contributing to a substantial worsening of disease, increased mortality, and increased health care costs [4]. Given the significance of this as a health issue and the scarcity of data to inform the scope of this problem in the local setting, the primary aim of this study was to evaluate adherence rates to antipsychotic medications, and secondarily to identify possible reasons for non-adherence to medications, among patients with psychosis in Jimma University Specialized Hospital in Southwest Ethiopia.

Methods

Study design

A cross-sectional study was conducted over a 2-month period in 2009 (January 15th to March 20th), on the internal medicine ward of the Jimma University Specialized Hospital (JUSH), which is the only referral hospital in the Oromia Regional State of South West Ethiopia. The adherence rate to anti-psychotic medications and identification of possible reasons for non- adherence was evaluated using patients self-reporting and pharmacy refill record. JUSH has four major in-patient wards: internal medicine (where psychiatric patients receive their treatment), surgery, pediatrics, and gynecology and obstetrics, and additionally provides ambulance/emergency services, pharmacy, outpatient services, blood bank, and diagnostics (e.g., laboratory, X-ray, ultrasound scanner, electrocardiogram).

Patient selection

Since psychiatric patients receive their treatment in the internal medicine ward of the hospital, patients of the internal medicine ward were eligible for inclusion. All patients who were prescribed antipsychotics within a 3-month time period were identified and consecutive patients meeting selection criteria were approached about inclusion in the study. The sample was restricted to patients with a diagnosis of schizophrenia, schizoaffective disorder, mood disorder with psychotic features, or psychosis not otherwise specified. Patients must have received maintenance therapy for at least 3 months to be included in the study. Excluded were patients who were taking anti-psychotic medication for non-psychotic mood disorders (e.g. disorders or behavioral disorders secondary to other diseases), patients who had started antipsychotic medication within the past 3 months, and patients below the age of 10.

Data collection

Adherence to prescribed medication regimens was determined with a quantitative, structured questionnaire. Face and content validity of the questionnaires were assessed through in-depth discussion with three experienced faculty colleagues and five senior internists in the internal medicine department at the study site. In addition, the questionnaires were pre-tested to minimize ambiguity and ensure the completeness of data capture. The result of the pretest was not included in the final analysis. Patients who were refilling a prescription were interviewed with the developed questionnaire. Using this questionnaire, a patient who reported that they had never missed either a daily dose or the time of taking a dose was considered to be adherent.

Medication adherence was also assessed by the compliant fill rate (CFR) method [23]. CFR represents the proportion of total fills that are adherent, i.e., filled at time-appropriate intervals over a specified time period. Adherence was assessed by comparing the number of days of medication supply with the number of calendar days between fills. A prescription fill was considered adherent if it took place before the completion of the previous prescription and there was no more than 20% of the medication still with the patient [23,24]. For example, if a patient received 60 tablets on a prescription and was instructed to take one tablet a day, the fill would be considered adherent if the patient collected the subsequent prescription within 48–60 days of the previous one. An exception was when a prescription became invalid because of a change in therapy. In such cases, the medication was either prematurely or delayed in being filled, but the fill was considered adherent.

Medication profiles were also examined to calculate the number of scheduled oral daily medications and the total number of prescribed tablets or capsules prescribed per day. If a patient was prescribed more than one agent for a disorder, adherence rates for all medications were calculated and the agent with the highest non-adherence was recorded and used for data analysis.

Sample size

Since there have been no previous study of medication adherence in Ethiopia, a prevalence rate (p) of 50%, confidence interval of 95% and margin of error (d) of 5% were used for sample size calculation. The sample size was calculated using the $[Z^2 * p * (1-p)]/d^2$ formula, where Z is the standard normal confidence internal (1.96). Accordingly, the appropriate sample size was calculated as 384.

Data analysis

Data were coded, checked for completeness and consistency, and analyzed using SPSS Version 16.0. Descriptive statistics were used to determine patient demographics, medication information, and adherence rates. The association between variables was calculated with Chi-square test of association and Pearsons r test where appropriate.

Ethics

The proposal was reviewed and approved by the ethical clearance committee of Jimma University. The aims of the study were provided to potential participants and informed consent was obtained prior to inclusion in the study.

Results

Socio demographic characteristics of patients

Among three hundred and eighty four participants who were approached regarding the study, 336 were included, resulting in a response rate of 87.5%. Of the remainder, 48 either did not fulfill the inclusion criteria, or give written consent for inclusion in the study. The cohort was comprised of 54.8% males with a mean age of 35 +/− 11.9 years. The majority of the study subjects were Orthodox Christian by religion and 26.5% were unemployed (Table 1).

Clinical characteristics of the patient

Amongst study participants, 75.6% were diagnosed with schizophrenia, 9.2% with schizoaffective disorder while the rest as mood disorder with psychotic features (11.9%) and psychosis not otherwise specified (3.3%). Most of the participants were taking only antipsychotics (88.1%), while 6.8% were taking antipsychotics and antidepressant, 3.9% antipsychotics and mood stabilizers and 1.2% a combination of antipsychotics, antidepressant and mood stabilizers. Participants attended for a medical checkup and prescription refill at 2 monthly intervals, during which time the pill counts, structured questionnaires and CFR analysis took place.

In relation to pill burden (in terms of the overall number of medications prescribed), the majority (74.0%) of patients were prescribed only one agent, 24.7% were taking two agents, and 1.4% were using three agents; the vast majority (96%) of doses were prescribed as once-daily dosing regimens.

In relation to the patients' experiences of side-effects with their medications, 44.1% reported ongoing depression, 14.7% experienced weight gain, 8.8% had extra-pyramidal side-effects; nearly a quarter (23.5%) of patients reported experiencing multiple side-effects. Among those patients who experienced side-effects, when asked about what measures they had taken to avoid the side-effects,

Table 1 Socio demographic characteristics of study participants

S.No.	Socio-demographic	Characteristics	Frequency	Percent
1	Gender	Male	185	54.8
		Female	151	45.5
2	Age (in years)	10-20	57	17.5
		21-30	109	33,6
		31-40	74	22.7
		41-50	58	18.0
		50+	37	8.1
3	Marital status	Never married	151	44.9
		Married	137	40.7
		Divorced	24	7.2
		Widowed	24	7.2
4	Living Condition	With family	300	89.9
		Living alone	19	5.5
		Others	17	4.5
5	Educational status	Diploma &above	62	18.3
		10-12 grade	117	34.7
		7-10 grade	71	21
		1-6 grade	33	9.6
		No formal schooling	53	13.2
6	Occupational status	Unemployed	89	26.5
		Private NGO	63	18.9
		Government	52	15.5
		Farmer	39	11.4
		Student	28	8.2
		Merchant	19	5.5
		Others	46	13.2
7	Religion	Orthodox	145	42.9
		Muslim	83	24.7
		Protestant	81	24. 2
		Catholic	13	3.7
		Others	14	4.6
8	Monthly income (In birr)	300+	108	32.1
		200-300	81	24.1
		100-200	72	21.5
		< 100	75	22.3

87.2% responded that they did nothing, 3.2% of them stopped taking their doses, 4.6% informed their health professional/s, 4.1% told their family members, and 0.5% stopped going to work. Most (95.9%) of patients responded that they felt comfortable in openly discussing their medication issues with their health professional/s (e.g., pharmacists, doctors, nurses and others).

Most patients (72.6%) reported that they had no previous exposure to any *social/ recreational* drugs. Among those who had been exposed to these agents, khat (n = 83), cigarette (n = 28), and alcohol (n = 20), were most commonly reported by the patients. Among social/ recreational drug users, 34% reported feeling depressed, 13.2% felt that their illness had worsened, and 18.9% reported feeling 'different' when they stopped using social/ recreational drugs.

Adherence rate and factors associated with non-adherence

Adherence to antipsychotic medications was measured when patients presented for prescription (medication) refills and medical check-ups (outpatient clinic visits) every two months.

Patient's self-reported adherence to medication

Approximately half (52.1%) of patients stated that they had *never* missed taking their prescribed medication, which included neither missing the daily dose outright nor missing the instructed time of dose administration. A small proportion (5.9%) of patients reported that they *sometimes* missed taking their medications in relation to either taking the daily dose outright and/or missing the instructed time of dose administration. Among those who reported that they had missed taking their medication, the most common reason (36.2%) for not taking doses was *forgetfulness* (Table 2).

Compliant fill rate (CFR)

Based upon the compliant fill rate, 57.5% of prescription fills were considered compliant. Of the subjects with 100% CFR (n = 66, 19.6%), the number of females (n = 35, 23.2% of all females) was greater than the number of males (n = 31, 16.8%). Accordingly, at CFR of 25% (n = 98), CFR 50% (n = 99) and CFR 75% (n = 68), the number of male patients was slightly greater. When CFR was analyzed by marital status, 86 of 150 never married participants (57.3%) had a CFR <50%, whereas among the 137 married patients, 86 (62.9%) had a CFR < 50%. Distribution of rate of adherence by education status indicated that among the 66 patients with CFR = 100%, the majority

Table 2 Patients reason for missing their anti-psychotic medication using self-report

Reasons	Frequency	Percent
Forgetfulness	59	36.2
Lack of information	17	10.5
Being busy	34	21.0
Decision to omit	20	12.4
Others	27	12.4
Both forgetfulness and being busy	7	3.8
Total	164	100.0

(34.9%) had an educational status of 10–12 grades. The number of patients with educational status of diploma and above who had 100% CFR was 9.8%, compared to 9 of 45 (20%) who did not have any formal schooling. Conversely among the 61 patients who had an educational status of diploma and above, a large proportion (n = 46, 75.4%) had a CFR < 50% (Table 3).

Amongst social drug users, 80, 72.2 and 76.9% respectively had CFR < 50% (P = 0.05 for the comparison of all social drug users vs non-social drug users). When the number of medications taken was compared with the rate of adherence, it was found that, amongst patients with high adherence (n = 66, CFR = 100%), 53.5% were taking one medication and 44.2% were taking two medications. Furthermore, amongst patients with CFR = 75% (n = 68), 84.1% were taking just one medication. The number of medications and rate of adherence was significantly associated - as the number of medication increased, the patients' adherence decreased (r = −0.12, p = 0.01).

One hundred eighty four patients (54.8%) took medications for more than a year and 152 for less than one year. When the rate of adherence was compared with the duration of antipsychotic drug use, it was found that those patients with a duration of maintenance therapy greater than a year had better adherence rate (r = 0.54, p = 0.04, Table 4).

Based on the association of different variables and rate of adherence, there was no statistically significant association between age, sex, regime, income, educational, and occupational status of the patients (P > 0.05), but the duration of antipsychotic medication use, experiencing a side effect of medications, exposure to social drugs and the total number of medications currently taken did show a significant association with rate of adherence (Table 4).

Discussion
Methods of assessing medication adherence
Medication adherence describes the extent to which the patient continues the agreed treatment or intervention as prescribed. In other words, adherence can be defined as the degree of conformity between treatment behavior and treatment standard [4]. Understanding adherence to pharmacotherapies is crucial in clinical practice to ensure optimal clinical outcomes. There is no single measure accepted as the "gold standard" for assessing adherence, as each of the commonly employed methods have distinct advantages and disadvantages [25-27].

Frequently used methods of assessing participant adherence to pharmacological interventions include self-report measures: participant interviews, questionnaires, and diaries [27-31]. These methods are simple and inexpensive, but they are limited as they are subjective, crude and relatively inaccurate [25,32]. Although some suggest that patient-recall and refill history assessments are accurate enough (especially if they are performed in combination with other methods [33,34]), it is generally accepted that they substantially overestimate medication adherence [29,35]. Additionally, the ability of patient recall and refill history to detect changes in adherence is unknown [32].

Pill counts are inexpensive and are frequently utilized; whilst they provide information about the number of pills taken, it is difficult to determine actual medication consumption, as they rely upon the assumption that medications missing from the pill bottle were taken [36], and patients can intentionally or unintentionally manipulate this measure [25]. In addition, pill counts are laborious and rely upon accurate reporting dates for starting prescriptions. However, it has shown that pill counts can be more precise when carefully performed [25,32], and they can show both differences in patient adherence to therapy and reported the rate of adherence (from which we can detect non-adherence), in addition to measuring the changes in adherence across time [32]. Pill counts are regarded as being the most common way to assess adherence [37]. They are more accurate than self-report or refill history [38], but are tedious and difficult to administer [32]. Other measures such as electronic bottle caps are sophisticated and may be more accurate, but are costly [20], whilst biological methods (eg urine analysis and biomarkers) are precise measures of ingestion, but are not always available and practical [37].

Medication adherence and factors associated with non-adherence
This study revealed that adherence to antipsychotic medications was low in our study population. Previously reported rates of adherence for anti-psychotic medications ranged from 25% to 75% [14,39-41], which is comparable to the reported adherence rate in this study, which showed that patients reported taking medications as prescribed and filled their medications at appropriate intervals just over half of the time. However, if we consider 100% CFR to represent the true rate of adherence, fewer than 20% of patients would have been considered adherent throughout the study period, which is quite low compared to these previous reports.

Given the consequences of antipsychotic discontinuation and haphazard antipsychotic use, the poor adherence rates demonstrated in this and other studies are troubling. Previous studies have reported that patients who discontinue antipsychotics may be two to five times more likely to relapse as other patients, leading to unnecessary suffering [22,42]. Robinson and colleagues [42] reported that 82% of first-episode patients experienced at least one relapse within 5 years of follow-up, and that

Table 3 Number of adherence of patients defined by socio- demographic characteristics

Socio-demographic Characteristic	Description	Compliant Fill Rate (CFR)			
		25%	50%	75%	100%
Gender	Male	61	57	35	31
	Female	37	48	32	35
Age (in years)	10-20	20	12	12	12
	21-30	26	37	22	25
	31-40	20	25	12	17
	41-50	11	6	6	6
Marital status	Never married	38	48	29	35
	Married	38	48	28	23
	Divorced	11	3	3	3
	Widowed	6	3	6	5
Educational status	Diploma &above	23	23	9	6
	10-12 grade	28	37	29	23
	7-10 grade	23	18	14	15
	1-6 grade	6	11	3	12
	No formal schooling	17	11	8	9
Occupational status	Unemployed	20	291	12	28
	Private NGO	12	17	12	11
	Government	26	20	12	5
	Farmer	18	8	8	5
	Student	11	6	6	5
	Merchant	5	9	3	2
	Others	5	15	12	12
Religion	Orthodox	46	43	29	26
	Muslim	20	26	14	20
	Protestant	23	28	18	15
	Catholic	6	3	2	2
	Others	3	5	5	3
Monthly income (In Ethiopian Birr)	>300	18	22	15	15
	200-300	23	20	14	11
	100-200	26	22	14	9
	< 100	22	28	18	17
		9	12	6	14

patients who discontinued medication were five times more likely to relapse. It might be speculated that after experiencing one relapse, patients would be substantially less likely to discontinue medication, so our study is particularly noteworthy in suggesting factors that might contribute to non-adherence.

In our study over the half of patients reported that they had never missed either a daily dose or the time of taking a dose, and while over half of all prescriptions were filled in an adherent manner, only 19.6% of the study population was 100% adherent according to the CFR method. This demonstrates the fundamental

Table 4 Association between rate of adherence and different variables

Variables	P- value	Pearson correlation coefficient (r)
Duration of medication	0.04	0.54
Side effect of medications	0.03	−0.19
Exposure to social drugs	0.05	−0.13
Number of different types of medication	0.01	−0.12

controversy regarding which is the most appropriate method to measure medication adherence. Patients' self-report may still represent an under-reporting of the magnitude of the problem [43], whereas methods such as CFR are less prone to manipulation, and may offer a better approximation of the true adherence status.

Whilst there was no association between adherence rates and age, gender, income, religion and educational status of the patients, we did find an association between the rate of adherence and duration of maintenance therapy. This is supported by some [14], but not other studies [11,43,44]. In a naturalistic sample, younger age is likely to be associated with a shorter duration of illness, which we observed to be associated with a lower rate of adherence. Two mechanisms may underlie this observation. The first involves patients early in the course of their illness being more willing to take risks to find out if they could remain well without medication, especially before they encounter repeated episodes of relapse. The second relates to a potential selection bias of our outpatient population, where patients with longer illness duration who attend clinic regularly are more likely to be compliant with their treatment. In our study, over half of our patients had received maintenance therapy for more than one year, and these patients had the highest rates of adherence. Investigators examining the course of schizophrenia have observed that positive symptoms show a modest improvement over time [45,46], and it may be that adherence improves along with the decline in these severe psychotic symptoms.

As with other studies [2,8,14], these results have shown an association between the quantity of medications taken and the adherence rate. This may be due to an association between an increasing number of medications with misunderstanding that may arise as a result of complex regimen and/or confusion of instructions from health professionals and health care givers.

Individuals noted to use social drugs (chat, cigarette, alcohol) were significantly less likely to be adherent to their antipsychotic medication. This finding is consistent with previous researches [45-50], and can be explained by the fact that social drugs themselves are a risk factor for several psychiatric manifestations. Similar research showed that active substance abuse has been found to have a nearly eight-fold higher risk of non-adherence [8]. These abusive substances may have an effect on the cognitive abilities of patients [51], which in turn may affect adherence.

Kozuki and Froelicher [51] demonstrated that comorbid situations may adversely affect medication adherence and prognosis. Since over three quarters of the participants in our study did not have additional medical illness, this was not assessed in this study, as the numbers were too small to draw accurate conclusions. Also, the

effect of the type of antipsychotic medication (typical versus atypical) on the adherence rate was not assessed, as atypical agents were not available at the hospital during the study period.

In the present study, communication between the patients and the health professional was excellent, as over 95% responded that they felt comfortable in openly discussing their medication issues with their health professional/s. This clarity of communication is very supportive in overcoming a significant barrier to adherence, because when misunderstanding occurs, treatment becomes more complex and side effects are not managed.

Knowledge of side effects, dosage regimen and the name of their medications had an effect on adherence in this study, which replicates previous results [9,14]. Similar to other studies [1,16], we have shown that confusion and forgetfulness are the major obstacles in achieving adherence to a medication regimen.

Limitation
The findings of this study should be interpreted with some acknowledgement of the limitations. Being a cross-sectional design conducted at a single university Hospital, the study findings might be non-representative of the broader patient population, particularly in view of the response rate. The self-report method used in this study to measure treatment adherence might substantially overestimate medication adherence, as it relies on patient recall. Furthermore, this approach might not fully identify all of the factors contributing to non-adherence, nor accurately measure incidence, or associations. Despite the above limitations, the study identifies issues for further in-depth investigation regarding medication adherence in psychosis in Ethiopia.

Conclusion
Adherence to antipsychotic medications is relatively low. Pill burden, exposure to social/recreational drugs, and experiencing side-effects from medication may decrease adherence to treatment. Prescribers need to more closely focus on implementing treatment plans that patients understand and to which they agree and commit. The pharmacist should provide appropriate counseling on medications, emphasizing the importance of adherence, to both patients and their careers.

Competing interests
The author(s) declare that they have no competing interests.

Acknowledgment
The study was financed by Students Research Project (SRP) of Jimma University. The author would like to express appreciation to patients, who participated in the study, for their time to participate in the study. Special thanks are due for research staff participated in data collection and write up.

Author details
[1]Regulatory Unit, Beker Pharmaceuticals General Business Plc, Lideta Kifle Ketema, Addis Ababa, Ethiopia. [2]Division of Health Sciences, School of Pharmacy and Medical Sciences, University of South Australia, Adelaide, Australia. [3]Clinical Pharmacy Unit, Pharmacy Department, College of Public Health and Medical Science, Jimma University, Jimma, Ethiopia. [4]School of Pharmacy, Graduate School of Health, The University of technology Sydney (UTS), Sydney, Australia.

Authors' contributions
MA and NTW were principal investigators. NTW, MDW and BVB participated in the sequence alignment and write up of the manuscript. MTA and MA performed the data analysis. EA participated in patient identification and design of the study. MDW and BVB are also involved in language copyediting of the manuscript and revised the manuscript for intellectual content. All authors read and approved the final manuscript.

References
1. Becker MH: **Patient adherence to prescribed therapies.** *Medical Care* 1985, **23:**539–555.
2. Cramer JA, Rosenheck R: **Compliance with medication regimens for mental and physical disorders.** *Psychiatr Serv* 1998, **49:**196–201.
3. Powsner S, Spitzer R: **Sex, lies, and medical compliance.** *Lancet* 2003, **361:**2003–2004.
4. Abula T: **Assessment of the magnitude and factors of non- compliance with therapeutic regimens prescribed for treatment of chronic disease.** *Ethiop J Health Dev* 2001, **15**(3):185–192.
5. Carpenter WT, Strauss JS, Bartko JJ: **Flexible system for the diagnosis of schizophrenia: report from the WHO international pilot study of schizophrenia.** *Science* 1973, **182:**1275–1278.
6. Bartko G, Herczeg I, Zador G: **Clinical symptomatology and drug compliance in schizophrenic patients.** *Acta Psychiatr Scand* 1988, **78:**74–76.
7. Ghaemi SN, Pope HG: **Lack of insight in psychotic and affective disorders: a review of empirical studies.** *Harv Rev Psychiatry* 1994, **2:**22–33.
8. McEvoy JP, Freter S, Everett G, *et al*: **Insight and the clinical outcome of schizophrenic patients.** *J Nerv Ment Dis* 1989, **177:**48–51.
9. Lysaker P, Bell M, Milstein R, *et al*: **Insight and psychosocial treatment compliance in schizophrenia.** *Psychiatry* 1994, **57:**307–315.
10. Babiker IE: **Noncompliance in schizophrenia.** *Psychiatr Dev* 1986, **186:**329–337.
11. Bebbington PE: **The content and context of compliance.** *Int Clin Psychopharmacol* 1995, **9**(5):41–50.
12. Marder SR, Mebane A, Chien C, *et al*: **A comparison of patients who refuse and consent to neuroleptic treatment.** *Am J Psychiatry* 1983, **140:**470–472.
13. Dekker FW, Dielemann FE, Kaptein AA, *et al*: **Compliance with pulmonary medication in general practice.** *European Respiration Journal* 1993, **6:**886–890.
14. Dolder CR, Lacro JP, Dunn LB, *et al*: **Antipsychotic medication adherence: is there a difference between typical and atypical agents?** *Am J Psychiatry* 2002, **159:**103–108.
15. Patel NC, Dorson PG, Edwards N, *et al*: **One-year rehospitalization rates of patients discharged on atypical versus conventional antipsychotics.** *Psychiatr Serv* 2002, **53:**891–893.
16. Weiden PJ, Zygmunt A: **Medication noncompliance in schizophrenia: I. assessment.** *Journal of Practical Psychiatry and Behavioral Health* 1997, **3:**106–110.
17. Terkelsen K, Menikoff A: **Measuring costs of schizophrenia: implications for the post-institutional era in the US.** *Pharmacoeconomics* 1995, **8:**199–222.
18. Weiden PJ, Olfson M: **Cost of relapse in schizophrenia.** *Schizophr Bull* 1995, **21:**419–429.
19. Allebeck P, Wistedt B: **Mortality in schizophrenia.** *Arch Gen Psychiatry* 1986, **43:**650–653.
20. Koranyi EK: **Morbidity and rate of undiagnosed physical illnesses in a psychiatric clinic population.** *Arch Gen Psychiatry* 1979, **36:**414–419.
21. Jeste DV, Gladsjo JA, Lindamer LA, Lacro JP: **Medical co morbidity in schizophrenia.** *Schizophr Bull* 1996, **22:**413–430.

22. Fenton WS, Blyler CR, Heinssen RK: **Determinants of medication compliance in schizophrenia: empirical and clinical findings.** *Schizophr Bull* 1997, **23:**637–651.
23. Steiner JF, Prochazka AV: **The assessment of refill compliance using pharmacy records: methods, validity, and applications.** *J Clin Epidemiol* 1997, **50:**105–116.
24. Hamilton RA, Briceland LL: **Use of prescription-refill records to assess patient compliance.** *Am J Hosp Pharm* 1992, **49:**1691–1696.
25. Benner JS, Glynn RJ, *et al*: **Long-term persistence in use of statin therapy in elderly patients.** *JAMA* 2002, **288:**455–461.
26. Garber MC, Nau DP, Erickson SR, *et al*: **The concordance of self-report with other measures of medication adherence: a summary of the literature.** *Med Care* 2004, **42:**649–652.
27. Vitolins MZ, Rand CS, Rapp SR, Ribisl PM, Sevick MA: **Measuring adherence to behavioral and medical interventions.** *Control Clin Trials* 2000, **21:**188S–194S.
28. Fletcher SW, Pappius EM, Harper SJ: **Measurement of medication compliance in a clinical setting. Comparison of three methods in patients prescribed digoxin.** *Arch Intern Med* 1979, **139:**635–638.
29. Grymonpre RE, Didur CD, Montgomery PR, *et al*: **Pill count, selfreport, and pharmacy claims data to measure medication adherence in the elderly.** *Ann Pharmacother* 1998, **32:**749–754.
30. Christensen DB, Williams B, Goldberg HI, *et al*: **Assessing compliance to antihypertensive medications using computer-based pharmacy records.** *Med Care* 1997, **35:**1164–1170.
31. Elm JJ, Kamp C, Tilley BC, Guimaraes P, Fraser D, Deppen P: **Self-Reported Adherence Versus Pill Count in Parkinson's Disease: The NET-PD Experience.** *Mov Disord* 2007, **22**(6):822–827.
32. Lee JK, Grace KA, Foster TG, Crawley MJ, Erowele GI, Sun HJ, *et al*: **How should we measure medication adherence in clinical trials and practice?** *Ther Clin Risk Manag.* 2007, **3**(4):x685–690.
33. DiMatteo MR, Giordani PJ, Lepper HS, *et al*: **Patient adherence and medical treatment outcomes: a meta-analysis.** *Med Care* 2002, **40:**794–811.
34. Farley J, Hines S, Musk A, *et al*: **Assessment of adherence to antiviral therapy in HIV-infected children using the Medication Event Monitoring System, pharmacy refi ll, provider assessment, caregiver self-report, and appointment keeping.** *J Acquir Immune Defi c Syndr* 2003, **33:**211–218.
35. Shalansky SJ, Levy AR, Ignaszewski AP: **Self-reported Morisky score for identifying nonadherence with cardiovascular medications.** *Ann Pharmacother* 2004, **38:**1363–1368.
36. Farmer KC: **Methods for measuring and monitoring medication regimen adherence in clinical trials and clinical practice.** *Clin Ther* 1999, **21:**1074–1090.
37. Pauler DK, Gower KB, Goodman PJ, Crowley JJ, Thompson IM: **Biomarker-based methods for determining noncompliance in a prevention trial.** *Control Clin Trials* 2002, **23:**675–685.
38. Choo PW, Rand CS, Inui TS, *et al*: **Validation of patient reports, automated pharmacy records, and pill counts with electronic monitoring of adherence to antihypertensive therapy.** *Med Care* 1999, **37:**846–857.
39. Valenstein M, Copeland LA, Blow FC, *et al*: **Pharmacy data identify poorly adherent patients with schizophrenia at increased risk for admission.** *Med Care* 2002, **40:**630–639.
40. Lehman AF, Kreyenbuhl J, Buchanan RW, *et al*: **The Schizophrenia Patient Outcomes Research Team (PORT): Updated Treatment Recommendations 2003.** *Schizophr Bull* 2004, **30:**193–217.
41. Lieberman JA, Stroup TS, McEvoy JP, *et al*: **Effectiveness of antipsychotic drugs in patients with chronic schizophrenia.** *N Engl J Med* 2005, **353:**1209–1223.
42. Robinson D, Woerner M, Alvir J, *et al*: **Predictors of relapse following response from a first episode of schizophrenia or schizoaffective disorder.** *Arch Gen Psychiatry* 1999, **56**(3):241–247.
43. Hui CLM, Chen YH, Kan CS, *et al*: **Anti-psychotics adherence among out-patients with schizophrenia in Hong Kong.** *Keio J Med* 2006, **55**(1):9–14.
44. Fleischhacker WW, Oehl MA, Hummer M: **Factors influencing compliance in schizophrenia patients.** *J Clin Psychiatry* 2003, **64**(Suppl 16):10–13.
45. Gilmer T, Dolder CR, Lacro JP, *et al*: **Adherence to Treatment With Antipsychotic Medication and Health Care Costs Among Medicaid Beneficiaries With Schizophrenia.** *Am J Psychiatry* 2004, **161:**692–699.
46. Olfson M, Mechanic D, Hansell S, Boyer CA, Walkup J, Weiden PJ: **Predicting medication noncompliance after hospital discharge among patients with schizophrenia.** *Psychiatr Serv* 2000, **51:**216–222.

47. Rosenheck R, Chang S, Choe Y, *et al*: Medication continuation and
     compliance: a comparison of patients treated with clozapine and
     haloperidol. *J Clin Psychiatry* 2000, **61**:382–386.
48. Owen RR, Fischer EP, Booth BM, Cuffel BJ: Medication noncompliance and
     substance abuse among patients with schizophrenia. *Psychiatr Serv* 1996,
     47:853–858.
49. Drake RE, Osher FC, Wallach MA: Alcohol use and abuse in schizophrenia:
     a prospective community study. *J Nerv Ment Dis* 1989, **177**:408–414.
50. Heyscue BE, Levin GM, Merrick JP: Compliance with depot antipsychotic
     medication by patients attending outpatient clinics. *Psychiatr Serv* 1998,
     49:1232–1234.
51. Kozuki Y, Froelicher ES: Lack of awareness and non-adherence in
     schizophrenia. *West J Nurs Res.* 2003, **25**(1):57–74.

14

Knowledge, attitudes and practice survey about antimicrobial resistance and prescribing among physicians in a hospital setting in Lima, Peru

Coralith García[1,2]*, Liz P Llamocca[1], Krystel García[1], Aimee Jiménez[1], Frine Samalvides[1,2], Eduardo Gotuzzo[1,2] and Jan Jacobs[3,4]

Abstract

Background: Misuse of antimicrobials (AMs) and antimicrobial resistance (AMR) are global concerns. The present study evaluated knowledge, attitudes and practices about AMR and AM prescribing among medical doctors in two large public hospitals in Lima, Peru, a middle-income country.

Methods: Cross-sectional study using a self-administered questionnaire

Results: A total of 256 participants completed the questionnaire (response rate 82%). Theoretical knowledge was good (mean score of 6 ± 1.3 on 7 questions) in contrast to poor awareness (< 33%) of local AMR rates of key-pathogens. Participants strongly agreed that AMR is a problem worldwide (70%) and in Peru (65%), but less in their own practice (22%). AM overuse was perceived both for the community (96%) and the hospital settings (90%). Patients' pressure to prescribing AMs was considered as contributing to AM overuse in the community (72%) more than in the hospital setting (50%). Confidence among AM prescribing was higher among attending physicians (82%) compared to residents (30%, p < 0.001%). Sources of information considered as very useful/useful included pocket-based AM prescribing guidelines (69%) and internet sources (62%). Fifty seven percent of participants regarded AMs in their hospitals to be of poor quality. Participants requested more AM prescribing educational programs (96%) and local AM guidelines (92%).

Conclusions: This survey revealed topics to address during future AM prescribing interventions such as dissemination of information about local AMR rates, promoting confidence in the quality of locally available AMs, redaction and dissemination of local AM guidelines and addressing the general public, and exploring the possibilities of internet-based training.

Keywords: Antimicrobial resistance - Antimicrobial use - Knowledge, attitude and practice survey

Background

Antimicrobial resistance (AMR) is a worldwide problem preferentially affecting low- and middle income countries [1,2]. Two main contributing factors are (i) excessive use of antimicrobials (AMs) adding to an increased selection pressure and (ii) insufficient infection control policies favouring the spread of resistant microorganisms [3]. Patients who receive AMs have an increased risk of acquiring infection from resistant microorganisms [4] and such infections may be associated with increased mortality and morbidity [5,6]. Reduction in AM use is a cornerstone in the containment of AMR and can be addressed through changes in prescribing behaviour. Therefore, knowledge about the driving forces behind AM prescription is needed, and such information can be obtained by means of so-called KAP-surveys (knowledge, attitudes and practice surveys). KAP-surveys about antimicrobial resistance have been conducted among medical doctors in the community setting, but at the time of submission, only five have been reported from the hospital setting,

* Correspondence: coralith.garcia@upch.pe
[1]Instituto de Medicina Tropical Alexander von Humboldt, Universidad Peruana Cayetano Heredia, Lima, Perú
Full list of author information is available at the end of the article

Table 1 Knowledge, attitudes and practices (KAP)-surveys about AMR in the hospital setting as reported in the English literature

Author	Country	Participants	Main findings
Pulcini et al., 2010	Scotland, France	Junior doctors (n = 139)	95% agreed AMR is a national problem, 63% agreed so for their own clinical practice. Only 26% knew the correct local prevalence of methicillin-resistant *S. aureus*
Guerra et al., 2007	Brazil	Mainly residents (n = 310)	95% agreed AMR is a problem and 87% that AMs are overprescribed
Giblin et al., 2004	USA	Health care workers (n = 117*)	95% agreed that AMR is a national problem, 65% agreed for in their own practice
Srinisavan et al., 2004	USA	House-staff physicians (other than paediatricians) (n = 179)	88% agreed that AMs are overused in general, 72% agreed so for their own hospital
Wester et al. 2002	USA	Internal medicine doctors (n = 490)	87% considered AMR as very important national problem

AMR: antimicrobial resistance AM: antimicrobial

* 33% of participants were physicians

including only one from a middle-income country [7-11] (Table 1).

The present study shows the results of a KAP-survey about AMR and AM prescribing among medical doctors from two hospitals in Lima, Peru. The survey was conducted in order to explore and target educational interventions about AM prescribing.

Methods

Study design, period and setting
The study consisted of a cross sectional survey of physicians from two public hospitals, Cayetano Heredia (CHH) and Arzobispo Loayza (ALH) during January 2009. Both hospitals are tertiary-level, teaching hospitals located in urban areas of Lima with 423 and 788 patient beds respectively.

Participants and survey instrument
A self-administered questionnaire was distributed in both hospitals among residents (*i.e.* physicians in training) and attending physicians (*i.e.* staff physicians after completion of training and specialization). Medical doctors from psychiatry, radiology, ophthalmology and anaesthesiology were not included as they do not routinely prescribe AMs. Questionnaires were distributed on site during working hours and participants were asked to respond immediately. There was no incentive for subjects to participate and no reminders were supplied. The questionnaire content was based on a previous survey described in the U.S. and adapted to the Peruvian system [9]. Prior to release, it was reviewed by a team of six Peruvian infectious diseases physicians to assess the relevance and wording of the questions as well as accuracy of the translation into Spanish. The 38-item questionnaire addressed the professional profile of the participants and frequency of AM prescription (5 questions), their awareness about the current scope of AMR (6 questions), sources of information and continuing education about AMs (2 questions), confidence and

seeking inputs (5 questions), factors influencing decisions around AM prescription (5 questions) and the acceptability and appropriateness of potential interventions (6 questions) (Additional file 1). Questions used a 4 or 5-point Likert scale (which included answers ranging from "strongly agree" to "strongly disagree", from "very useful" to "not useful at all" and from "always" to "never"). The survey also included seven questions that assessed basic knowledge about the clinical indications, spectrum, administration and pharmacology of AMs. Three case-based questions addressed the choice of AMs for treating acute diarrhoea, an upper respiratory tract infection and sepsis in a patient with impaired renal function; one question addressed safety of AMs during pregnancy, and three questions addressed the spectrum of AMs and their ability to cross the blood-brain barrier. Finally, in order to evaluate physician awareness about AMR rates within local hospitals, participants were asked to estimate the proportion of *Klebsiella pneumoniae* resistance to cephalosporins and *Pseudomonas aeruginosa* resistance to ciprofloxacin (answer options "20% or less", "20%-50%", "more than 50%" or "don't know"). The true rate was obtained from a surveillance study on AMR in Lima hospitals in 2008.

Ethical clearance
The study was approved by the Institutional Review Board from Universidad Peruana Cayetano Heredia, Lima, Peru, and by the Ethical Committees in each hospital. Based on the anonymous nature of the collected data, informed consent form was not taken.

Statistical analysis
A sample size of 234 was calculated using the Epi Info 3.5.3 software (CDC, Atlanta, USA) considering a total population of 1050 physicians and the expected correct answer on the questions about knowledge of local AMR rates. This was set at 27% according to a previous publication [7] and a 95% of confidence level was applied.

Participants were not sampled randomly. Proportions were calculated for categorical variables and their significance assessed by the Chi square or Fisher's exact test. Means and standard deviations were calculated for continuous variables. Unless otherwise stated, we used Likert items by combining the data into two categories, "strongly agree/agree", "very useful/useful" and "very confident/confident" versus the remaining options of the scale. Data were analysed with the software STATA 10.1 (Statacorp, Texas, USA).

Results
Demographics and professional profile
A total of 260/317 physicians filled in the questionnaire (response rate 82%). Four were excluded since they did not specify which department they were affiliated to. The vast majority of participants (97%) agreed that knowledge about AMs and their adequate use are important in their daily work and 49% declared to prescribe AMs more than once a day. Table 2 gives an overview of the professional profile of the 256 participants; the profiles were similar within the two hospitals except for the proportion of surgeons. Unless otherwise stated, there were no significant differences between the participants belonging to different professional categories and levels, departments or hospitals for the results presented below.

Knowledge on AM use and AMR rates
The average score to the questions regarding knowledge of AMs was 6 out of 7(SD ± 1.3). For the case-based questions about acute diarrhoea and upper respiratory tract infection, the vast majority of participants agreed that there was no need to start an AM (238, 93% and 194, 76%, respectively). The knowledge about the need to reduce the dose of AM in a patient with severe renal impairment was assessed by presenting a sepsis case

where ceftriaxone and gentamicin were prescribed. About three quarters (n = 194, 76%) correctly identified that AMs would need to be reduced in this case. Furthermore, nearly all participants (n = 250, 99%) correctly replied that metronidazole has activity against anaerobes and 213 (83%) participants correctly answered that methicillin resistant *Staphylococcus aureus* (MRSA) is not susceptible to cephalosporins, the remaining participants (n = 41, 16%) incorrectly responded that it is susceptible to cefalotine, cefuroxime or ceftriaxone. The majority (n = 237, 93%) of participants agreed that amoxicillin is safe during the first three-month period of pregnancy whereas 17 (7%) incorrectly answered that ciprofloxacin or gentamicin are safe. A total of 180 (70%) participants correctly answered that ceftriaxone is the most effective drug crossing the blood-brain barrier where as 62 (24%) and 10 (4%) of participants incorrectly chose vancomycin and clindamycin above ceftriaxone. With regard to the estimate about local AMR rates, it was striking that only 51 (20%) of participants correctly estimated that > 50% of *K. pneumoniae* isolates are resistant to cephalosporins, whilst half, 129 (50%) answered that the resistance rate was 20%-50% and 47 (18%) answered 'don't know'. In response to the question about resistance rates of *P. aeruginosa* to ciprofloxacin, 82 (32%) of participants gave correct estimates (*i.e.* 20-50%), 118 (46%) answered that the rate was higher than 50% and 39 (15%) answered 'don't know'.

Awareness about the current scope of AMR
Almost all participants considered that AMR is a problem (98%). There were fewer residents than attending physicians who strongly agreed that AMR is a worldwide problem (58% versus 81%, p < 0.001). A similar scenario was observed in relation to the perception of AMR at the national level as 54% of residents strongly agreed that AMR was a problem compared to 78% of

Table 2 Professional profile of the participants in the two hospitals of Lima, Peru

Characteristic	Cayetano Heredia hospital (n = 132)	Arzobispo Loayza Hospital (n = 124)	Total (n = 256)
Working time in hospitals			
0 - 4 years	74 (56)	66 (53)	140 (55)
≥ 5 years	58 (44)	58 (47)	116 (45)
Hospital department			
Medicine	66 (50.0)	76 (61)	142 (55)
Surgery	39 (30)*	14 (11)*	53 (21)
O&B	15 (11)	17 (14)	32 (13)
Paediatrics	12 (9)	17 (14)	29 (11)
Position			
Resident (in training)	64 (48)	71 (57)	135 (53)
Attending physician	68 (52)	53 (43)	121 (47)

Data represent numbers (%).
*p < 0.05 O&B: Obstetrics and Gynaecology

attending physicians (p < 0.001). However, whilst a mere 22% strongly agreed AMR is a problem in their own practice (Figure 1), Further, there was agreement upon the perception of overuse of AMs in both the Peruvian community and hospitals (96% and 90% combined "strongly agree" and "agree" answers for both settings respectively).

Confidence and seeking of inputs

Nearly half (63/135, 47%) of residents revealed they were very confident about the optimal use of antimicrobials compared to 99/121 (82%) of attending physicians (p < 0.001). A total of 78 (31%) participants agreed that it is difficult for them to select the correct AM, this was recorded for 36% participants from the medical departments versus 20% from the surgical departments (p = 0.014). Moreover, it should be noted that almost a quarter of participants (n = 58, 23%), strongly agreed and agreed that prescribing AMs when they are not required does not cause any harm. With regard to seeking inputs, when participants were asked about the frequency of reviewing their decision to prescribe AMs with a senior colleague, 15% replied 'never' and 57% 'sometimes'; only 6% answered 'always'. More than half (74/135, 55%) of residents declared that they never or only sometimes reviewed their decision with a senior colleague compared to 89% (108/121) of attending physicians (p < 0.001). This was seen more frequently among participants from surgical

departments compared to those from medical departments (80% versus 67%, p = 0.03). Among the 219 participants who declared to review their decision to prescribe AMs with a senior colleague at least sometimes, nearly three quarters (161, 74%) reported that senior colleagues sometimes recommended a different AM.

Sources of information and continuing education about AMs

Overall, 88 (34%) participants declared that there had been no lectures about AM use as part of academic activities within their departments during the previous year, although there was a slight difference between the medical and surgical departments (29% versus 45%; p = 0.015). Likewise, 37% (95/256) of participants had not participated in a course on AM use during the previous year; the rate was 65% among residents versus 35% among attending physicians (p = 0.003). Regarding sources of information, two-thirds (173, 68%) of participants reported having readily available sources of information on AMs. The "Sanford Guide on Antimicrobial Therapy" was considered as a very useful source (n = 129, 50%), although preferentially among residents (n = 78, 58%) compared to attending physicians (n = 51, 42%, p = 0.013). Internet sources were considered as very useful or useful by nearly two-thirds (159, 62%) of participants. Thirty six (14%) participants did not

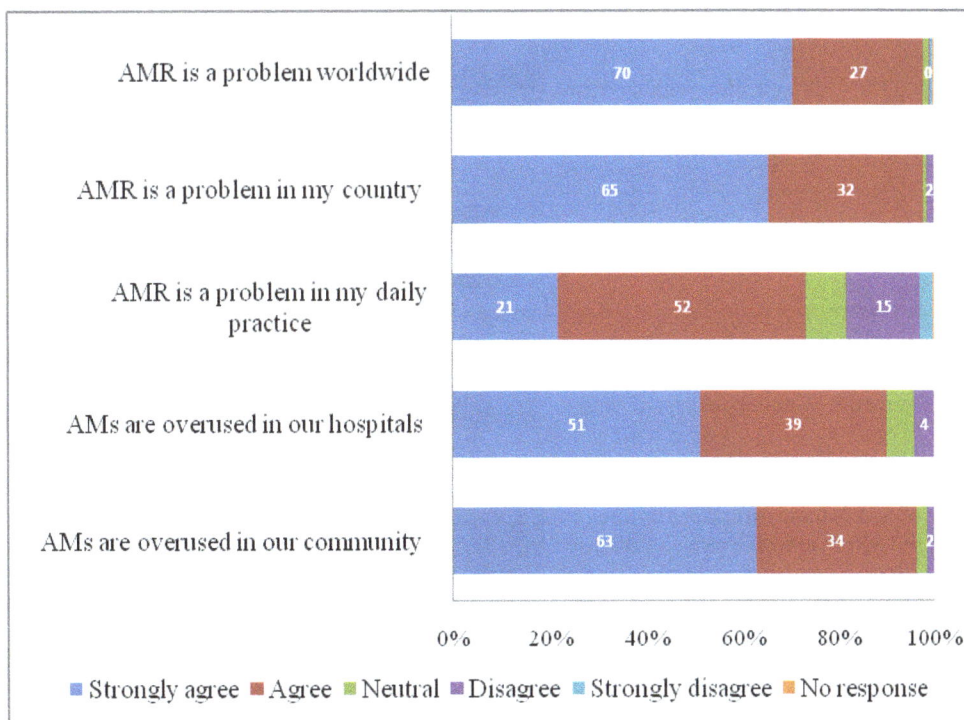

Figure 1 Awareness of the scope of AMR among 256 participants (data in the graphs represent percentages). AM: Antimicrobial, AMR: Antimicrobial resistance

consider the national guidelines useful and a quarter (65, 25%) noted that they were not familiar with these guidelines. Advice from colleagues of higher rank or same rank were considered useful or very useful in 98 (38%) and 71 (28%) of participants respectively.

Factors influencing decisions around AM prescription

Nearly three quarters (183/256, 72%) of participants strongly agreed or agreed that patients' demand for AMs contributes to their overuse in the community, but only half (n = 128, 50%) did so for the hospital setting (Figure 2). Almost 40% (n = 102) of participants declared that they were unaware of the AMs available in their hospital because of continuously changing formulations. Surprisingly, more than half (146, 57%) agreed with the statement that the AMs available in their hospitals are of poor quality and are not effective.

Acceptability and appropriateness of potential interventions

The vast majority of participants strongly agreed and agreed with the development of AM prescribing educational programs (n = 247, 97%) and confirmed that a

local AM guideline would be more useful than an international one (n = 235, 92%). Moreover, 224 (88%) participants strongly agreed and agreed that knowledge about local AMR rates should be considered when prescribing AMs. Ninety-six participants (38%) strongly agreed and agreed that the need to apply for approval to prescribe restricted AMs caused them to seek an alternative AM (Figure 3). More participants from Arzobispo Loayza hospital (88%) strongly disagreed or disagreed with the statement that AM guidelines and AM committees are an obstacle to patient care compared to participants from Cayetano Heredia hospital (45%) (p < 0.001).

Discussion

The present study describes the results of a KAP-survey among 256 medical doctors (both residents in training and attending physicians) practicing in two large public teaching hospitals in the Lima area, Peru.

Knowledge on AMs and AMR

Overall, the theoretical knowledge about AMs including indications, administration and side effects ranged from

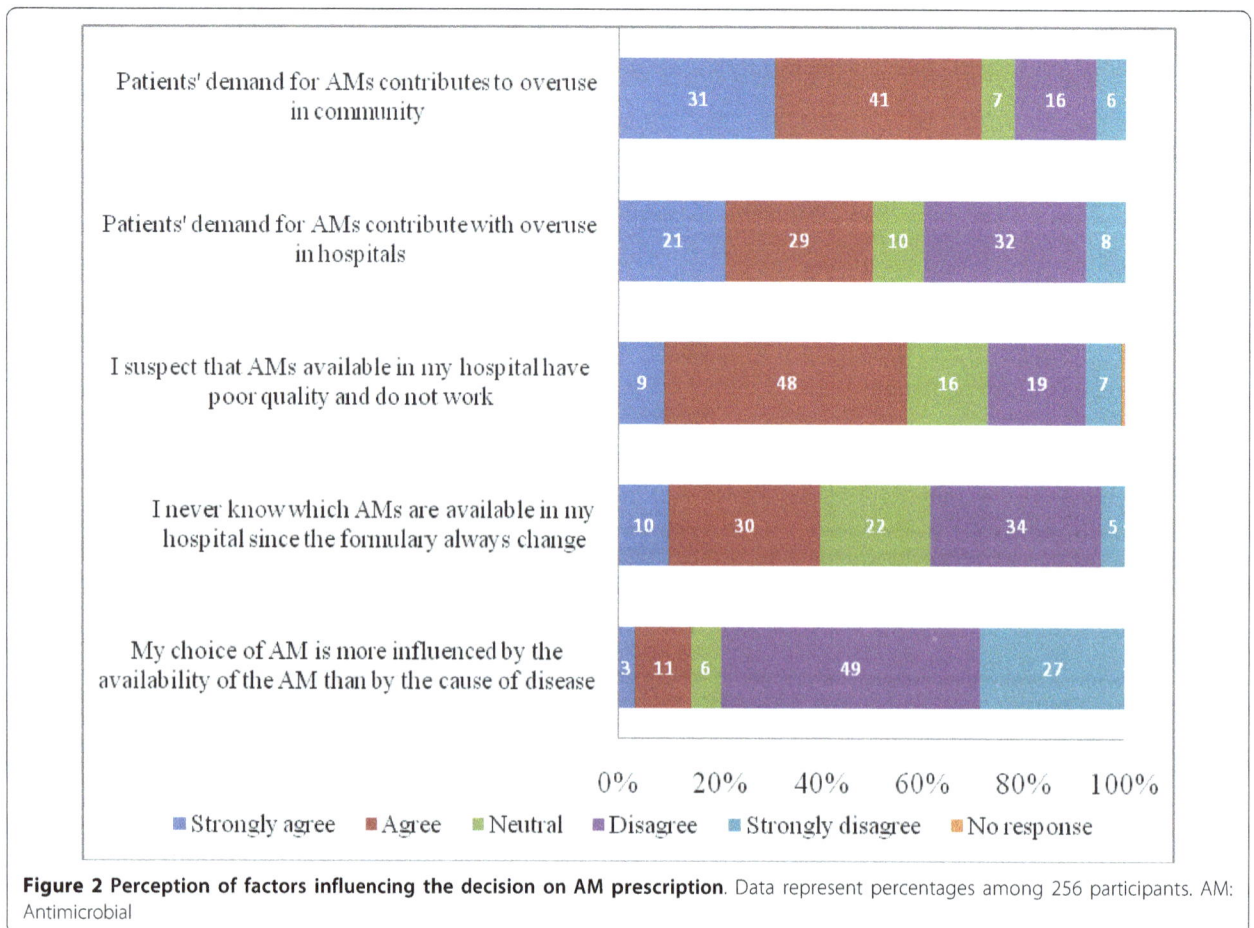

Figure 2 Perception of factors influencing the decision on AM prescription. Data represent percentages among 256 participants. AM: Antimicrobial

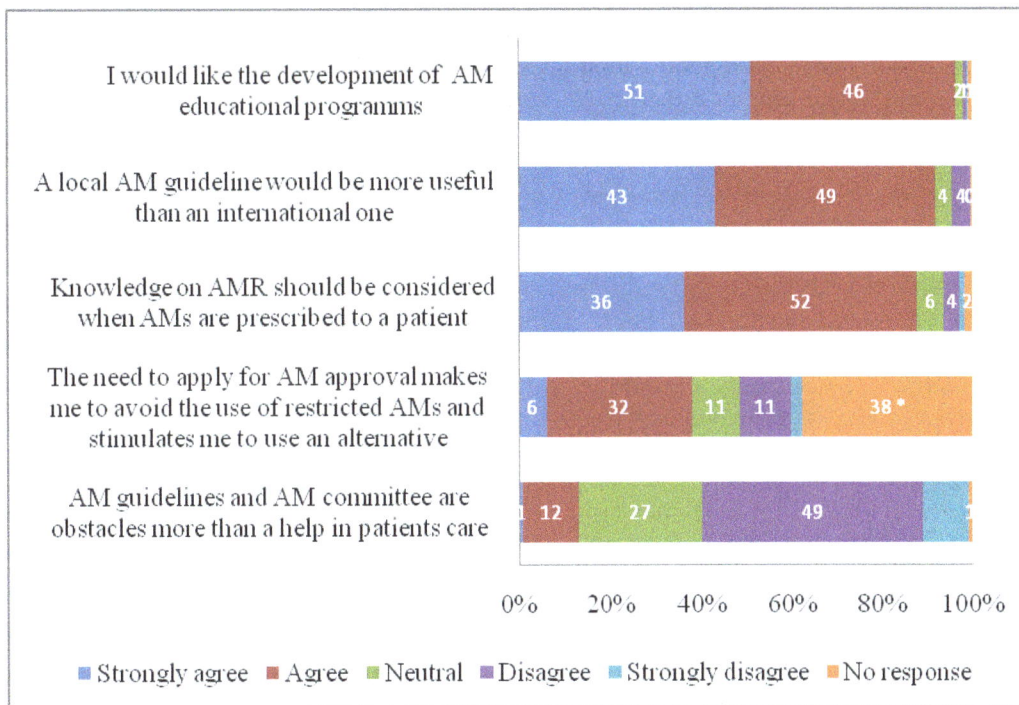

Figure 3 **Acceptability and appropriateness of potential interventions on AM prescribing as surveyed among 256 participants**. Data represent percentages. AM: antimicrobial, AMR: Antimicrobial resistance, *38% answered 'There is no a restrictive policy in my hospital'

very good to excellent. Despite this apparently good score for these questions, it should be noted that a quarter of participants still considered that it was correct to use AMs for upper respiratory tract infections. This suggests that this issue should be targeted in future educational interventions. Furthermore, it is known that in practice AM use may not reflect these results, and this can be illustrated by a recent study: in a rural Peruvian village, 58% of children with acute upper respiratory symptoms or watery diarrhoea (for which AMs are not recommended) were given AMs when they went to see a doctor [12]. This contrasts with the survey's results, in which the majority of participants answered correctly that AMs are unnecessary for either of these conditions. Likewise, it should be noted that a quarter of participants agreed with the statement that unnecessary prescribing of AMs does not cause any harm. Although the participants' overall knowledge about AMs was appropriate, most of them incorrectly estimated the local resistance rates of two key-pathogens in the hospital setting, *K. pneumoniae* and *P. aeruginosa*. Similar findings have been described in other studies [7,8]: Pulcini *et al.* showed that only 16% of young doctors in a French hospital knew the actual proportion of community acquired-*Escherichia coli* resistant to fluoroquinolones. Local microbiology laboratories are encouraged to maintain a database about the levels of resistance of key

pathogens and diffuse it to prescribers: when reinforced by the local antibiotic committee, information may orient prescribing doctors [13].

Awareness about current scope of AMR

The awareness of AMR as a worldwide and national problem was very high among the participants. However, in contrast, AMR was much less recognised as a problem in participants' own practice. This trend has also been observed among physicians surveyed in the U. S. (Table 1) [9-11]. On the other hand, qualitative research among general practitioners in the U.S. showed that most of the physicians interviewed were aware that inappropriate use of AM in their own practice contributes to increasing AMR [14]. Interestingly, the majority of participants recognized excessive use of AMs as a factor contributing to AMR in the community, but only half did so for the hospital settings.

Confidence and seeking of inputs

Compared to attending physicians, residents in training were less confident about AM prescribing. This correlates with the findings of Srinivasan *et al.*: in this study, senior residents were more confident about optimal use of antimicrobials compared with first year-residents [9]. Moreover, residents tended to seek advice from their senior colleagues when prescribing, irrespective of their specialization (department) or hospital affiliation, compared with attending physicians who have more years of clinical experience. However, more residents declared that they consulted internet-based sources rather than approaching senior colleagues for advice. It is surprising than more than 50% of residents declared that they did not consult senior colleagues considering that both institutions were teaching hospitals. Other sources of AM guidance are discussed below.

Sources of information and continuing education about AMs

The present survey also revealed information about the sources of information for AM use. The popularity of the Sanford Guide illustrates the accessibility of pocket-based treatment guidelines. Internet sources were ranked as the second most useful source. In this scenario, distant learning technologies which have been used successfully in Peru for other disciplines [15,16] may have a place in promoting educational AM prescribing programs. The poor appreciation of and familiarity with the national guidelines among the participants is striking and contrasts with the seemingly large demand for local AM guidelines.

Factors influencing decisions around AM prescription

Three quarters of participants identified patient demand for AMs as a key factor contributing to the overuse of AMs in the community, with half doing so for the hospital setting. Pressure from patients is indeed an important factor particularly in the middle- and low-income settings. A study among parents and paediatricians in Venezuela revealed that 87% of doctors felt pressured by parents into prescribing AMs; 48% of parents said that they had requested AMs and 33% revealed that they had obtained a prescription [17].

The high expectation about AM use from patients is very probably a consequence of their minimal understanding of AMR and AM side effects. Education of the general public through community-targeted media information is extremely important

More than half of participants agreed that AMs in their hospitals are of poor quality. Although we have not explored in detail the definition of "poor quality" according to the prescribers, there are several issues. Firstly, despite regional and national regulations for drug marketing, counterfeit (and probably substandard) drugs have been detected in Peru, but information was mainly distributed by the lay press and as such, it is difficult to estimate the magnitude of this problem. Secondly, in our experience, generic drugs are also frequently perceived to be less effective, an idea reinforced by recent studies from Colombia showing that generic vancomycin and oxacillin had a less therapeutic

effect in animal subjects [18,19]. This is of concern, as a lack of confidence in generic and locally market drugs may similarly affect confidence in following standard treatment guidelines and in the implementation of essential drug lists and may deflect patients and prescribers towards the private sector. The Peruvian Ministry of Health should build confidence in the quality of locally available AMs by circulating adequate information about locally marketed AMs. In line with the need to diffuse data on AMR rates among key-pathogens, it is clear from the present results that the hospital pharmacy should diffuse timely and accessible information about the availability of AMs.

Acceptability and appropriateness of potential interventions

Formal programs about AMR and AM prescribing were welcomed by the vast majority of participants suggesting a gap in knowledge about infectious diseases, microbiology and AM prescribing in university programs [20]. There was also strong agreement about the usefulness of local AM guidelines, although concerns about the acceptability of the local antibiotic committee and its steering measures should be addressed in the future.

One of the main limitations of KAP-surveys is the fact that participants may tend to give socially desirable answers rather than expressing their true opinions. The present setting of teaching hospital may contribute to this bias. In order to minimize this potential bias anonymous participation was ensured and the case-based questions about AM prescription (which might have been suggestive) were presented at the end of the survey. The fact that this survey was based on a survey conducted among U.S. physicians may be another limitation, but it was countered by the pre-release validation. In addition, the survey was extended to the local context by adding questions relevant to the Peruvian situation. Another issue was that physicians working in hospitals were also questioned about their knowledge and attitudes towards community infections. However, the majority of doctors in the two hospitals were practicing in both the hospital and the community setting. Further studies should be done to study the knowledge, attitudes and practice surrounding AM use among physicians from community centres. Finally, one may question whether the attitude of doctors in other parts of Peru to AMs is reflected by the results of this survey. As this study was conducted in two large, public, tertiary-level teaching institutions and involved a large number of prescribing doctors, we are confident that the results may be applied to other public general hospitals in Peru. However, the generalizability of the results to other health care settings remains to be demonstrated.

Conclusion

The present KAP-survey has generated information about the prescribing attitudes and practices of medical doctors from public hospitals of a middle-income country. It identified topics to address in the containment of AMR, such as the dissemination of information about local AMR rates, the importance of renewing public confidence in the quality of locally available AMs, the revision and dissemination of local AM guidelines, addressing the general public and exploring the possibilities of internet-based trainings.

Additional material

Additional file 1: Knowledge, attitudes and practice survey about antimicrobial resistance and prescribing. This is a 38-item questionnaire that evaluated the knowledge, attitudes and practice of antimicrobial use and antimicrobial resistance among physicians.

Acknowledgements
This study was sponsored by the Directorate General for Development Cooperation (DGCD) of the Belgian Government (framework agreement 3, project 95502). We want to thank Dr. Arjun Srinisavan for sharing with us the questionnaire used in reference 9 and Dr. Alexander Baron, Jennifer Hulme, Jair Medina, and Dr. Dalila Martinez for editing the manuscript.

Author details
[1]Instituto de Medicina Tropical Alexander von Humboldt, Universidad Peruana Cayetano Heredia, Lima, Perú. [2]Hospital Nacional Cayetano Heredia, Lima, Perú. [3]Institute of Tropical Medicine Antwerp, Antwerp, Belgium. [4]Department of Medical Microbiology, Faculty of Health, Life Sciences and Medicine, Maastricht University, The Netherlands.

Authors' contributions
CG designed the protocol and survey, obtained ethical approval, analysed the database and drafted the manuscript. LL, AJ and KG validated the questionnaire, collected data and completed the database. FS and EG assisted with preparation of research protocol and review of the manuscript. JJ collaborated with the preparation protocol and survey, analysis and redaction of the manuscript. All authors read and approved the final manuscript.

Competing interests
The authors declare that they have no competing interests.

References
1. Levy SB: The challenge of antibiotic resistance. Sci Am 1998, 278:46-53.
2. Okeke IN, Laxminarayan R, Bhutta ZA, Duse AG, Jenkins P, O'Brien TF, Pablos-Mendez A, Klugman KP: Antimicrobial resistance in developing countries. Part I: recent trends and current status. Lancet Infect Dis 2005, 5(8):481-493.
3. Okeke IN: Poverty and root causes of resistance in developing countries. In Antimicrobial resistance in developing countries.. First edition. Edited by: Sosa AB, DK; Amabile-Cuevas, CF; Hsueh, PR; Kariuki, S; Okeke. IN New York: Springer; 2010:27-36.
4. Costelloe C, Metcalfe C, Lovering A, Mant D, Hay AD: Effect of antibiotic prescribing in primary care on antimicrobial resistance in individual patients: systematic review and meta-analysis. BMJ 2010, 340:c2096.
5. Shanthi M, Sekar U: Multi-drug resistant Pseudomonas aeruginosa and Acinetobacter baumannii infections among hospitalized patients: risk factors and outcomes. J Assoc Physicians India 2009, 57:636, 638-640, 645.
6. Woodford N, Livermore DM: Infections caused by Gram-positive bacteria: a review of the global challenge. J Infect 2009, 59(Suppl 1):S4-16.
7. Guerra CM, Pereira CA, Neves Neto AR, Cardo DM, Correa L: Physicians' perceptions, beliefs, attitudes, and knowledge concerning antimicrobial resistance in a Brazilian teaching hospital. Infect Control Hosp Epidemiol 2007, 28(12):1411-1414.
8. Pulcini C, Williams F, Molinari N, Davey P, Nathwani D: Junior doctors' knowledge and perceptions of antibiotic resistance and prescribing: a survey in France and Scotland. Clin Microbiol Infect 2011, 17(1):80-87.
9. Srinivasan A, Song X, Richards A, Sinkowitz-Cochran R, Cardo D, Rand C: A survey of knowledge, attitudes, and beliefs of house staff physicians from various specialties concerning antimicrobial use and resistance. Arch Intern Med 2004, 164(13):1451-1456.
10. Wester CW, Durairaj L, Evans AT, Schwartz DN, Husain S, Martinez E: Antibiotic resistance: a survey of physician perceptions. Arch Intern Med 2002, 162(19):2210-2216.
11. Giblin TB, Sinkowitz-Cochran RL, Harris PL, Jacobs S, Liberatore K, Palfreyman MA, Harrison EI, Cardo DM: Clinicians' perceptions of the problem of antimicrobial resistance in health care facilities. Arch Intern Med 2004, 164(15):1662-1668.
12. Kristiansson C, Reilly M, Gotuzzo E, Rodriguez H, Bartoloni A, Thorson A, Falkenberg T, Bartalesi F, Tomson G, Larsson M: Antibiotic use and health-seeking behaviour in an underprivileged area of Peru. Trop Med Int Health 2008, 13(3):434-441.
13. World Health Organization: Drug and therapeutics committee: a practical guide. Geneva: World Health Organization; 2003.
14. Simpson SA, Wood F, Butler CC: General practitioners' perceptions of antimicrobial resistance: a qualitative study. J Antimicrob Chemother 2007, 59(2):292-296.
15. Garcia PJ, Vargas JH, Caballero NP, Calle VJ, Bayer AM: An e-health driven laboratory information system to support HIV treatment in Peru: E-quity for laboratory personnel, health providers and people living with HIV. BMC Med Inform Decis Mak 2009, 9:50.
16. Martinez A, Villarroel V, Seoane J, del Pozo F: A study of a rural telemedicine system in the Amazon region of Peru. J Telemed Telecare 2004, 10(4):219-225.
17. Nweihed L ML, Martin A: Influencia de los padres en la prescripcion de antibioticos hecha por los pediatras. Arch Venez Pueric Pediatr 2002, 65:21-27.
18. Vesga O AM, Salazar BE, Rodriguez CA, Zuluaga AF: Generic vancomycin products fail in vivo despite being pharmaceutical equivalents of the innovator. Antimicrob agents chemother 2010, 54(8):3271-3279.
19. Rodriguez CA, Agudelo M, Zuluaga AF, Vesga O: In vitro and in vivo comparison of the anti-staphylococcal efficacy of generic products and the innovator of oxacillin. BMC Infect Dis 2010, 10:153.
20. Amabile-Cuevas CF: Global perspectives of antibiotic resistance. In Antimicrobial resistance in developing countries.. First edition. Edited by: Sosa AB, DK; Amabile-Cuevas, CF; Hsueh, PR; Kariuki, S; Okeke, IN. New York: Springer; 2010:3-14.

Inappropriate long-term use of antipsychotic drugs is common among people with dementia living in specialized care units

Maria Gustafsson[1*], Stig Karlsson[2] and Hugo Lövheim[3]

Abstract

Background: Antipsychotic drugs are widely used for the treatment of Behavioral and Psychological Symptoms of Dementia (BPSD), despite their limited efficacy and concerns about safety. The aim of this study was to describe antipsychotic drug therapy among people with dementia living in specialized care units in northern Sweden.

Methods: This study was conducted in 40 specialized care units in northern Sweden, with a total study population of 344 people with dementia. The study population was described in regard to antipsychotic drug use, ADL function, cognitive function and BPSD, using the Multi-Dimensional Dementia Assessment Scale (MDDAS). These data were collected at baseline and six months later. Detailed data about antipsychotic prescribing were collected from prescription records.

Results: This study showed that 132 persons (38%) in the study population used antipsychotic drugs at the start of the study. Of these, 52/132 (39%) had prescriptions that followed national guidelines with regard to dose and substance.

After six months, there were 111 of 132 persons left because of deaths and dropouts. Of these 111 people, 80 (72%) were still being treated with antipsychotics, 63/111 (57%) with the same dose. People who exhibited aggressive behavior (OR: 1.980, CI: 1.515-2.588), or passiveness (OR: 1.548, CI: 1.150-2.083), or had mild cognitive impairment (OR: 2.284 CI: 1.046-4.988), were at increased risk of being prescribed antipsychotics.

Conclusion: The prevalence of antipsychotic drug use among people with dementia living in specialized care units was high and inappropriate long-term use of antipsychotic drugs was common.

Keywords: Antipsychotic prescribing, Dementia, BPSD, Inappropriate prescribing, Aggression, Passiveness

Background

Dementia is a disorder that causes permanent and progressive impairment of cognitive functions such as memory and other cognitive abilities [1]. Behavioral and Psychological Symptoms of Dementia (BPSD) is the term applied to the various problems that complicate dementia and prevalence is high. It is estimated that up to 90% of patients with Alzheimer's disease may present at least one BPSD during the course of the disease [2]. BPSD include behaviors such as aggression, screaming, rest-lessness, and also symptoms such as anxiety, hallucinations and depressive mood [3].

Antipsychotic drugs are widely used for the treatment of certain BPSDs; one study showed that 40% of elderly people with cognitive impairment living in group dwellings took antipsychotic drugs [4]. However, antipsychotic drugs have demonstrated only limited efficacy in the treatment of BPSD. A systematic review found that first generation antipsychotics had little efficacy at best, and that the benefits may not outweigh the risk of side effects [5]. The same review showed that olanzapine and risperidone had a modest, statistically significant efficacy with minimal adverse effects at lower doses [5]. However, in another study, adverse effects offset the clinical

* Correspondence: maria.gustafsson@pharm.umu.se
[1]Maria Gustafsson, Department of Pharmacology and Clinical Neuroscience, Umeå University, 901 85, Umeå, Sweden
Full list of author information is available at the end of the article

benefit of second generation antipsychotics for the treatment of BPSD [6].

Older people tend to experience side-effects more frequently and with greater severity than younger people, and antipsychotic drugs have a number of side-effects. First generation antipsychotics are associated with a high prevalence of extrapyramidal side-effects (EPS) and tardive dyskinesia due to their high affinity for D_2-receptors [7]. Second generation antipsychotics have a different receptor-binding profile. Since they interact with both D_2 and $5HT_2$-receptors, they cause EPS to a lesser extent [8]. The use of antipsychotic drugs appears to be associated with accelerated cognitive decline in people with Alzheimer's disease; treatment with haloperidol over 6–8 weeks was associated with a decline in cognition measured using the Mini-Mental State Examination (MMSE) [9]. However, one study showed that the MMSE score did not worsen after treatment with risperidone among people with dementia [10], which might be due to the lack of anticholinergic activity of risperidone [11]. All antipsychotics seem to cause metabolic side-effects. However, it appears that second generation antipsychotics are worse in this regard, even if there is variation among substances in this group [12].

Second generation antipsychotics have also been associated with an increased risk of cerebrovascular events and increased mortality, and first generation antipsychotics seem to carry the same risk [13,14].

Support for the long-term use of antipsychotics in this patient population is limited. There is some evidence favoring short-term use, [1,15] even if it is considered an option of last resort. Even short-term use of antipsychotics increases the risk of serious adverse events [16]. According to the Swedish Medical Products Agency, the dose should initially be low and then titrated upwards and treatment should be time-limited and regularly reviewed [1]. Only two recent studies have described long-term antipsychotic treatment among people with dementia [17,18] and both found relatively high rates of long-term treatment. There is still a need for detailed study of the long-term use of antipsychotic in this population. The aim of this retrospective study was to describe the prevalence, associated factors and long-term use of antipsychotic drugs among people with dementia living in specialized care units.

Methods
Subjects and settings
The study population for this project has previously been used in a research study concerning use of physical restraint [19]. This was an intervention study conducted in 2005-2006, which included 40 specialized care units (353 people) in nine communities in northern Sweden. These units are designed to provide care for six to eight persons with dementia in homelike environments. All specialized care units in these communities were inventoried, i.e. 99 units were contacted - and units with the highest prevalence of physical restraint use (≥20%) were selected. In the present study, 9 people were excluded due to incomplete data. The study was approved by the Regional Ethical Review Board in Umeå (registration number 02-105).

Procedures
Data were collected by means of a questionnaire completed by care unit staff, the Multi-Dimensional Dementia Assessment Scale (MDDAS) [20]. The MDDAS has good intra- and inter-rater reliability [20]. This instrument includes assessment of the level of functioning in activities of daily living (ADL), cognition and behavioral and psychological symptoms. ADL function score ranges from 4-24, where a higher score indicates greater ADL independence. This score is based on the person's ability to cope with hygiene, dressing, eating and bladder and bowel control. Cognitive function was measured using an assessment scale developed by Gottfries and Gottfries [21]. This scale ranges from 0-27 points and a score of less than 24 is considered to indicate cognitive impairment, correlating with a sensitivity of 90% and a specificity of 91% to the usual cut-off point of the MMSE (24/30) [21,22]. The scale is further subdivided into three groups - mild cognitive impairment (16-23), moderate cognitive impairment (8-15) and severe cognitive impairment (0-7). The MDDAS contains 25 behavioral items and 14 psychological symptom items. Each item is rated on a three-point scale indicating that the symptom was present at least once a day, once a week, or never during the observation period of one week. These variables are dichotomized between at least once a week and less than once a week in the present study.

All persons' prescription records were collected at the start of the study and six months later. The majority of people dispensing service where the used an automated multidose dispensing service where the persons' drugs are dispensed in one dose unit bag for each dose occasion.

The prescription records were searched to identify those people from the study population treated with antipsychotic drugs. All people were listed by age, sex, and treatment with antidepressants (N06A), anxiolytics, hypnotics and sedatives (N05B&C), anti-dementia drugs (N06D), and antipsychotics (N05A). The WHO ATC (Anatomical Therapeutic Chemical Index) classification system was used.

Information about dose and type of antipsychotic drugs was collected, and also indication for treatment when this was reported in the prescription records. These indications are written by the prescribing physicians to describe for the patient and nursing staff why the patient is prescribed the drug. Also, the pharmacy uses the indication to check the appropriateness of drug choice and dose.

Lithium (N05AN01) was not included since it differs from antipsychotics regarding both mechanism of action and use. Pro re nata (PRN) drugs were also not included, as information was lacking on the actual use of these drugs, and furthermore very few people used PRN antipsychotics.

To be able to compare antipsychotic doses between baseline and follow-up, we calculated all antipsychotics in haloperidol equivalents. Recommendations concerning antipsychotic use vary slightly in different guidelines [1,15]. Since this study was conducted in Sweden, we used the guidelines from the Swedish Medical Products Agency to evaluate the appropriate use of antipsychotics [1]. These guidelines state that risperidone is the only antipsychotic drug that is labeled for use in combating BPSD in Sweden, and the recommended dose is ≤1.5 mg daily. According to the same guidelines, the indications that justify the prescribing of antipsychotic drugs in people with BPSD are psychotic symptoms and aggressive behavior that causes suffering or potential danger for the person or others.

Statistics and calculations

People who did and did not take antipsychotics were compared using the Pearson chi-square test and t-test for dichotomous and continuous variables respectively. SPSS 18 for MacOS X was used for data handling and statistical calculations. A p-value of < 0.05 was considered statistically significant. A multiple logistic regression model was constructed to find factors independently associated with antipsychotic drug use. The behavioral and the psychological symptom items of the MDDAS were grouped and weighted (in each group every symptom was multiplied with the calculated factor loading and then added with next symptom) according to a factor analysis previously described by Lövheim et al [23]. The factors were then normalized and included in a logistic regression model which also included age, sex and level of cognitive impairment. As many of the behavioral and psychological symptoms correlated strongly, the behaviors and symptoms were tested in the regression model in a stepwise procedure, where the behavior that had the strongest bivariate correlation (aggressive behavior) was included first, and all other behaviors and symptoms were included subsequently one by one to see if any of them contributed independently. These behaviors and factors, apart from aggressive behavior, were: wandering behavior, restless behavior, verbally disruptive/ attention-seeking behavior, passiveness, hallucinatory symptoms, depressive symptoms, disoriented symptoms and regressive/inappropriate behavior. Ultimately, all significant behaviors and symptoms were included in a final model.

Survival among people who were treated with antipsychotic drugs at the start of the study was compared with those who were not treated with antipsychotics, using a Cox regression, also including age, sex and level of cognitive impairment.

Results

The study population comprised 344 people with dementia whose characteristics are presented in Table 1. One hundred and thirty-two (38%) of these people used antipsychotic drugs at the start of the study; 118 people were prescribed one antipsychotic drug, 13 took two, and 1 person had three antipsychotic drugs prescribed concomitantly. Ninety prescriptions were for second generation antipsychotics, and 57 for first generation antipsychotics. There were no associations between antipsychotic drug use and antidepressant drug use, or between antipsychotic drug use and anti-dementia drug use. However, there was an association between antipsychotic drug use and anxiolytic, hypnotic and sedative drug use, as shown in Table 1. An association was found between antipsychotic drug prescribing and age, but no difference between men and women.

The multiple logistic regression analysis showed that those who exhibited an aggressive behavior, or passiveness, were younger or had mild cognitive impairment as compared to severe cognitive impairment, were at increased risk of being prescribed an antipsychotic drug (Table 2).

After six months, 111 people remained to be evaluated of those who were treated with antipsychotics at baseline (7 dropouts, 14 deceased), as presented in Figure 1. Of these 111 people, 80 (72%) were still being treated with antipsychotics, 63 of these with the same dose. Seventy-eight people of 80 were taking the same antipsychotics as before. Of those who were not treated with antipsychotics at baseline, 10 people were receiving antipsychotics at the 6- month follow-up. After six months, 31 persons had ended their treatment with antipsychotics. The mean age of this group was 83.1, compared to 80.0 among those who still were using antipsychotics after six months (80 persons). However, this difference was not significant. No significant differences were seen concerning ADL, cognitive score or sex.

The mortality analysis showed no difference in mortality between those who received antipsychotics at the start of the study and those who did not (OR 0.69, CI 0.36-1.32, p-value 0.26).

At the start of the study, 132 people were prescribed antipsychotic drugs; 62 of these received risperidone, the only antipsychotic drug that is labeled for use in BPSD in Sweden, as shown in Table 3. Of these 62, 52 received the recommended dose, i.e. ≤1.5 mg daily. Hence, 52/ 132 (39%) received both recommended antipsychotic

Table 1 Characteristics of study population and comparison between people with and without antipsychotics

	With AP	Without AP	Total	p-value
Cases, n (%)	132 (38.4)	212 (61.6)	344	
Women, n (%)	92 (69.7)	153 (72.2)	245 (71.2)	0.62
Mean age ± SD	80.9 ± 8.6	82.9 ± 7.2	82.1 ± 7.8	0.02
ADL score (4-24) mean ± SD	11.9 ± 5.2	12.2 ± 5.4	12.1 ± 5.3	0.63
Cognitive score (0-27) mean ± SD	10.6 ± 7.4	10.0 ± 7.2	10.2 ± 7.3	0.47
Antidepressant (N06A) use, n (%)	73 (55.3)	107 (50.5)	180 (52.3)	0.38
Anxiolytics, hypnotics and sedatives (N05B&C) use, n (%)	72 (54.5)	84 (39.6)	156 (45.3)	0.007
Anxiolytics (N05B) use, n (%)	28 (21.2)	18 (8.5)	46 (13.4)	0.001
Hypnotics and sedatives (N05C) use, n (%)	63 (47.7)	76 (35.8)	139 (40.4)	0.029
Anti-dementia drugs (N06D) use, n (%)	26 (19.7)	45 (21.2)	71 (20.6)	0.733

SD= Standard Deviation, ADL= activities of daily living, AP= Antipsychotic drug.

drug and the recommended dose, assuming that antipsychotics were used solely for the treatment of BPSD.

The indications for prescribing antipsychotic drugs to this patient group are listed in Table 4. The most common indication was "treatment of disturbed and restless behavior/sedative". No indication was listed for 19 prescriptions. After six months, ten people who did not receive antipsychotics at baseline, had been started on antipsychotic drugs. Of these ten, one received risperidone and nine people received other antipsychotics. The dose of risperidone of this one person, however, was higher than the recommended dose. The most common indication was "treatment of disturbed and restless behavior/sedative", similar to those having antipsychotics at study start.

Discussion

This study showed that many people with dementia who lived in specialized care units were prescribed antipsychotic drugs for long periods. It seems that in most

Table 2 Multiple logistic regression of antipsychotic drug use

	Odds Ratio	95% confidence interval	p-value
Male sex	0.969	0.546-1.719	0.913
Higher age	0.958	0.924-0.993	0.018
Moderate cognitive impairment[a]	1.802	0.973-3.338	0.061
Mild cognitive impairment[a]	2.284	1.046-4.988	0.038
Aggressive behavior	1.980	1.515-2.588	<0.001
Passiveness	1.548	1.150-2.083	0.004

Model Cox and Snell R^2: 0.129, concordance between observed and predicted value: 67.6%. [a] Cognitive score ranges from 0-27 points and a score of less than 24 is considered to indicate cognitive impairment. The scale is subdivided into three groups, 0-7 (severe cognitive impairment), 8-15 (moderate cognitive impairment) and 16-23 (mild cognitive impairment). Severe cognitive impairment is reference category.

cases the doses were probably not regularly adjusted; a majority of the people appeared to be on stable doses for six months or possibly longer. There were also few people in our study who had been prescribed the drugs in agreement with current recommendations concerning dosage and drug choice. The study showed that people who exhibited aggressive behavior, or passiveness, or had a higher cognitive score, were at increased risk of being prescribed antipsychotics. Those who received antipsychotics were also significantly younger. We found no difference between men and women concerning antipsychotic drug use.

Furthermore, the use of more than one psychotropic drug seemed to be common, 72/344 had anxiolytics/hypnotics/sedatives and an antipsychotic drug prescribed simultaneously and 73/344 had antidepressants and an antipsychotic drug prescribed simultaneously. In addition, 14 persons had more than one antipsychotic drug prescribed.

The present results are in accordance with previous studies. One study found that people received psychotropic drugs over at least one year despite uncertainty about symptom improvement and another study showed that most antipsychotic prescriptions remained unchanged over a six-month period [17,18]. In the present study, 63/111 (57%) received exactly the same antipsychotic dose after six months. The high prevalence of long-term use is not in line with current recommendations which emphasize that treatment should be time-limited and regularly reviewed [15]. Selbæk et al also demonstrated that most symptoms show an intermittent course which does not support long-term treatment with antipsychotics [18]. O'Connor et al discuss the fact that the person's symptoms are classified as present when in reality they occur only occasionally [17]. These findings stress the importance of reviewing antipsychotic use regularly to ensure that the indication remains. One study also showed that dementia persons' symptoms

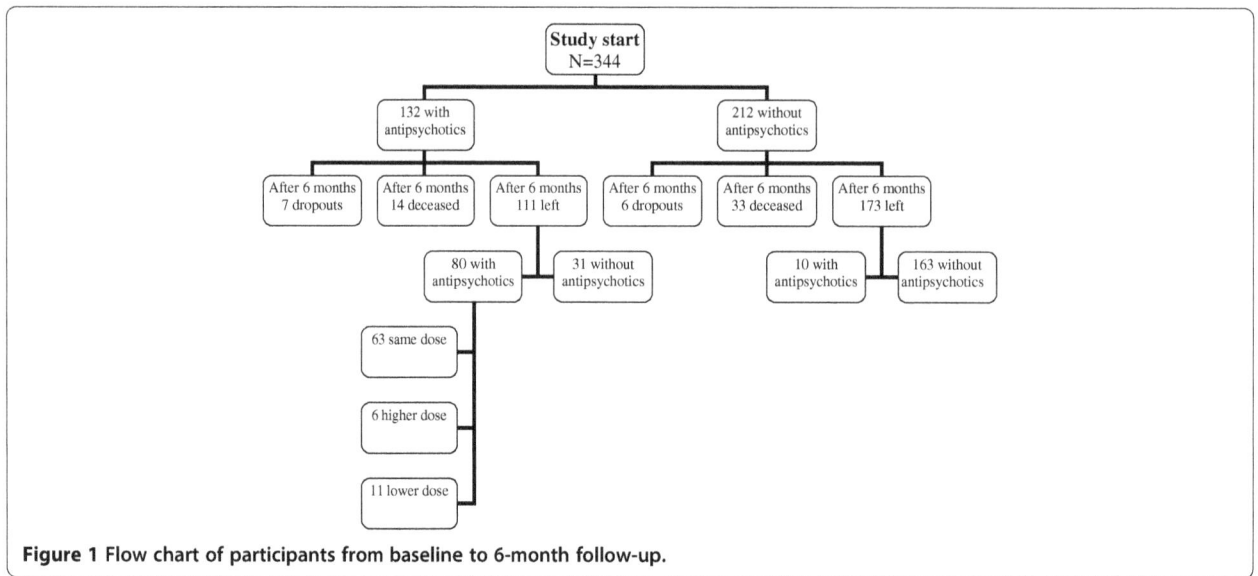

Figure 1 Flow chart of participants from baseline to 6-month follow-up.

remain stable when they are withdrawn from first generation antipsychotics, and another study found that people actually improved when second generation antipsychotics were withdrawn [25,26].

Furthermore, the indications that were given for the prescriptions in our study were not in line with the recommendations. By far the most common indication in this study was "treatment of disturbed and restless behavior/sedative", and this is not an approved indication, according to the guidelines. Some indications were doubtful and in many cases were missing. However, these results should be interpreted with caution since the indications often overlap and the way of expression

might differ between physicians. The choice of antipsychotic drugs among prescribers in this study was somewhat surprising considering that the second generation antipsychotics risperidone and olanzapine seem to have the best evidence-base for effectiveness, compared to placebo for physical aggression, agitation and psychosis [27,28]. Risperidone and haloperidol were the most commonly used antipsychotics in our study, which is to be expected. Haloperidol has little anticholinergic activity and was by many considered the most preferable antipsychotic to people with dementia before the introduction of the second generation antipsychotics. An established treatment tradition might possibly have

Table 3 Characteristics of antipsychotic drugs at the start of the study

Drug	n	Percent (%) of prescribings	Dose, mean ± SD	Median Dose (mg)	Range (mg)	Mean Dose (mg) Haloperidol equivalents	Halo-peridol 1 mg equivalent doses[a]
First generation AP							
Haloperidol	25	17.0	2.1±3.1	1.0	0.5-16	2.1	1
Levomepromazine	12	8.1	19.6±15.6	15.0	5-50	0.4	50
Zuclopenthixol	6	4.1	3.7±2.0	3.0	2-6	0.7	5
Dixyrazine	5	3.4	32.0±38.3	20.0	10-100	1.1	30
Melperone	4	2.7	33.8±11.1	30.0	25-50	0.8	40
Perphenazine	4	2.7	7.8±5.9	6.0	3-16	1.9	4
Chlorpromazine	1	0.7	100.0			2.0	50
Second generation AP							
Risperidone	62	42.2	1.1±1.1	0.8	0.25-8	1.1	1
Olanzapine	18	12.2	6.9±5.1	5.0	3-20	2.3	3
Ziprasidone	6	4.1	60.0±31.0	50.0	40-120	1.5	40
Clozapine	3	2.0	216.7±332.0	25.0	25-600	4.3	50
Quetiapine	1	0.7	50.0			0.3	150

Number of prescriptions=147, number of persons taking AP=132, AP=antipsychotic drugs. [a][24].

Table 4 Indications for antipsychotic treatment at the start of the study

Treatment of disturbed and restless behavior/sedative n (%)	67 (42.9)
Delusions/hallucinations/paranoia n (%)	16 (10.3)
Treatment of mood/irritability/anxiety, n (%)	14 (9.0)
Treatment of aggression, n (%)	13 (8.3)
Treatment of insomnia, n (%)	12 (7.7)
Treatment of psychosis, n (%)	7 (4.5)
Treatment of confusion, n (%)	3 (1.9)
To combat behavioral disorders/BPSD, n (%)	2 (1.3)
Other indications, n (%)	3 (1.9)
No indication, n (%)	19 (12.2)

Indication at baseline. Number of prescriptions=147, number of persons taking antipsychotics=132. The number of indications (156) is higher since there were sometimes more than one indication per prescription.

delayed the switch to second generation drugs and explain why many old people with dementia were still treated with haloperidol in 2006. Haloperidol has some efficacy against behavioral problems in higher doses, but its use is limited by side-effects [1]. Risperidone on the other hand is a well-tolerated alternative among people with dementia in lower doses [29] and is, as stated above, the only antipsychotic drug that is labeled for use in BPSD in Sweden. The proportion of people with antipsychotics treated with second generation drugs will probably continue to increase [30].

A more unexpected finding was the fact that these two drugs did not account for a larger share of the antipsychotic prescriptions. Many older first generation antipsychotics and also some of the newest second generation antipsychotics were used to treat BPSD in this patient group. The reason prescribing physicians deviated from current guidelines is unclear. This study was conducted in 2005 and 2006, i.e. 2-3 years before the guideline was issued. Possibly, the prescription may have changed due to new recommendations, however, we still find it relevant to compare the treatment with what is now considered to be appropriate medication.

However, there are other possibilities for treating BPSD in persons with dementia. Primarily, non-pharmacological approaches are recommended, such as investigation /survey of symptoms, possible causes and triggering moments. It is also important to review current pharmacological treatment and consider discontinuation of drugs with potentially adverse effects on the central nervous system and finally, to optimize the care environment and treatment [1,31]. For example, it has been shown that music, physical exercise and recreation might have some effect considering psychological symptoms in people with dementia [32]. When it comes to pharmacological treatment, memantine, cholinesterase inhibitors and SSRI have shown positive efficacy in various studies [33-39]. Among anti-

dementia drugs, memantine appears to reduce specific problems such as agitation and irritability [34]. Concerning cholinesterase inhibitors, one meta-analysis showed that rivastigmine had positive effects on nonpsychotic and psychotic symptoms associated with Alzheimer's disease [35]. Among antidepressants, citalopram has for example showed significant efficacy against behavioral disturbances in individuals with dementia [36,37], and sertraline has showed efficacy against aggressive behavior [38]. Selective serotonin reuptake inhibitors are also recommended as first line treatment for irritability, agitation and anxiety among people with dementia [1].

The association found between antipsychotics and aggressive behavior, as well as the association between antipsychotic use and lower age, confirms the results of an earlier study [4]. The increased risk of receiving antipsychotic treatment among people with aggressive behavior might be expected since this is one of the approved indications for antipsychotics. We also found an association between use of antipsychotics and a higher cognitive score. It has been shown that the prevalence of the behaviors and symptoms decline in those with severe cognitive impairment, and this might possibly lead to less use of antipsychotics [23]. There was also an association between passiveness and use of antipsychotics in the present study. It has been shown that passiveness increases almost linearly with the severity of cognitive impairment [23]. It can be difficult to know what is cause and what is effect, but the passiveness shown among those who use antipsychotic drugs might also, in some cases, be a side-effect of the antipsychotics.

This study did not show any difference in mortality between those who received antipsychotics at the start of the study and those who did not. Several studies have reported an increased mortality among people prescribed antipsychotics, [13,14] while other studies have not - for example one study that found no association between antipsychotics and cerebrovascular events compared to benzodiazepines [40]. A selection effect, where the healthier persons were possibly prescribed antipsychotics more frequently, might have contributed to our results considering mortality and antipsychotics. We did not know the length of exposure to antipsychotics, only that a person was treated with an antipsychotic drug at the start of the study and this have possibly influenced the results. Also, in this study we lacked information about the prevalence of cerebrovascular diseases and other co-morbidities that might have impacted on mortality.

In this study we have been able to describe in detail long-term use of antipsychotics among people with dementia. The registration of drugs and doses in the present study was of high quality. We can also assume that compliance was high since the vast majority of patients used an automated dose dispensing system.

The study also has some methodological limitations. The selection of specialized care units was not random but based on the prevalence of physical restraint use. It could be that people in these homes have severe problems with BPSD and, therefore, receive long-term treatment to a greater extent. In the physical restraint study [19] there was no difference in antipsychotic use within groups or between groups at baseline and after six months, but we have not been able to compare data with non-selected units since we do not have that information. However, the proportion of those who were on antipsychotic drugs does not appear to differ from those found in other studies [4]. We believe that this does not affect the main results of the study, but it should be borne in mind when interpreting the results.

Data were registered at the start of the study and six months later, but what happened between those times is not known, except for mortality. We do not know the duration of antipsychotic treatment at the time of recruitment into the study, and we also do not know if any attempts of dose reduction or attempts of non-pharmacological treatment of BPSD have been made. Further, we do not know the background or other diseases of the participants, and we lack information about adverse effects of antipsychotics e.g. extrapyramidal effects or falls.

In our study, there could possibly have been reasons other than BPSD for prescribing antipsychotics. Some people might have schizophrenia or other chronic psychotic illnesses where recommendations about dose and substance differ from recommendations among people with dementia. This might, to some extent, explain the use of other antipsychotic drugs or higher doses.

Still, the reason for prescribing antipsychotics is probably related to BPSD in the vast majority of cases, among old people with dementia living in specialized care units.

Conclusion

The prevalence of antipsychotic drug use among people with dementia living in specialized care units was high and inappropriate long-term use of antipsychotic drugs was common. The prescriptions were often not in agreement with current recommendations.

Competing interests

The authors declare no conflict of interests.

Authors' contributions

SK was responsible for the study concept, design and acquisition of subjects. MG reviewed the data for a second time and HL made the statistical analysis. MG and HL analyzed and interpreted the data and prepared the manuscript. All authors critically revised the manuscript, added their comments and approved the final version.

Acknowledgements

This study was supported financially by grants from the Swedish Academy of Pharmaceutical Sciences, the Lions Research Foundation for Age-Related Diseases, Swedish Brain Power, the Swedish Dementia Association and the County Council of Västerbotten.

Author details

[1]Maria Gustafsson, Department of Pharmacology and Clinical Neuroscience, Umeå University, 901 85, Umeå, Sweden. [2]Stig Karlsson, Department of Nursing, Umeå University, Umeå, Sweden. [3]Hugo Lövheim, Department of Community Medicine and Rehabilitation, Geriatric Medicine, Umeå University, Umeå, Sweden.

References

1. Läkemedelsverket: *Beteendemässiga och psykiska symtom vid demenssjukdom – BPSD [In English: Drug therapy and treatment for Behavioral and Psychological Symptoms of dementia – BPSD. Information from the Medical Products Agency].* Retrieved June 10, 2012 from http://www.lakemedelsverket.se/upload/halso-och-sjukvard/behandlingsrekommendationer/BPSD_bakgrund_webb.pdf.
2. Liperoti R, Pedone C, Corsonello A: **Antipsychotics for the treatment of Behavioral and Psychological Symptoms of Dementia (BPSD).** *Current Neuropharmacology* 2008, **6:**117–124.
3. Cerejeira J, Lagarto L, Mukaetova-Ladinska EB: **Behavioral and psychological symptoms of dementia.** *Frontiers in Neurology* 2012, **3:**73.
4. Lövheim H, Sandman PO, Kallin K, Karlsson S, Gustafson Y: **Relationship between antipsychotic drug use and behavioral and psychological symptoms of dementia in old people with cognitive impairment living in geriatric care.** *Int Psychogeriatr* 2006, **18:**713–26.
5. Sink KM, Holden KF, Yaffe K: **Pharmacological treatment of neuropsychiatric symptoms of dementia: a review of the evidence.** *J Am Med Assoc* 2005, **293:**596–608.
6. Schneider LS, Tariot PN, Dagerman KS, Davis SM, Hsiao JK, Ismail MS, Lebowitz BD, Lyketsos CG, Ryan JM, Stroup TS, Sultzer DL, Weintraub D, Lieberman JA, CATIE-AD Study Group: **Effectiveness of atypical antipsychotic drugs in patients with Alzheimer's disease.** *N Eng J Med* 2006, **355:**1525–1538.
7. Neil W, Curran S, Wattis J: **Antipsychotic prescribing in older people.** *Age Ageing* 2003, **32:**475–483.
8. Gareri P, De Fazio P, Stilo MA, Ferreri G, De Sarro G: **Conventional and atypical antipsychotics in the elderly: a review.** *Clin Drug Investig* 2003, **23:**287–322.
9. Gareri P, Cortoneo A, Marchisio U, Curcio M, De Sarro G: **Risperidone in the treatment of behavioral disorders in elderly patients with dementia.** *Arch Gerontol Geriatr Suppl* 2001, **7:**173–82.
10. Gareri P, De Fazio P, De Fazio S, Marigliano N, Ferreri Ibbadu G, De Sarro G: **Adverse effects of atypical antipsychotics in the elderly: a review.** *Drugs Aging* 2006, **23:**937–56.
11. Devanand DP, Sackeim HA, Brown RP, Mayeux R: **A pilot study of haloperidol treatment of psychosis and behavioral disturbance in Alzheimer's disease.** *Arch Neurol* 1989, **46:**854–857.
12. Melkersson KI, Dahl ML, Hulting AL: **Guidelines for prevention and treatment of adverse effects of antipsychotic drugs on glucose-insulin homeostasis and lipid metabolism.** *Psychopharmacology* 2004, **175:**1–6.
13. Schneider LS, Dagerman KS, Insel P: **Risk of death with atypical antipsychotic drug treatment for dementia: meta-analysis of randomized placebo-controlled trials.** *J Am Med Assoc* 2005, **294:**1934–1943.
14. Gill SS, Bronskill SE, Normand SL, Anderson GM, Sykora K, Lam K, Bell CM, Lee PE, Fischer HD, Herrmann N, Gurwitz JH, Rochon PA: **Antipsychotic drug use and mortality in older adults in dementia.** *Ann Intern Med* 2007, **146:**775–786.
15. National Institute for Health and Clinical Excellence (NICE): *Dementia - Supporting people with dementia and their careers in health and social care.* Retrieved June 24, 2012 from: http://www.nice.org.uk/nicemedia/live/10998/30318/30318.pdf.
16. Rochon PA, Normand SL, Gomes T, Gill SS, Anderson GM, Melo M, Sykora K, Lipscombe L, Bell CM, Gurwitz JH: **Antipsychotic therapy and short-term serious events in older adults with dementia.** *Arch Intern Med* 2008, **168:**1090–1096.

17. O'Connor DW, Griffith J, McSweeney K: Changes to psychotropic medications in the six month after admission to nursing homes in Melbourne, Australia. *Int Psychogeriatr* 2010, **22**:1149–53.

18. Selbæk G, Kirkevold Ø, Engedal K: The course of psychiatric and behavioural symptoms and the use of psychotropic medication in patients with dementia in Norwegian nursing homes a 12-month follow-up study. *Am J Geriatr Psychiatry* 2008, **16**:528–536.

19. Pellfolk TJ, Gustafson Y, Bucht G, Karlsson S: Effects of a restraint minimization program on staff knowledge, attitudes, and practice: a cluster randomized trial. *J Am Geriatr Soc* 2010, **58**:62–9.

20. Sandman PO, Adolfsson R, Norberg A, Nyström L, Winblad B: Long-term care of the elderly. A descriptive study of 3600 institutionalized patients in the county of Vasterbotten, Sweden. *Compr Gerontol A* 1988, **2**:120–132.

21. Adolfsson R, Gottfries CG, Nyström L, Winblad B: Prevalence of dementia disorders in institutionalized Swedish old people. The work load imposed by caring for these patients. *Acta Psychiatr Scand* 1981, **63**:225–244.

22. Folstein MF, Folstein SE, McHugh PR: "Mini-mental state": a practical method for grading the cognitive state of patients for the clinican. *J Psychiatr Res* 1975, **12**:189–198.

23. Lövheim H, Sandman PO, Karlsson S, Gustafson Y: Behavioral and psychological symptoms of dementia in relation to level of cognitive impairment. *Int Psychogeriatr* 2008, **20**:777–89.

24. Eriksson L, Pelling H: Psykoser [In English: Psychoses]. In *Läkemedelsboken. 2005/2006*. Stockholm: Apoteket AB; 2005:806–814.

25. Cohen-Mansfield J, Lipson S, Werner P, Billig N, Taylor L, Woosley R: Withdrawal of haloperidol, thioridazine, and lorazepam in the nursing home: a controlled, double-blind study. *Arch Intern Med* 1999, **159**:1733–1740.

26. Ruths S, Straand J, Nygaard HA, Aarsland D: Stopping antipsychotic drug therapy in demented nursing home patients: a randomized, placebo-controlled study – The Bergen District Nursing Home Study (BEDNURS). *Int J Geriatr Psychiatry* 2008, **23**:889–895.

27. Brodaty H, Ames D, Snowdon J, Woodward M, Kirwan J, Clarnette R, Lee E, Lyons B, Grossman F: A randomized placebo-controlled trial of risperidone for the treatment of aggression, agitation, and psychosis of dementia. *J Clin Psychiatry* 2003, **64**:134–143.

28. Street JS, Clark WS, Gannon KS, Cummings JL, Bymaster FP, Tamura RN, Mitan SJ, Kadam DL, Sanger TM, Feldman PD, Tollefson GD, Breier A, The HGEU Study Group: Olanzapine treatment of psychotic and behavioral symptoms in patients with Alzheimer disease in nursing care facilities: a double-blind, randomized, placebo-controlled trial. *Arch Gen Psychiatry* 2000, **57**:968–76.

29. Gareri P, Cotroneo A, Lacava R, Seminara G, Marigliano N, Loiacono A, De Sarro G: Comparison of the efficacy of new and conventional antipsychotic drugs in the treatment of behavioral and psychological symptoms of dementia (BPSD). *Arch Gerontol Geriatr Suppl* 2004, **9**:207–15.

30. Lövheim H, Gustafson Y, Karlsson S, Sandman PO: Comparison of behavioral and psychological symptoms of dementia and psychotropic drug treatments among old people in geriatric care in 2000 and 2007. *Int Psychogeriatr* 2011, **23**:1616–22.

31. Fossey J, Ballard C, Juszczak E, James I, Alder N, Jacoby R, Howard R: Effect of enhanced psychosocial care on antipsychotic use in nursing home residents with severe dementia: cluster randomised trial. *Br Med J* 2006, **332**:756–61.

32. O'Connor DW, Ames D, Gardner B, King M: Psychosocial treatments of psychological symptoms in dementia: a systematic review of reports meeting quality standards. *Int Psychogeriatr* 2009, **21**:241–251.

33. Maidment ID, Fox CG, Boustani M, Rodriguez J, Brown RC, Katona CL: Efficacy of memantine on behavioral and psychological symptoms related to dementia: a systematic meta-analysis. *Ann Pharmacother* 2008, **42**:32–38.

34. Gauthier S, Cummings J, Ballard C, Brodaty H, Grossberg G, Robert P, Lyketsos C: Management of behavioral problems in Alzheimer's disease. *Int Psychogeriatr* 2010, **22**:346–72.

35. Finkel SI: Effects of rivastigmine on behavioral and psychological symptoms of dementia in Alzheimer's disease. *Clin Ther* 2004, **26**:980–990.

36. Pollock BG, Mulsant BH, Rosen J, Sweet RA, Mazumdar S, Bharucha A, Marin R, Jacob NJ, Huber KA, Kastango KB, Chew ML: Comparison of citalopram, perphenazine, and placebo for the acute treatment of psychosis and behavioral disturbances in hospitalized, demented patients. *Am J Psychiatry* 2002, **159**:460–465.

37. Nyth AL, Gottfries CG: The clinical efficacy of citalopram in treatment of emotional disturbances in dementia disorders. A Nordic Multicentre study. *Br J Psychiatry* 1990, **157**:894–901.

38. Lanctôt KL, Herrmann N, van Reekum R, Eryavec G, Naranjo CA: Gender, aggression and serotonergic function are associated with response to sertraline for behavioral disturbances in Alzheimer's disease. *Int J Geriatr Psychiatry* 2002, **17**:531–541.

39. Pollock BG, Mulsant BH, Rosen J, Mazumdar S, Blakesley RE, Houck PR, Huber KA: A double-blind comparison of Citalopram and Risperidone for the Treatment of Behavioral and Psychotic Symptoms Associated With Dementia. *Am J Geriatr Psychiatry* 2007, **15**:942–52.

40. Finkel S, Kozma C, Long S, Greenspan A, Mahmoud R, Baser O, Engelhart L: Risperidone treatment in elderly patients with dementia: relative risk of cerebrovascular events versus other antipsychotics. *Int Psychogeriatr* 2005, **17**:617–29.

16

Use of antipsychotic and antidepressant within the Psychiatric Disease Centre, Regional Health Service of Ferrara

Stefano Bianchi*, Erica Bianchini and Paola Scanavacca

Abstract

Background: This study aimed at describing the type and dosage of psychopharmaceuticals dispensed to patients with psychiatric disorders and to assess the percentage of patients treated with antipsychotics and antidepressants, the associated therapies, treatment adherence, and dosages used in individuals registered at the Psychiatric Disease Center (PDC), Regional Health Service of Ferrara.

Methods: The analysis focused on therapeutic programmes presented to the Department of Pharmacy of the University Hospital of Ferrara of 892 patients treated by the PDC (catchment area of 134605 inhabitants). All diagnoses were made according to International Classification of Diseases (ICD-9). The analysis focused on prescriptions from September 2007 to June 2009. Data on adherence to prescribed therapy have were processed by analysis of variance.

Results: Among the patients 63% were treated with antipsychotics and 40% with antidepressants. Among patients receiving antipsychotics 92% used second-generation antipsychotics (SGAs) whereas the remaining 8% used first generation antipsychotics (FGAs). Antipsychotic doses were lower than Daily Defined Dose (DDDs), and SGAs were often given with anticholinergics to decrease side effects. Mean adherence to antipsychotic therapy was 64%. Among antidepressants, selective serotonin reuptake inhibitors (SSRIs) were the most often prescribed, 55%. Dosages of these were within the limits indicated by the technical datasheet but higher than DDDs. Only 26% of patients underwent monotherapy. In antidepressants polytherapy, medication was associated with another antidepressant, 6% or with an antipsychotic, 51%. Mean adherence to the antidepressant therapy was 64%.

Conclusions: Patients treated with antipsychotics tend to use doses lower than DDDs. The opposite tendency was noted in patients treated with antidepressants. Only a small percentage of patients (14%) modified their neuroleptic therapy by increasing the dosage. On the contrary, patients treated with antidepressants mainly tended to reduce the doses of their drugs. This study highlights the tendency to follow combination therapies, prescribing SGAs together with anticholinergics in order to minimize extrapyramidal side effects or by combining two antidepressants. The study showed low adherence for both pharmaceutical therapies, which is typical in the setting of the analyzed diseases.

Background

Psychiatric disorders including different forms of depression and psychosis are highly debilitating conditions that generate strong discomfort in affected patients and a heavy burden on society as a whole; drugs indicated for these are expensive and treatment for these patients costs more than the average cost of care for other common diseases such as diabetes and hypertension.

Several studies [1,2] demonstrated good efficacy of antipsychotics and antidepressants in alleviating mental disorders such as schizophrenia, depression, and bipolar disorder. However, the efficacy of controlling the symptoms of these disorders clearly depends on patient adherence to treatments, which is typically unsatisfactory [3].

* Correspondence: s.bianchi@ospfe.it
Department of Pharmacy, University Hospital of Ferrara, Corso Giovecca 203, 44123 Ferrara (Italy

Literature reports [4,5] show significant differences between prescriptions in the clinical setting of psychiatric disorders and recommendations in official guidelines. In particular, studies on prescription of drugs have highlighted the frequent co-prescription of two or more medications [6-10], including anticholinergics [11,12], antidepressants, and antiepileptic drugs. Moreover, further studies [13] have shown that a high percentage of users receive drugs that affect the CNS above defined therapeutic ranges [14,15].

In this study, we looked at the patterns of antipsychotic and antidepressant use within the Psychiatric Disease Centre (PDC), Regional Health Service of Ferrara, Italy.

Method

Study design

This was a descriptive, retrospective single-centre study focusing on drugs prescribed by the psychiatrists of the PDC, with a catchment area of 134605 inhabitants, and dispensed by the Department of Pharmacy of the University Hospital of Ferrara.

The study mainly focused on patients treated at the PDC with antipsychotics (Anatomical Therapeutic Chemical [ATC] N05) and antidepressants (ATC N06), even when associated with CNS-active drugs (ATC N). ATC is a classification system in which drugs are divided into different groups depending on the organ and their chemical, pharmacological, and therapeutic properties. Drug prescriptions including CNS-inactive drugs were not taken into account.

The observation period was 26 months from March 2007 to 31 May 2009. The number of patients evaluated during the evaluation period was 911.

Since the diagnoses for 21% of patients were incomplete, it was not possible to obtain definitive diagnoses for all patients considered in the study. Furthermore, 19 patients (2%) were ineligible for the study because they did not take drugs specified in the inclusion criteria mentioned above. Therefore, the total number of patients eligible for this study was 892 (98%). Drugs prescribed to patients treated by the PDC were all dispensed by the hospital pharmacy.

Subjects

This study was approved by the Ethics Committee of Ferrara on 28/07/2011 and conducted by applying the legislative decree of June 24, 2003, no. 211 of Good Clinical Practice in clinical trials of medicines for clinical use. The study was conducted in accordance with the Declaration of Helsinki.

Efficacy and safety assessment

This study aimed to assess the use of antipsychotic agents (ATC N05) and antidepressants (ATC N06) dispensed to patients treated at the PDC, Regional Health Service of Ferrara. More specifically, it aimed to assess:

- clinical characteristics of patients;
- type of drugs prescribed and their dosage;
- doses used compared with those indicated by drug technical datasheets (Summary Product Characteristics; SPC) and the Daily Defined Dose (DDD) [16];
- potential modifications to therapy (change of active drugs and their doses or addition of other active drugs);
- percent patients treated with polytherapy and analysis of the most frequent combinations;
- patient adherence to prescribed therapies, calculated as percentage drugs consumed versus quantity prescribed.

Description of instruments

Patients treated at the PDC obtained drugs prescribed by psychiatrists from the Department of Pharmacy of the University Hospital of Ferrara. The pharmacist completed the dispensation database including the following information: patient data (name, date of birth); prescribing specialist; diagnosis (coded as ICD-9), prescription (limitation period; prescribed medication; dosage; pharmaceutical form; routes of administration; active substance or drug); and amount of medication dispensed calculated on the basis of previous drug dispensations.

From that database, we analyzed the following data: overview of patient data, pathology according to ICD-9, prescribing centre, number of tablets/capsules/vials distributed, duration of prescription, daily dosage, quantity consumed. All variations made by doctors on patients' prescriptions concerning routes and time of administration were also taken into account.

We calculated the minimum, average, and maximum doses of the psychopharmaceuticals used in therapies and compared them with the DDDs as well as the minimum and maximum dosages of typical and atypical drugs listed in the SPCs.

Being the only daily average dosage internationally recognized, the DDD value was chosen as a parameter to compare daily dosages of therapy. Moreover, the dosage corresponding to the maximum frequency used in therapy was calculated for each drug.

Patient level of adherence to prescribed therapies was also assessed, calculated as the ratio between the amount of drug they actually withdrew to that prescribed by the doctor.

Statistics

Data on adherence to prescribed therapy were assessed by analysis of variance (ANOVA). Adherence was reported as the mean and its confidence interval 95% to asses whether is a difference in adherence of the various molecules. For statistical analysis we used SPSS 18 software.

A t-test was performed on the average adherence of patients treated with FGAs compared with SGAs.

Results

Patients

A total of 892 patients were eligible for the study (M/F, 362/530); their clinical characteristics are shown in Table 1.

Mood disorders (especially major depressive disorder and bipolar disorder) and schizophrenia were the most frequently diagnosed conditions, accounting for 36% and 35%, respectively, for a combined total of 72% of all diagnoses (Table 2).

Antipsychotics

In all, 63% of patients (564/892) were prescribed antipsychotics; 42% of them (235/564) were men and 58% (329/564) women. Their age range was 15-98 years and most (40% of the total) were in the age range 41-60 years, although a few prescriptions were made to patients aged <20 years (0.5%) and in their 90s (1%). Mean age of the analyzed population was 55 years (SD % ± 17).

Type of prescribed drugs

In patients on antipsychotics, 520/564 (92%) took second-generation antipsychotics (SGAs) whereas the remaining 8% (44/564) took first-generation antipsychotics (FGAs). The distribution is shown in Table 3.

Drug doses

Mean doses were consistently lower than those indicated by the DDDs. Namely, drugs with prescribed doses slightly

Table 1 Features of patients eligible for the study

Parameter	n	%
Men	362	40.58
Women	530	59.42
Age group		
10-20	8	0.93
21-30	50	5.61
31-40	124	13.90
41-50	190	21.30
51-60	167	18.72
61-70	154	17.26
71-80	133	14.91
81-90	61	6.84
91-100	5	0.56
Mean age, years	56 ± 10.09	

SD, standard deviation.

Table 2 Diagnosis reported in therapeutic programs and coded with the ICD-9 system

ICD-9	Correspondence	%
296	Mood disorders	36.4
295	Schizophrenia	35.4
298	Non-organic psychosis	5.6
299	Pervasive developmental disorders	4.7
297	Delusional disorders	4
290	Dementia	3.9
294	Persistent mental illnesses caused by pathologic conditions	3
292	Mental disorder caused by substances	2.4
293	Temporary mental illnesses caused by pathologic conditions	2
300	Anxiety disorders	1.42
309	Adaptation reactions	0.85
318.1	Severe mental retardation	0.28
307.1	Anorexia nervosa	0.14

ICD, International Classification of Diseases.

lower than the DDDs were: aripiprazole 13.2 mg (DDD, 15 mg); olanzapine 8.6 mg (DDD, 10 mg); risperidone 3.7 mg (DDD, 5 mg); and haloperidol 3.7 mg (DDD, 8 mg) (Table 4). Drugs with prescribed doses much lower than the DDDs were: quetiapine 230.6 mg (DDD, 400 mg); clozapine 179.5 mg (DDD, 300 mg); clotiapine 38.6 mg (DDD, 80 mg); levomepromazine 25 mg (DDD, 300 mg); chlorpromazine 62.5 mg (DDD, 300 mg) (Table 4).

Moreover, the following drugs were prescribed at doses lower than those described in the SPCs: clozapine 179.5 mg (SPC, 200-450 mg); haloperidol 3.71 mg (SPC, 60 mg); clotiapine 38.6 mg (SPC, 100-120 mg); and levomepromazine 25 mg (SPC 75-300 mg) (Table 4).

Variations in therapy

In all, 16% of the analyzed population (95/564 patients) changed their drug dosage during therapy: 44/564 patients (8%) reduced it while 51/564 patients (9%) increased it. More specifically, increases in prescribed doses of the following drugs were noted: quetiapine (24/51), olanzapine (17/51), aripiprazole (4/51), haloperidol (3/51) and risperidone (3/51). Antipsychotics that were dose-reduced were olanzapine (25/44), aripiprazole (7/44), quetiapine (6/44), risperidone (5/44), and haloperidol (1/44).

The originally prescribed drug was switched to other medication in 14% of patients (81/564). As such, the following antipsychotics were switched: olanzapine 0.8%; risperidone 4%; quetiapine 3%; aripiprazole 1%; clotiapine 0.4%; haloperidol 0.4%; and chlorpromazine 0.2%.

Concomitant medications used with antipsychotics

In all, 427/564 patients (76%) were treated with antipsychotics and other concomitant therapies. Concomitant

Table 3 Patients treated with antipsychotics and treatment adherence

Drug	n	% patients	Adherence			CI 95%	P-value
			Minimum	Mean	Maximum		
SGAs							
Aripiprazole	43	7.6	7.78	62.07	100	22.6 - 80.1	0.01
Olanzapine	193	34.2	7.78	59.15	100	25.9 - 81.2	0.01
Quetiapine	156	27.7	8.33	66.68	100	27.9 - 88.5	0.01
Risperidone	109	19.3	8.33	59.75	100	29.3 -84.3	0.01
Clozapine	19	3.4	7.8	51.80	100	29.7 - 85.2	0.01
FGAs							
Haloperidol	26	4.6	8.33	63.99	100	17.4 - 59.2	0.01
Clotiapine	8	1.4	16	66.38	100	24.3 - 96.5	0.01
Levomepromazine	6	1.1	33.33	68.06	100	32.8 - 87.9	0.01
Clorpromazine	4	0.7	22.22	69.44	100	20.4 - 80.0	0.01

SGA, second-generation antipsychotics;
FGA, first-generation antipsychotic.

therapies prescribed with antipsychotics included the following: antidepressants 40% (228/564); antiepileptics 16% (88/564); anticholinergic 9% (48/564); antiepileptic and antidepressant 7% (40/564); anticholinergic and antidepressant 2% (12/564); anticholinergic and antiepileptic 1% (8/564); and anticholinergic, antidepressant, and antiepileptic 0.5% (3/564).

Among patients taking an antipsychotic with an antidepressant, 83% were on SGAs. Moreover, SGAs were frequently given with anticholinergics (73%).

Adherence to therapy

Patient adherence to therapy is shown in Table 3; this parameter was calculated ranging from a minimum of 60% for risperidone to a maximum of 69% for chlorpromazine. Mean adherence to treatments was 64% (SD% ± 28).

We used the statistical t-test to evaluate and compare the average value of first-generation antipsychotic adherence to that of the second generation. For FGAs, the adherence mean was 66.97 (SD% ± 2.35), while for SGAs it was 59.89 (SD% ± 5.37). This statistical testing

Table 4 Antipsychotic dosages in milligrams used in therapy

Drug	DDD	Dosage			SPC	Most commonly prescribed dosage, mg	% Patients with add-on anticholinergic
		Minimum	Mean	Maximum			
SGAs							
Aripiprazole	15	2.5	13.16	30	10-30	10	2.3
Olanzapine	10	1.3	8.6	20	5-20	5	6.7
Quetiapine	400	12.5	230.6	1200	200-800	200	2.6
Risperidone	5	0.5	3.7	9	2-16	2	11
Clozapine	300	25	179.5	450	200-450	100	10.5
FGAs							
Haloperidol	8	1	3.71	8	60	2	27
Clotiapine	80	14	38.6	100	100-120	50	87.6
Levomepromazine	300	12.5	25	50	75-300	25	0
Chlorpromazine	300	62.5	62.5	100	30-75	50	50.4

Trascrizione fonetica
DDD, Defined Daily Dose;
SPC, Summary of Product Characteristics;
SGA, second-generation antipsychotic;
FGA, first-generation antipsychotics.

(95% confidence interval) resulted in a significant p-value equal to.038, showing a difference of treatment adherence among patients receiving the two categories of antipsychotics, slightly higher for patients using FGAs compared with patients treated with SGAs.

Antidepressants
Among patients treated with psychopharmaceuticals, 40% (361/892) took antidepressants, among whom 63% (228/361) were women and 37% (133/361) men. Their mean age was 55 years (SD% ± 9). The most frequently observed age group was 41-60 years (43%). However, a small number of prescriptions to patients aged 21-30 years (5%) and 81-90 years (4%) were also made.

Type of prescribed drugs
Prescribed antidepressants are shown in Table 5. The most prescribed antidepressant was venlafaxine (24%) whereas the most prescribed drug category was selective serotonin reuptake inhibitors (SSRIs) at 55%.

Drug doses
Minimum, mean, and maximum dosages of antidepressants and their comparison versus the DDDs and the SPCs are displayed in Table 6. The following antidepressants were given at higher doses versus the DDD: citalopram 44.3 mg (DDD, 20 mg); mirtazapine 44.2 mg (DDD, 30 mg); paroxetine 29.5 mg (DDD, 20 mg); sertraline 73.8 mg (DDD, 50 mg); venlafaxine 129.2 mg (DDD, 100 mg).

Variations in therapy
In all, 52 of 361 patients (14%) modified the dose of their therapy: 56% (29/52) of patients reduced it, while the remaining 44% (23/52) increased it.

The following drugs were dose-decreased during the observation period: 19/361 (5%) cases for venlafaxine; 3/361 (0.8%) each for citalopram and paroxetine; 2/361

(0.6%) for amitriptyline; and 1/361 (0.3%) each for sertraline and clomipramine.

On the other hand, patients who increased their drug doses were: 10/361 (3%) for citalopram; 4/361 (1%) for venlafaxine; 3/361 (0.8%) for paroxetine; 2/361 (0.6%) for sertraline; 1/361 (0.3%) each for mirtazapine, fluoxetine, trazodone, and clomipramine.

In all, 6% of patients (22/361) switched their originally prescribed medication to other drugs. More specifically, the following medications were switched to other drugs during the observation period: citalopram 23%; mirtazapine 18%, sertraline and venlafaxine both 14%; trazodone, reboxetine, and fluoxetine all 9%; and paroxetine 5%.

Concomitant therapies with antidepressants
Only 26% of patients took antidepressants as monotherapy. Drugs taken in addition to antidepressants were: another antidepressant 6% (22/361); antipsychotic 51% (184/361); antipsychotic and antiepileptic 9% (32/361); anticholinergic 0.5% (2/361); antiepileptic 4% (13/361); two antipsychotics 3% (11/361); antipsychotic and anticholinergic 0.3% (1/361); and antipsychotic, anticholinergic, and antiepileptic 0.3% (1/361).

Mean adherence to therapy
Mean adherence to therapy was: 81% for reboxetine; 77% for citalopram; 76% for trazodone; 59% for mirtazapine; 58% for paroxetine; 63% for sertraline; 62% for venlafaxine; and 52% for fluoxetine. Mean overall adherence to treatments was 64% (SD % ± 34).

Discussion
Antipsychotics
Atypical antipsychotics were most frequently prescribed (92%). Among atypical antipsychotics, olanzapine, quetiapine, and risperidone were the most prescribed, whereas among typical antipsychotics haloperidol was by far the most taken.

Table 5 Patients treated with antidepressants and treatment adherence

Drug	n	% patients	Adherence			CI 95%	P-value
			Minimum	Mean	Maximum		
Paroxetine	75	20.83	7.78	57.7	100	23.8 - 76.5	0.03
Citalopram	83	23.06	7.78	77.2	100	26.0 - 83.6	0.03
Venlafaxine	87	24.17	8.33	61.65	100	24.1 - 81.2	0.03
Sertraline	29	8.06	8.33	62.80	100	23.7 - 85.3	0.03
Mirtazapine	32	8.89	59.14	59.14	100	25.8 - 82.2	0.03
Trazodone	25	6.94	11.11	75.94	100	24.5 - 83.5	0.03
Fluoxetine	10	2.78	13.33	52.18	93.33	18.9 - 73.1	0.03
Amitriptiline	4	1.11	35.71	43.42	50	37.2 - 49.5	0.03
Clomipramine	6	1.67	14.81	67.72	100	23.1 - 84.3	0.03
Reboxetine	10	2.78	33.33	81.07	100	38.6 - 92.5	0.03
Total	**361**						

Table 6 Antidepressants dosages in milligrams used in therapy

Drug	DDD	Dosage			Most commonly prescribed dosage, mg	SPC
		Minimum	Mean	Maximum		
Citalopram	20	10	44.25	60	20	20-60
Mirtazapine	30	15	44.23	45	30	15-45
Paroxetine	20	5	29.54	60	40	20-60
Sertraline	50	30	73.82	180	100	50-200
Venlafaxine	100	37.5	129.2	300	150	75-375

DDD, Defined Daily Dose;
SPC, Summary of Product Characteristics.

Mean doses of atypical antipsychotics were within the limits indicated by the SPCs. When compared with the DDDs, although of limited use in such investigations, doses lower than the DDDs and within the limits indicated by the SPCs can mean two different things: on the one hand, low doses can be therapeutically successful, while on the other, their concomitant use allows the reduction of each individual drug dosage as well as of side effects. Moreover, we observed one case of a patient treated with quetiapine at a dosage 1200 mg/day higher than that suggested in the technical datasheet (200-800 mg).

Our analysis of typical neuroleptic daily dispensations showed that prescribed mean dosages were nearly all within the limits indicated by technical datasheets and the DDDs [17] except for two drugs. Once again, this suggests that therapeutic results are achievable at low dosages and that attempts are made to minimize side effects. The only exception here was chlorpromazine, for which maximum doses were higher than those indicated by technical datasheets and the DDDs.

The greatest dosage variations with antipsychotics during the therapy were seen for quetiapine and olanzapine.

The study showed that 14% (81/564) of patients on antipsychotics replaced the initial drug. More specifically, 74/81 (91%) patients initially treated with SGAs were switched to other drugs; only 2/81 (2%) patients replaced the SGAs with FGAs whereas 6% (5/81) of patients switched from FGAs to SGAs. The most often replaced drugs were olanzapine, risperidone, and quetiapine.

The most frequently noted combination therapy was an antipsychotic (mainly SGAs) and an anticholinergic.

SGA dosages used with anticholinergics were consistently lower than the DDDs. Since the risk of extrapyramidal side effects is very low when atypical drugs are taken, the combination use with anticholinergics would be unnecessary. However, the combined use of these drugs was very common and usually higher than FGAs. This therapeutic choice probably aims at further reducing the onset of side effects.

The majority of patients followed prescribed antipsychotic therapy [18] with a low adherence range of 51-66%.

The difference in adherence to treatment (slightly higher among patients treated with FGAs compared with patients treated with SGAs) was statistically significant; however, we recognize the limits of the different types of patients in terms of disease severity. SGAs are currently the first choice of treatment; it often happens that FGAs are reserved to patients as a second choice or where SGAs are contraindicated. Probably for this reason, these patients are the most monitored by the specialists and this could be a reason for greater adherence to therapy for patients treated with FGAs.

In a study by Magliano et al. [6] carried out in 30 Italian mental health services which included 682 patients (M/F 469/213), the data, when compared with our results, revealed some differences. Their study included patients aged 18-60 years (mean age 37 years) and among them, 98% of the subjects used antipsychotics (63% treated with FGAs and 35% with SGAs). In our study, the recruited patients had a wider age range of 15-98 years (and therefore the average age was 55 years old) and only 63% used antipsychotic drugs, with a lower percentage of patients using FGAs (8%) while 92% were treated with SGAs. In our study, the use of combination therapy was more widespread than in the data obtained from the Magliano study, where only 5% of patients were prescribed an antipsychotic and an antidepressant (versus 40% of patients in Ferrara) and 7% were receiving an antipsychotic and an anticholinergic (versus 9% in Ferrara).

Antidepressants

The most prescribed antidepressant was venlafaxine whereas the most prescribed category of antidepressants, 55% of all antidepressants, was the SSRI class. These data confirm the results highlighted by other studies [19], which showed that SSRIs are the most prescribed antidepressants in Italy. This figure has also been confirmed by other European studies such as those by Finder [19] and Serna [20]. Our analysis shows that doses were almost always within the limits indicated by the technical sheets but consistently above those indicated by the DDDs.

During the therapy, a small proportion (14%) of patients modified their dosage of prescribed drug: 8% of them reduced it while the remaining 6% increased it. The most frequently up-titrated antidepressant was citalopram (19% of the total of patients who increased their therapy) followed by venlafaxine (8%) and paroxetine (6%). On the other hand, it emerged that the prescribed dosage of venlafaxine was usually reduced (in 37% of patients).

Citalopram was apparently not very efficacious based on our finding that it was dose-increased more than other drugs despite having a good adherence.

In most cases, antidepressants were prescribed concomitantly with an antipsychotic or another antidepressant, suggesting quite a high comorbidity of depression and psychosis in patients in this study. The presence of a number of patients taking two antidepressants concomitantly also suggests that depression symptoms are difficult to treat successfully with just a single drug.

Conclusion

This retrospective study evaluated the prescription profiles of 892 patients treated by the PDC. SGAs were the most commonly prescribed antipsychotic agents. Dosages prescribed were usually within those recommended by the drug manufacturers and international standards. These agents were often used with concomitant therapies, especially with anticholinergics, despite the reduced risk of extrapyramidal side effects. SSRIs were the most commonly prescribed antidepressants, at dosages within the range recommended by suppliers but higher than the DDDs. Antidepressants were mainly prescribed in association with a second antidepressant or an antipsychotic. For both classes of drugs, we observed an average level of patient adherence to their therapies, although there have not been many studies that have investigated adherence to therapy of antipsychotics and antidepressants. Unfortunately, this may represent a limitation to our study because it does not allow comparison of our results to those obtained in other populations.

List of abbreviations

ATC: Anatomical Therapeutic Chemical; PDC: Psychiatric Disease Centre; SPC: Summary Product Characteristic; DDD: Daily Defined Dose; ICD-9: International Statistical Classification of Diseases and Related Health Problems; SD: standard deviation; SSRI: selective serotonin reuptake inhibitor; SGA: second-generation antipsychotic; FGA: first-generation antipsychotic.

Acknowledgements

The authors thank the staff of the mental health centre and the health statistics service at the University Hospital of Ferrara, whose assistance allowed the realization of this study.

Authors' contributions

SB defined the design of this study, establishing the number of patients to be enrolled, the number of prescriptions by therapeutic analysis, and the type of data needed to achieve the defined objectives. SB submitted the study to the Ethics Committee of Ferrara, established the protocols for statistical data analysis, continuously monitored the data obtained, and contributed to the writing and revision of the article. SB defined operating modes, introducing the DDD for comparison of treatments in the dosage given. EB analyzed the requirements of patients and processed the data to obtain patient characteristics, types of drugs prescribed, dosages used in therapy, changes of drug or dosing and possible associations. He participated in drafting and revising the article.
PS evaluated the data obtained and the execution of the study, also participating in the drafting and revision of the article.
All authors read and approved the final manuscript.

Competing interests

The authors declare that they have no competing interests.

References
1. Hirsch SR, Kissling W, Bauml J, Power A, O'Connor R: A 28-week comparison of ziprasidone and haloperidol in outpatients with stable schizophrenia. *J Clin Psychiatriy* 2002, **63**:516-523.
2. Kane JM, Carson WH, Saha AR, *et al*: Efficacy and safety of aripiprazole and haloperidol versus placebo in patient with schizophrenia and schizoaffective disorder. *J Clin Psychiatriy* 2002, **63**:763-771.
3. Ren XS, Herz L, Qian S, Smith E, Kazis LE: Measurement of treatment adherence with antipsychotic agents in patient with schizophrenia. *Neuropsychiatric Disease and Treatment* 2009, **5**:491-498.
4. American Psychiatric Association: Practice Guideline for the Treatment Of Patients With Schizophrenia. American Psychiatric Press, Washington DC; 2007.
5. National Institute for Clinical Excellence-Nice: Schizophrenia-Full National Clinic Guideline On Core Intervention In Primary And Secondary Care. Gaskell Press e British Psychological Society, London; 2003.
6. Magliano L, Fiorillo A, Guarneri M, Marasco C, De Rosa C, Malangone C, Maj M: Prescription of psychotropic drugs to patients with schizophrenia: an Italian national survey. *Eur J Clin Pharmacol* 2004, **60**:513-522.
7. Schmidt LG, Lammers V, Stockel M, Muller-Oerlinghausen B: Recent trends in prescribing psychotropic drugs at a psychiatric university hospital 1981-1984. *Pharmacopsychiatry* 1998, **21**:126-130.
8. Tognoni G: Pharmacoepidemiology of psychotropic drugs in patients with severe mental disorders in Italy: Italian Collaborative Study Group on the Outcome of Severe Mental Disorders. *Eur J Clin Pharmacol* 1999, **55**:685-690.
9. Williams CL, Johnstone BM, Kesterson JG, Yavor KA, Schmetzer AD: Evaluation of antypsychotics and concomitance medication use patterns in patients with schizophrenia. *Care Med* 1999, **4**:AS81-AS86.
10. Brunot A, Lachaux B, Sontag H, Casadebaig F, Philippe A, Rouillon F, Clery-Melin P, Hergueta T, Llorca PM, Moreaudefarges T, Guillon P, Lebrun T: Pharmaco-epidemiological study on antipsychotic drug prescription: in French psychiatry: patient characteristics, antyphichotic treatment and care management for schizophrenia. *Encephale* 2002, **28**:129-138.
11. Keks NA, Altson K, Hope J, Krapivensky N, Culhane C, Tanaghow A, Doherty P, Bootle A: Use of antipsychotics and adjunctive medications by an inner urban community psychiartic service. *Aust NZJ Psychiatriy* 1999, **33**:896-901.
12. Yip KC, Ungvari GS, Cheung HK, Ng FS, Lau ST: A survey of antipsychotic treatment for schizophrenia in Hong Kong. *Chin Med J* 1997, **110**:792-796.
13. Lesli DL, Rosenheck RA: Use of pharmacy date to assess quality of pharmacotherapy for schizophrenia in a national health care system: individual and facility predictors. *Med Care* 2001, **39**:907-907.
14. Lehman AF, Steinwachs DM, the Co-Investigators of the Port Project: Translating research into practice: the schizophrenia Patient Outcomes Research Team (PORT) treatment recommendations. *Schizophr Bull* 1998, **24**:1-10.

15. Bardui C, Danese A, Guaiana G, Mapelli L, Miele L, Monzani E, Percudani M, on behalf of the study group: **Prescribing second generation antipsychotics and the evolving standard of care in Italy.** *Phacopsychiatry* 2002, **35**:239-243.
16. **WHO Collaborating center for Drug Statistics Methodology.** *Guidelines for ATC classification and DDD assignment 2010* Oslo; 2009.
17. **Compendio Farmaceutico Ospedaliero.** Farmadati Italia; 2010, Updating n ° 97,.
18. Ren XS, Herz L, Qian S, Smith E, Kazis LE: **Measurement of treatment adherence with antipsychotic agents in patient with schizophrenia.** *Neuropsychiatric Disease and Treatment* 2009, **5**:491-498.
19. Bauer M, Monz BU, Montejo AL, Quail D, Dantchev N, Demyttenaere K, Garcia CA, Grassi L, Perahia DGS, Reed C, Tylee A: **Prescribing patterns of antidepressants in Europe: results from the Factors Influencing Depression Endpoints Research (FINDER) study.** *European Psychiatry* 2008, **23**:66-73.
20. Serna MC, Cruz I, Real J, Gascò E, Galvan L: **Duration and adherence of antidepressant treatment (2003 to 2007) based on prescription database.** *European Psychiatry* 2009, 7-12.

17

First human dose-escalation study with remogliflozin etabonate, a selective inhibitor of the sodium-glucose transporter 2 (SGLT2), in healthy subjects and in subjects with type 2 diabetes mellitus

Anita Kapur[1][*], Robin O'Connor-Semmes[1], Elizabeth K Hussey[1], Robert L Dobbins[1], Wenli Tao[1], Marcus Hompesch[2], Glenn A Smith[1], Joseph W Polli[1], Charles D James Jr[3], Imao Mikoshiba[4] and Derek J Nunez[1]

Abstract

Background: Remogliflozin etabonate (RE) is the prodrug of remogliflozin, a selective inhibitor of the renal sodium-dependent glucose transporter 2 (SGLT2), which could increase urine glucose excretion (UGE) and lower plasma glucose in humans.

Methods: This double-blind, randomized, placebo-controlled, single-dose, dose-escalation, crossover study is the first human trial designed to evaluate safety, tolerability, pharmacokinetics (PK) and pharmacodynamics of RE. All subjects received single oral doses of either RE or placebo separated by approximately 2 week intervals. In Part A, 10 healthy subjects participated in 5 dosing periods where they received RE (20 mg, 50 mg, 150 mg, 500 mg, or 1000 mg) or placebo (4:1 active to placebo ratio per treatment period). In Part B, 6 subjects with type 2 diabetes mellitus (T2DM) participated in 3 dose periods where they received RE (50 mg and 500 mg) or placebo (2:1 active to placebo per treatment period). The study protocol was registered with the NIH clinical trials data base with identifier NCT01571661.

Results: RE was generally well-tolerated; there were no serious adverse events. In both populations, RE was rapidly absorbed and converted to remogliflozin (time to maximum plasma concentration [$C_{max};T_{max}$] approximately 1 h). Generally, exposure to remogliflozin was proportional to the administered dose. RE was rapidly eliminated (mean $T_{1/2}$ of ~25 min; mean plasma $T_{1/2}$ for remogliflozin was 120 min) and was independent of dose. All subjects showed dose-dependent increases in 24-hour UGE, which plateaued at approximately 200 to 250 mmol glucose with RE doses ≥150 mg. In T2DM subjects, increased plasma glucose following OGTT was attenuated by RE in a drug-dependent fashion, but there were no clear trends in plasma insulin. There were no apparent effects of treatment on plasma or urine electrolytes.

Conclusions: The results support progression of RE as a potential treatment for T2DM.

Trial registration: ClinicalTrials.gov NCT01571661

Keywords: Remogliflozin etabonate, Sodium-dependent glucose transporter 2 inhibitor, Pharmacokinetics, Pharmacodynamics, Type 2 diabetes mellitus

* Correspondence: anita.x.kapur@gsk.com
[1]GlaxoSmithKline, 5 Moore Drive, Research Triangle Park, NC 27709, USA
Full list of author information is available at the end of the article

Background

Type 2 diabetes mellitus (T2DM) is characterized by abnormalities of glucose and lipid homeostasis, which drive secondary micro- and macrovascular complications. Clinical evidence indicates that maintaining glycemic control and reducing postprandial glucose excursions can lower the risk of diabetic complications, e.g. reduce the risk of myocardial infarction, renal disease and retinopathy [1,2]. Despite the availability of multiple classes and combinations of antidiabetic agents, the clinical management of T2DM remains challenging, with the majority of patients failing to achieve and maintain target glycemic levels in practice [3]. There is a continued need for novel therapeutic approaches, particularly those with complementary modes of action that will enable further improvement of glycemic control.

Glucose homeostasis is a complex process controlled by gastrointestinal absorption, tissue utilization, hepatic/renal gluconeogenesis and renal filtration/reabsorption/excretion. Under normal physiological conditions when the glomerular filtrate reaches the proximal tubule, glucose is primarily reabsorbed through the active sodium-dependent glucose transporter 2 (SGLT2) located on the apical or luminal membrane of the epithelial cell in the S1 segment [4-6].

SGLT1 is a high-affinity, low-capacity glucose/galactose co-transporter primarily expressed in the intestine and in the kidney [7,8]. In contrast, SGLT2 is a low-affinity, high-capacity glucose transporter selectively expressed in the kidney. Together, SGLT1 and SGLT2 are responsible for the active reabsorption of glucose across the renal luminal membrane [9,10]. Once reabsorbed by the renal epithelial cell, glucose is transported to the blood by facilitated diffusion via the sodium-independent glucose transporter 2 (GLUT-2). The uptake of glucose in the proximal tubules by SGLT1 and SGLT2 is highly efficient, resulting in complete reabsorption of glucose. In humans, genetic alterations in SGLT2 increase renal glucose excretion (up to 200 g/day) with no apparent adverse effects on renal function or carbohydrate metabolism [11].

SGLT2 is currently the focus of interest as a potential therapeutic target for reducing hyperglycemia in T2DM, and several selective SGLT2 inhibitors have been developed [12-16]. In diabetic animal models, pharmacological inhibition of SGLT2 leads to glucosuria, and improvement of plasma glucose levels, followed by a reduction of insulin resistance [17-19].

SGLT2 inhibitors have the potential to offer distinct advantages over currently available diabetic treatments. Because SGLT2 inhibitors work by an insulin-independent mechanism, this class of compounds may be of benefit as adjunctive therapy in patients whose pancreatic function is diminished or in patients who have insulin resistance. Thus, treatment with SGLT2 inhibitors may be appropriate in all stages of T2DM, provided the patient still has adequate renal function to deliver the drug to the site of action in the kidney. Another advantage is that SGLT2 inhibitors cause calorie wasting by loss of glucose in the urine, thus offering the potential for promoting weight loss, whereas some other anti-diabetic treatments such as sulfonylureas and insulin promote weight gain.

Remogliflozin etabonate is the ester prodrug of remogliflozin [20], which is the active entity that selectively inhibits SGLT2. Remogliflozin undergoes further transformation to GSK279782, an active metabolite. The structures of remogliflozin etabonate, remogliflozin and GSK279782 are presented in Figure 1.

Remogliflozin etabonate causes a concentration-dependent increase in urinary glucose excretion in mice and rats [20,21]. Unlike earlier SGLT inhibitors, such as phlorizin and T-1095, remogliflozin displays a high level of selectivity for SGLT2 over SGLT1 [22]. This single-dose evaluation was the first study to be conducted with remogliflozin etabonate in humans and was designed to provide safety, tolerability, PK and pharmacodynamic information.

Methods

This single center study was conducted at Profil Institute for Clinical Research (Chula Vista, CA, USA) and was conducted in accordance with Good Clinical Practice and the principles of the Declaration of Helsinki. The study protocol and subject information were reviewed and approved by Biomedical Research Institute of America investigational reviewer board (San Diego, CA, USA) and all subjects provided written, informed consent prior to start of study-related procedures.

Subjects

Ten healthy male and female subjects followed by a separate group of 6 subjects with T2DM were enrolled in this study. Enrollment of women was restricted to those who were postmenopausal or surgically sterile. All subjects gave written informed consent prior to participation in any study-related procedures. Healthy subjects were required to be 18–55 years of age, and have a body mass index (BMI) of 19.0 to 30.0 kg/m^2 inclusive. Subjects with T2DM were required to be 30–60 years of age, have a BMI of 22–35 kg/m^2, to be healthy other than having been diagnosed with T2DM at least 6 months prior to entry in the study, and to have been maintained on a stable treatment regimen for at least 3 months. Diabetic subjects were required to have hemoglobin A1c (HbA1c) ≤10% and fasting plasma glucose <280 mg/dL at screening. Participants with diabetes were required to be on a stable treatment regimen using a single oral antidiabetic agent (either sulfonylureas, rosiglitazone, metformin or acarbose) or management by diet and exercise. All T2DM subjects

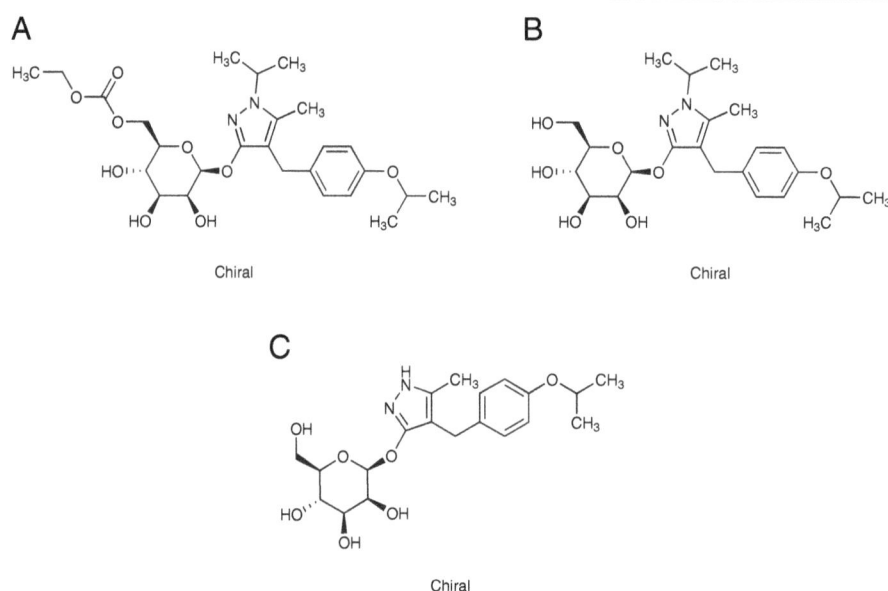

Figure 1 Structures of remogliflozin etabonate, remogliflozin, and GSK279782. Structures of (**A**) remogliflozin etabonate, (**B**) remogliflozin and (**C**) GSK279782).

also had to be willing and medically able to discontinue their diabetes medications for up to 72 h during each treatment period. Subjects were excluded if they had been taking diuretics, corticosteroids or other medications that might result in electrolyte depletion; had required insulin during the last 3 months; had significant renal disease; or if their participation would have resulted in donation of blood in excess of 550 mL within an 8-week period.

Study design

This double-blind, randomized, placebo-controlled, single escalating-dose crossover study was conducted in two parts: Part A consisted of a randomized, dose-escalation in healthy subjects; Part B was of similar design, but conducted in subjects with T2DM and included an evaluation of pharmacodynamics using a 50 g oral glucose tolerance test (OGTT).

Part A

Ten healthy subjects were evaluated in 5 study sessions, each separated by approximately 2 weeks. At each study session, subjects received either an oral dose of remogliflozin etabonate or placebo after an overnight fast. Remogliflozin etabonate doses were 20 mg, 50 mg, 150 mg, 500 mg and 1000 mg. Over the course of participation in the study, each subject received 4 of the 5 active remogliflozin etabonate doses and 1 dose of placebo (4:1 active to placebo ratio per treatment period). The available safety and PK results from each dosing period were evaluated before proceeding to the next dose level.

Part B

Six subjects with T2DM received two doses of remogliflozin etabonate and a placebo dose, in a randomized, dose escalating, crossover design, along with an oral glucose load on three study sessions separated by 7–14 days. Full PK and safety profiles were measured on Day 1 of each dosing period. The doses selected for this portion of the study, 50 mg and 500 mg, were based on data obtained in Part A. In each dosing period, subjects were assigned to active vs placebo in a 2:1 ratio.

All subjects were admitted to the unit two nights prior to receiving study drug to establish baseline safety parameters and fluid intake levels over a 36 h period. Subjects remained in the unit for at least 24 h after doses were administered for monitoring of clinical laboratory parameters exploratory biomarkers, vital signs, ECGs and adverse events. While confined to the clinical research unit, all subjects received meals standardized with respect to calories, fat, protein, carbohydrate, and sodium content; however, detailed dietary information was not captured in this study. In Part A, subjects were dosed following an overnight fast; lunch and dinner were provided at 4 and 10 h after dosing, respectively. Fifteen minutes after dosing in each treatment period in Part B, a fasting OGTT was performed using 50 g glucose (administered as 50 g Glucola™). A 50 g glucose load was chosen since the OGTT was being performed in subjects already known to have diabetes. The glucose drink was consumed by subjects within approximately 5 minutes. Blood samples for the measurement of glucose, insulin, and intact glucagon-like peptide 1 (GLP-1) were collected for 24 hours following dose administration. Provided that there were no safety or tolerability concerns, subjects were released from the clinic on day 2 of each treatment period until their return for the next treatment or follow-up period. Each subject was involved in the study for approximately 8 weeks (from screening to follow-up).

Pharmacokinetic assessments
Blood collections and analysis
On each dosing day, a series of 2.0 mL blood samples were collected at pre-dose and 10, 20, 30 and 45 min, and 1, 1.25, 1.5, 2, 2.5, 3, 4, 6, 8, 12, 16, and 24 h post-dose for the determination of remogliflozin etabonate, remogliflozin and GSK279782 in plasma by using high-performance liquid chromatography with tandem mass spectrometry (MS/MS) as described [23].

Pharmacokinetic calculations
Non-compartmental PK analysis of plasma concentration–time data was performed using WinNonlin Version 4.1 (Pharsight Corporation, Mountainview, CA, USA). The C_{max} and T_{max} were obtained directly from the data. Areas under the plasma concentration–time curves from time zero to the last quantifiable time point ($AUC_{[0-last]}$) and extrapolated to infinity ($AUC_{[0-\infty]}$) were calculated using the log-linear trapezoidal method. The terminal plasma elimination rate-constant (λz) was estimated from log-linear regression analysis of the terminal phase of the plasma concentration–time curve, and the $T_{1/2}$ was calculated as $T_{1/2} = \ln2/\lambda z$. Ratios of $AUC_{(0-\infty)}$ remogliflozin to $AUC_{(0-last)}$ remogliflozin etabonate were calculated including molecular weight corrections.

Pharmacodynamic assessments
Plasma pharmacodynamics
Blood samples for glucose were taken at 0 (pre-dose), and 1, 2, 4, 8 and 12 h after dosing in each treatment period (Part A). For Part B, blood samples for glucose, insulin and GLP-1 were taken at check-in on day -2, and at 0 h (pre-dose), and 0.5, 1, 1.5, 2, 4 h (prior to lunch), 4.5, 5, 6, 8, 10, 12 and 24 h after dosing on day 1 of each treatment period.

Glucose and insulin sample handling For glucose, plasma was analyzed using a YSI 2300 Glucose Analyzer (Yellow Springs International Life Sciences, Yellow Springs, OH, USA). For insulin, plasma was rapidly prepared and frozen at -70°C until analyzed by LabCorp (San Diego, CA, USA) using a chemiluminescent immunometric assay method (Siemen's Immulite 2000 analyzer with Immulite Insulin Kit L2KIN2).

GLP-1 sample handling For assay of intact GLP-1, blood was collected into a chilled EDTA tube and protease

inhibitors (DPP4 inhibitor obtained from EMD Millipore, St. Charles, MO) were immediately added. Samples were then spun down and plasma split into two separate tubes and frozen at -70°C until analyzed by Pathway Diagnostics (Malibu, CA, USA) by ELISA (kit # EGLP-35 K, EMD Millipore). The lowest level of intact GLP-1 this assay can detect is 2 pM (with a minimum plasma sample size of 0.4 mL).

Urine pharmacodynamics
Sample collection
Urine samples were collected at pre-dose, and over a series of intervals (0–2, 2–4, 4–6, 6–8, 8–12 and 12–24 h post-dose) for the analysis of creatinine, glucose and electrolytes (Na, K and Cl). All fluid intake was recorded, as well as urine volume, over the 24 hours before and after dosing in each treatment period. Urine was tested for protein on the first morning void of day -1 and 24 h after dosing.

Calculations
Creatinine clearance (CL_{CR}) was calculated as the amount of creatinine excreted in 24 h ($Ae_{0-24\,h}$) divided by the mean of the pre-dose and 24-h post-dose plasma creatinine levels. The percentage of filtered glucose excreted in the urine for each individual time period was calculated as the amount of glucose excreted during that time period divided by ($CL_{CR} \times PG \times$ time interval length), where CL_{CR} is the creatinine clearance for the time interval, PG is the plasma glucose concentration closest to the midpoint of the time interval, and the time interval is the period (min) of urine collection ($CL_{CR} \times PG$ represents the glucose filtered load). For the 24-h period, the percentage of filtered glucose excreted was calculated as the amount of glucose excreted over 24 h divided by the sum over the individual time intervals of ($CL_{CR} \times PG \times$ time interval length).

Statistical analysis
Safety and pharmacodynamic data were summarized using descriptive statistics. This was a small exploratory study and no formal hypothesis-testing was conducted. Dose proportionality with respect to C_{max}, and AUC was assessed using the power model $y = \alpha\, dose^{\beta}$, where $y = C_{max}$ or AUC, and α denotes a random subject effect. The exponent β in the power model will be estimated by regressing the $\log_e$-transformed PK parameters on $\log_e$ dose, i.e. $\ln(\text{PK parameter}) = \ln(\alpha) + \beta * \ln(dose)$. Dose proportionality implied that $\beta = 1$ and was assessed by estimating β and its corresponding 90% confidence interval. The power model was fitted by restricted maximum likelihood using SAS Proc Mixed.

Results

Subject demographics

In Part A, 10 subjects (8 males, 2 females, mean age of 39 years, mean BMI of 24.5 mg/kg^2, and mean baseline fasting plasma glucose 4.7 mmol/L [range 4.2 to 5.1 mmol/L, SD 0.29 mmol/L]) were randomized; 9 completed the study (1 subject participated in all the study visits but did not return for the follow up visit). In Part B, 6 T2DM subjects (2 males, 4 females, mean age of 53 years, mean BMI of 30.5 mg/kg^2, and mean baseline fasting plasma glucose 8.9 mmol/L [range 5.81 to 12.1 mmol/L, SD 2.47 mmol/L]) were randomized and all completed the dosing period.

Safety and tolerability

Remogliflozin etabonate was generally well-tolerated by all subjects. There were no obvious patterns suggesting an effect of remogliflozin etabonate on clinical laboratory results, urine electrolytes, vital signs or ECGs. There were no deaths, serious adverse events or adverse events (AEs) leading to withdrawal. The most frequently reported AE was headache. AEs are summarized in Table 1.

Urine beta-2 microglobulin levels, an exploratory bio-marker that was measured as a potential early indicator

of renal toxicity, were within the normal range at both baseline and after treatment for all subjects except for two subjects with diabetes.

One of these subjects had normal beta-2 microglobulin values at 1 and 4 days after dosing with 500 mg remogliflozin etabonate. However, 11 days after dosing, this subject returned to the clinic for the Day -2 visit of the 3rd treatment period. At this time, the subject's beta-2 microglobulin levels were elevated to 2.5 µg/mL. The values returned to normal (<0.3 µg/mL) within 2 days. The investigator attributed the elevated pre-placebo levels to other concomitant disease. A second subject, however, did have what was considered by the investigator to be a drug-related elevation of beta-2 microglobulin of 1.62 µg/mL on day 1 after dosing with 500 mg remogliflozin etabonate. The value returned to normal levels within 4 days. No associated changes in serum creatinine and urea or urine microalbumin were observed.

Pharmacokinetics

Healthy subjects

PK parameters are summarized in Table 2 (remogliflozin etabonate), and Table 3 (remogliflozin and GSK279782). Remogliflozin etabonate was rapidly absorbed and

Table 1 Summary of adverse events

| | Placebo | Remogliflozin etabonate dose | | | | | Total |
		20 mg	50 mg	150 mg	500 mg	1000 mg	
Healthy Subjects	n = 10	n = 8	n = 8	n = 8	n = 8	n = 8	n = 10
	n (%)	n (%)	n (%)	n (%)	n (%)	n (%)	n (%)
At least one adverse event	4 (40)	2 (25)	3 (38)	1 (13)	3 (38)	1 (13)	8 (80)
Adverse events reported by >1 subject in total							
Headache	1 (10)	1 (13)	1 (13)	0	2 (25)	1 (13)	4 (40)
Blood creatine phosphokinase increased	1 (10)	0	0	0	1 (13)	0	2 (20)
Drug-related adverse events							
Headache	1 (10)	1 (13)	1 (13)	0	0	1 (13)	3 (30)
Dizziness	0	0	0	0	0	1 (13)	1 (10)
Diarrhea	0	1 (13)	0	0	0	0	1 (10)
Hot flush	0	0	0	0	0	1 (13)	1 (10)
T2DM subjects	n = 6		n = 6		n = 6		n = 6
	n (%)		n (%)		n (%)		n (%)
At least one adverse event	3 (50)		1 (17)		2 (33)		4 (67)
Adverse events reported by >1 subject in total							
Muscle cramp	1 (17)		1 (17)		0		2 (33)
β$_2$-microglobulin increased	0		0		2 (33)		2 (33)
Drug-related adverse events							
Nausea	0		0		1 (17)		1 (17)
β$_2$-microglobulin increased	0		0		1 (17)		1 (17)
Pain in extremity	0		0		1 (17)		1 (17)

n = number of subjects reporting event.
% = percentage of subjects reporting event.

Table 2 Summary of plasma remoglifozin etabonate pharmacokinetic parameters in healthy subjects[a,b]

Remogliflozin etabonate dose	20 mg	50 mg	150 mg	500 mg	1000 mg
$AUC_{(0-\infty)}$ (ng·h/mL)	NQ^c	$3.70 (46)^d$	$9.77 (48)^d$	$36.8 (67)^e$	$126 (44)^f$
$AUC_{(0-t)}$ (ng.h/mL)	$1.61 (67)^g$	3.56 (56)	9.51 (42)	35.4 (62)	107 (53)
C_{max} (ng/mL)	1.89 (78)	4.98 (61)	17.6 (48)	41.6 (81)	144 (59)
T_{max} (h)	0.625	0.625	0.515	1.25	0.625
	0.33-2.03	0.17-1.50	0.17-1.50	0.33-2.50	0.33-2.50
$T_{\frac{1}{2}}$ (h)	NQ^c	$0.353 (56)^d$	$0.256 (35)^d$	$0.263^e (27)$	$0.707^f (56)$

a. Geometric mean and CV% except for T_{max} (median and range).
b. n = 8 unless otherwise specified.
c. NQ, not quantifiable because concentrations at later time points were below the limit of quantification.
d. n = 6.
e. n = 4.
f. n = 7.
g. n = 5.

extensively hydrolyzed to the active entity in all dose groups. The median T_{max} estimates for the prodrug ranged from 0.52 to 1.25 h and median $T_{\frac{1}{2}}$ estimates ranged from 0.26 to 0.71 h. The concentration–time profiles are shown for the 50 mg dose in Figure 2 illustrating low circulating plasma concentrations of prodrug relative to active entity.

Remogliflozin appeared in plasma at relatively high concentrations within 10 min of remogliflozin etabonate dosing. Mean remogliflozin C_{max} of the active entity occurred within 1.5 h of prodrug dosing and was eliminated from plasma more slowly than prodrug. The mean $T_{\frac{1}{2}}$ estimates ranged from 1.38 to 2.86 h. The AUC(0-∞) ratios of remogliflozin to prodrug (or AUC(0-t) when AUC(0-∞) not available for prodrug), ranged from 81 to 105 indicating

extensive conversion to active entity. The ratios were consistent across all doses.

An active metabolite of remogliflozin, GSK279782, was monitored in this study and found to be present in relatively high concentrations in plasma. An estimated mean AUC(0-∞) ratio of GSK279782 to remogliflozin was 40 to 45%. The median T_{max} estimates for GSK279782 ranged from 1.0 to 1.5 h and median $T_{\frac{1}{2}}$ estimates ranged from 1.54 to 3.50 h. The concentration profiles of GSK279782 followed a similar time course to those of remogliflozin with only a small delay in appearance of C_{max} and slightly longer $T_{\frac{1}{2}}$.

The statistical analysis showed AUC(0-∞) and C_{max} for all three analytes increased nearly dose proportionally over the 50-fold dose range of 20 to 1000 mg in healthy

Table 3 Summary of plasma remogliflozin and GSK279782 PK parameters in healthy subjects[a]

Remogliflozin etabonate dose	20 mg		50 mg		150 mg		500 mg		1000 mg	
Analyte	R^b	279782	R^b	279782	R^b	279782	R^b	279782	R^b	279782
$AUC_{(0-\infty)}^c$ (ng·h/mL)										
Geometric mean (CV%)	133 (45)	51.8 (48)	324 (29)	145 (48)	991 (25)	447 (44)	3721 (29)	1523 (40)	10257 (17)	3995 (22)
C_{max} (ng/mL)										
Geometric mean (CV%)	61 (54)	17.5 (72)	158 (44)	50.2 (62)	515 (37)	155 (50)	1703 (45)	498 (44)	4822 (37)	1286 (28)
T_{max} (h)										
Median	0.89	1.26	1.14	1.38	0.66	1.00	1.50	1.50	1.25	1.25
(range)	(0.50–1.5)	(0.75–2.5)	(0.50–1.5)	(1.00–2.0)	(0.33–2.0)	(0.75–2.0)	(0.50–3.0)	(1.00–4.0)	(0.50–3.0)	(0.75–3.0)
$T_{\frac{1}{2}}$ (h)										
Geometric mean (CV%)	1.38 (21)	1.54 (11)	1.47 (15)	2.19 (17)	1.59 (13)	2.28(13)	2.57 (29)	3.07 (13)	2.86 (17)	3.50 (12)
AUC ratio (remogliflozin/ remogliflozin etabonate)										
Geometric mean	84^d	—	81	—	102	—	105	—	95	—
CV%	(39)		(34)		(53)		(86)		(69)	

a. n = 8 unless otherwise specified.
b. R = remogliflozin.
c. The median percentage of AUC(0-∞) extrapolated for R was low ranging from 0.07% to 2.1% across all doses and for 279782 ranging from 0.29% to 4.51%.
d. n = 5.

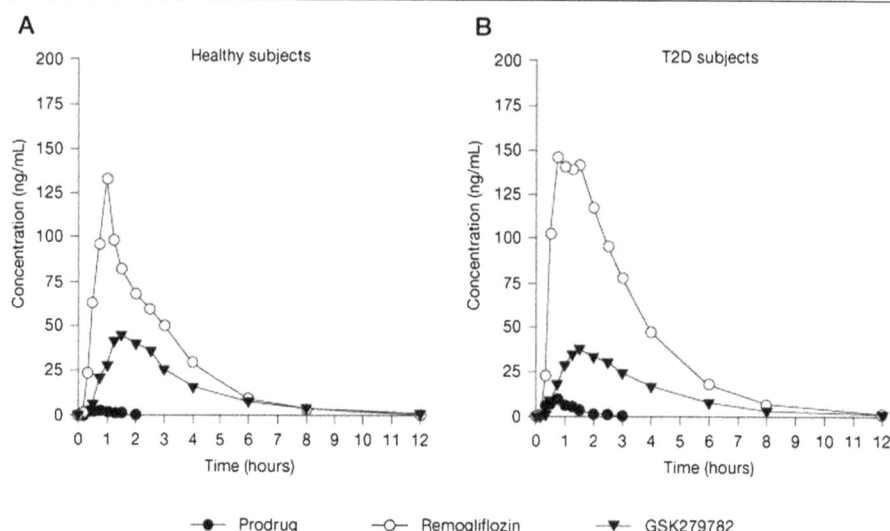

Figure 2 Mean plasma concentration-time profiles for remogliflozin etabonate (prodrug), remogliflozin (active entity), and GSK279782 (metabolite) following a 50 mg dose of remogliflozin etabonate to subjects.

subjects. For remogliflozin etabonate, the mean slopes and 90% confidence intervals (CI) for AUC(0-∞) and Cmax were 1.17 (1.04, 1.30) and 1.04 (0.94, 1.14). For remogliflozin, the mean slopes and 90% CIs for AUC(0-∞) and Cmax were 1.09 (1.06, 1.12) and 1.08 (1.02, 1.14). For GSK279782, the mean slopes and 90% CIs for AUC(0-∞) and Cmax were 1.08 (1.05, 1.12 and 1.07 (1.01, 1.12).

Type 2 diabetes subjects

The PK parameters for remogliflozin etabonate, remogliflozin, and GSK279782 in subjects with T2DM are shown in Table 4. The prodrug was rapidly absorbed and extensively hydrolyzed to the active entity in patients as well as non-diabetic subjects. There were no discernable

differences in mean T_{max} or $T_{1/2}$ values of remogliflozin or GSK279782 between patients and healthy subjects. The apparent differences in AUCs for remogliflozin and AUC ratios between populations are potentially the result of small sample size and variability rather than differences in absorption or metabolism.

Pharmacodynamics
Urine glucose

In both populations, the total amount of glucose excreted in urine from 0–24 h increased in a dose-dependent manner; however, urine glucose excretion increased less than proportionally with increasing doses of remogliflozin etabonate (Table 5), suggesting a plateau of effect. The

Table 4 Summary of plasma remogliflozin etabonate, remogliflozin, and GSK279782 PK parameters in T2DM subjects[a]

Remogliflozin etabonate dose	Remogliflozin etabonate		Remogliflozin		GSK279782	
	50 mg	500 mg	50 mg	500 mg	50 mg	500 mg
$AUC_{(0-\infty)}^{c}$(ng·h/mL)						
Geometric mean (CV%)	8.91 (58)	91.9 (46) [b]	523 (38)	5176 (44)	130 (50)	1293 (45)
C_{max} (ng/mL)						
Geometric mean (CV%)	9.56 (39)	83.9 (89)	195 (46)	1891 (49)	34.6 (39)	314 (39)
T_{max} (h)						
Median	0.58	0.75	1.46	2.50	1.74	2.75
(range)	(0.33–0.78)	(0.33–2.50)	(0.33–2.00)	(0.33–4.00)	(0.75–4.00)	(0.75–4.00)
$T_{1/2}$ (h)						
Geometric mean (CV%)	0.61 (32)	0.82 (69) [b]	1.59 (27)	3.93 (25)	2.05 (24)	3.28 (23)
$AUC_{(0-\infty)}$ ratio						
(Remogliflozin/remogliflozin etabonate) Geometric mean (CV%)	—	—	59 (62)	54 (38)	—	—

a. n = 6 unless otherwise specified.
b. n = 2.
c. The median percentage of AUC(0-∞) extrapolated for remogliflozin etabonate ranged from 10% to 11% and for remogliflozin was low ranging from 0.14% to 0.42% and for GSK279782 was 0.47% to 2.0%.

Table 5 24-h urinary glucose and electrolyte excretion, after single-dose administration of remogliflozin etabonate (20–1000 mg) in healthy volunteers (n = 8 per remogliflozin etabonate group and n = 10 for placebo) and subjects with T2DM (n = 6)

Parameter	Placebo	Remogliflozin etabonate dose, mg				
		20	50	150	500	1000
Healthy subjects						
Urinary glucose excretion (mmol)	6.5 (18.6)[a]	67.1 (17.9)	96.7 (17.1)[b]	168 (49.4)[b]	223 (49.5)	304 (137)
Filtered glucose excreted in urine (%)	0.9 (2.4)[a]	9.0 (2.2)	12.7 (3.7)[b]	25.5 (7.8)[b]	34.2 (5.0)	26.4 (11.7)
Urinary sodium excretion (mmol)	162 (49.4)[a]	148 (64.0)	212 (67.6)[b]	176 (38.7)[b]	143 (55.0)	207 (62.9)
Urinary chloride excretion (mmol)	141 (39.8)[a]	136 (56.6)	189 (51.4)[b]	179 (49.6)[b]	126 (55)	201 (61.5)
Urinary potassium excretion (mmol)	62.2 (15.7)[a]	66.6 (27.7)	75.2 (21.3)[b]	59.7 (20.3)[b]	55.8 (17.2)	89.1 (24.7)
T2DM subjects						
Urinary glucose excretion (mmol)	40.4 (62.4)[c]		384 (210)		642 (256)	
Filtered glucose excreted in urine (%)	2.3 (3.6)[c]		15.9 (5.9)[c]		21.6 (9.1)	
Urinary sodium excretion (mmol)	196 (39.2)[c]		173 (35.5)[c]		301 (128)	
Urinary chloride excretion (mmol)	181 (48.3)[c]		168 (23.9)[c]		287 (147)	
Urinary potassium excretion (mmol)	71.7 (12.1)[c]		65.8 (4.5)[c]		108 (65.8)	

Results are expressed as mean (SD).
a. n = 9.
b. n = 7.
c. n = 5.

urine glucose excretion was higher in the T2DM subjects due to higher plasma glucose concentrations. When urine glucose excretion was corrected for circulating plasma glucose concentrations and CL_{CR} (to provide an estimate of percentage filtered glucose load or FGL%), the FGL% was similar between the populations. Figure 3 illustrates the similarity between populations and the saturation of urine glucose excretion with increasing doses. The saturation is related to maximal SGLT2 transporter inhibition. Figure 4 shows the cumulative mean values

for the amount of glucose excreted in healthy subjects over time for each dose.

Urine electrolytes

Urine electrolytes are also summarized in Table 5. Urine excretion of electrolytes was highly variable, and no treatment-related changes were observed. Much of the variability in the 500 mg dose period can be attributed to one subject (#12) whose values for all three electrolytes were roughly 2-fold higher than those of the other participants during that period.

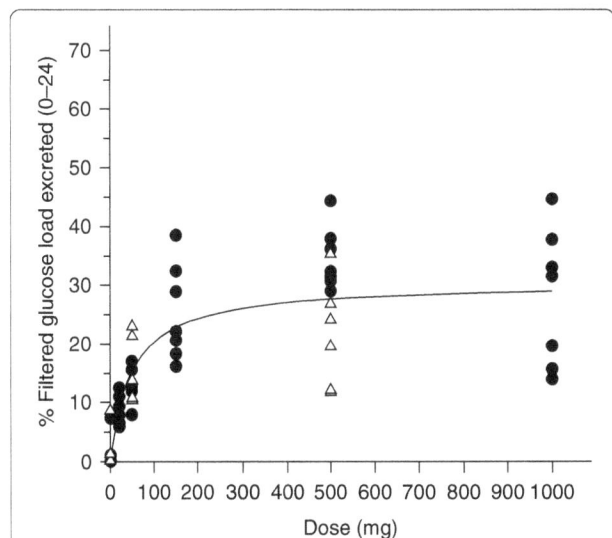

Figure 3 The filtered glucose load (%) vs dose in healthy volunteers (filled circles) and subjects with T2DM (open triangles).

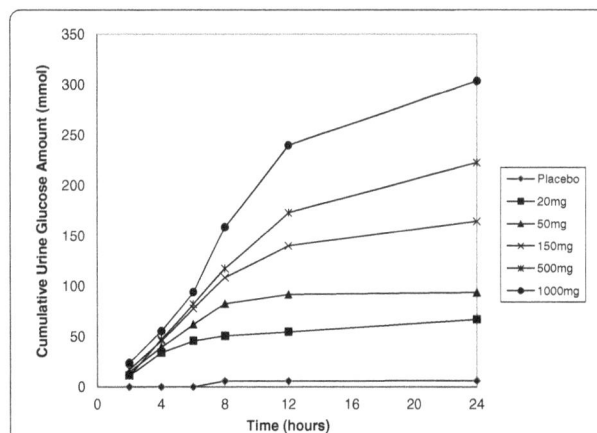

Figure 4 Mean cumulative 24-h urine glucose excretion following single-dose administration of remogliflozin etabonate (20 to 1000 mg) in healthy subjects.

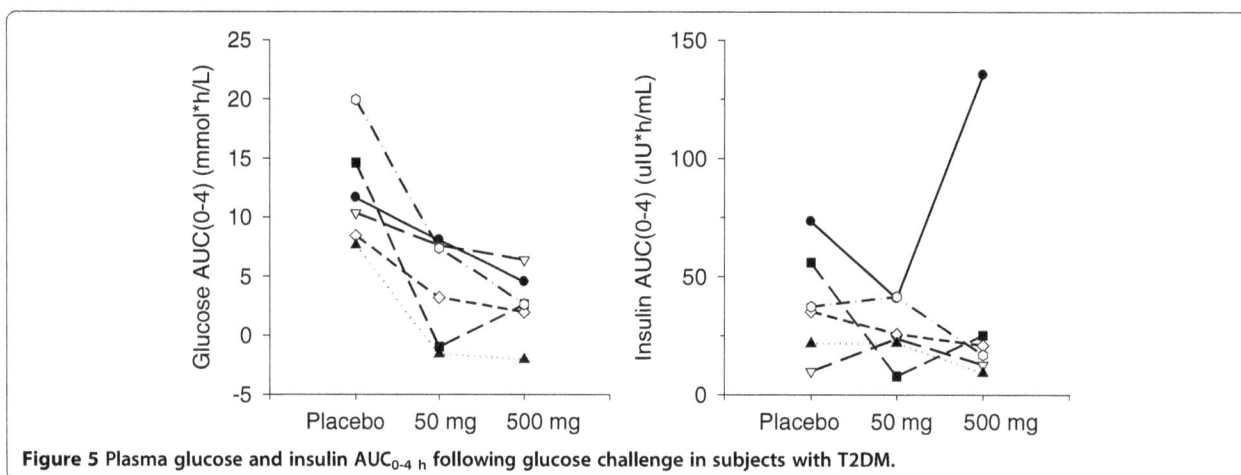

Figure 5 Plasma glucose and insulin AUC$_{0-4\,h}$ following glucose challenge in subjects with T2DM.

Plasma glucose and insulin

For healthy subjects, AUC values for plasma glucose were very similar between placebo and remogliflozin etabonate periods at both 0–4 h (mean of approximately 18 mmol•h/L) and 0–12 h (mean of approximately 55–59 mmol•h/L) following study drug administration.

For T2DM subjects, the increases in plasma glucose following an OGTT were clearly attenuated between placebo and 50 mg RE; the effect on glucose was altered little by increasing the dose from 50 mg to 500 mg RE. There were no clear trends in plasma insulin following the glucose load. The baseline adjusted AUC$_{(0-4)}$ values for plasma glucose and insulin following an OGTT, are depicted in Figure 5.

Plasma intact GLP-1

In T2DM subjects, the median baseline adjusted AUC$_{(0-4)}$ for plasma GLP-1 following an OGTT was 6.36 pM*h (range, 0 to 16.6) for placebo, -8.85 pM*h (range, -46.7 to 33.4) for remogliflozin etabonate 50 mg, and -1.95 pM*h (range, -11.6 to 7.0) for remogliflozin etabonate 500 mg. These data are difficult to interpret because the ranges for placebo, 50 mg, and 500 mg groups contain zero,

and also because the analytical method likely did not include extraction of the samples, which can confound the analysis of intact GLP-1 [24,25].

Fluid balance

Fluid balance data for both healthy and T2DM subjects are shown in Table 6.

On the day prior to dosing in healthy subjects, fluid balance (total fluid intake minus total urine volume) was negative (mean volumes in the range of -126 to -512 mL). In the 0–12 h interval after dosing, fluid balance shifted to positive for the placebo (+163 mL) and 20 mg remogliflozin etabonate (+242 mL) periods, while the 50 to 1000 mg remogliflozin etabonate treatment periods remained negative. For the 12 to 24 h post-dose interval, all regimens had a fluid balance that was negative. There was no evidence of a clear dose–response.

In T2DM subjects, fluid balance was variable in the 24 h prior to dosing; T2DM subjects assigned to placebo and remogliflozin etabonate 50 mg had a negative fluid balance (mean volumes ranging from -312 mL to -504 mL), while those assigned to remogliflozin etabonate 500 mg had a positive fluid balance (mean volume +188 mL). From

Table 6 Summary of fluid balance data (mL)

	Placebo	Remogliflozin etabonate dose				
		20 mg	50 mg	150 mg	500 mg	1000 mg
Healthy Subjects	(n = 10)	(n = 8)	(n = 8)	(n = 8)	(n = 8)	(n = 8)
−24 h to pre-dose	−462 (605)	−460 (1311)	−338 (525)	−512 (731)	−278 (1250)	−126 (798)
0–12 h post-dose	163 (668)	243 (1161)	−570 (582)	−86 (909)	−159 (531)	−273 (331)
12–24 h post-dose	−739 (423)	−581 (387)	−551 (530)	−564 (478)	−424 (334)	−495(367)
T2DM subjects	n = 6		n = 6		n = 6	
−24 h to pre-dose	−312 (457)		−504 (294)		188 (1879)	
0–12 h post-dose	569 (400)		−78(433)		−29 (749)	
12–24 h post-dose	−908 (524)		−803 (658)		−1088(679)	

Fluid balance = total fluid intake minus total urine volume.
Results are expressed as mean (SD).

0–12 h after dosing, fluid balance was positive for the placebo regimen and negative for the remogliflozin etabonate 50 mg and 500 mg regimens. For the 12–24 h interval, all regimens had negative fluid balance (mean volumes ranging from -802 mL to -1087 mL). As with the healthy subjects, there was no clear dose–response.

Discussion

By promoting urinary glucose excretion, SGLT2 inhibitors offer a novel mechanism of antidiabetic action that is complementary to currently available classes of drugs which reduce hepatic gluconeogenesis (e.g. metformin), increase glucose flux into muscle and fat (e.g. insulin sensitizers such as thiazolidinediones) or stimulate β-cell insulin secretion (e.g. GLP-1-based therapies).

In both healthy and T2DM subject populations, the prodrug, remogliflozin etabonate was extensively converted to its active entity, remogliflozin, and to an active metabolite, GSK279782, which is as potent as remogliflozin in inhibiting SGLT-2 in vitro [23]. The PK parameters (C_{max} and AUC) of all three analytes (remogliflozin etabonate, remogliflozin, and GSK279782) increased nearly dose proportionally over the 50-fold dose range, 20 to 1000 mg, of remogliflozin etabonate in healthy subjects. Although limited data are available, there appeared to be dose proportionality in subjects with T2DM between 50 and 500 mg doses as well. The PK parameters were similar between the healthy subjects and T2DM subjects.

Evidence of the desired pharmacological effect was seen in the dose-dependent increase in urinary glucose excretion in healthy subjects and in T2DM subjects following administration of remogliflozin etabonate. The total amount of glucose excreted in the 24 h after dosing increased less than proportional to the dose and exposure to remogliflozin in healthy subjects. The plateau in glucose excretion was observed between exposures associated with single doses of 150 mg and 500 mg, suggesting maximal inhibition of the SGLT2 transporter at this dose range. Subjects with T2DM showed increased glucose excretion over 24 hours with increasing doses of remogliflozin etabonate, but the percentage of filtered glucose excreted was similar between the two study groups. This amount of urine glucose excretion has been predicted to provide clinically meaningful reduction in plasma glucose [26]. For subjects with T2DM, the increase in plasma glucose following an oral glucose load appeared to be blunted in a drug-dependent fashion following dosing with remogliflozin etabonate, suggesting that SGLT2 inhibition is an appropriate mechanism for glucose lowering in these patients.

Conclusions

This single-dose evaluation is the first clinical study to be conducted with remogliflozin etabonate, and it provides safety, tolerability, pharmacokinetic and pharmacodynamic information in both healthy subjects and those with T2DM. In this study, single oral doses of remogliflozin etabonate (20 mg to 1000 mg for healthy subjects; 50 mg and 500 mg for subjects with T2DM) were generally safe and well-tolerated. Clinically significant fluid and electrolyte imbalances were not seen in this study, but longer repeat dose studies will be required to establish the safety profile. Remogliflozin etabonate increased urinary glucose excretion in a dose dependent fashion and also blunted increases in plasma glucose following an oral glucose load, which suggests that remogliflozin etabonate could be useful as a treatment for T2DM.

Competing interests
AK, ROCS, EKH, RLD, WT, GAS, JWP, CJ, and DN are/were all employees of GlaxoSmithKline at the time of the study; IM is an employee of Kissei Pharmaceutical Company.

Authors' contributions
AK, ROCS, EKH, RLD, WT, GAS, JWP, CJ, and DN participated in the design of the study, its co-ordination and performed the statistical analysis. IM contributed to study design and the analysis, and MH contributed to study conduct. All authors have been involved in critically revising the drafts of the manuscript and read and approved the final manuscript.

Acknowledgements
The authors thank Laurene Wang-Smith for her assistance with PK analyses. Editorial assistance in the preparation of this manuscript was provided by Katie Green, International Medical Press, funded by GlaxoSmithKline.

Author details
[1]GlaxoSmithKline, 5 Moore Drive, Research Triangle Park, NC 27709, USA. [2]Profil Institute for Clinical Research, Chula Vista, CA, USA. [3]Tandem Labs, Durham, NC, USA. [4]Kissei Pharmaceutical Company LTD, Matsumoto City, Japan.

References
1. Holman RR, Paul SK, Bethel MA, Matthews DR, Neil HA: 10-year follow-up of intensive glucose control in type 2 diabetes. N Engl J Med 2008, 359:1577–1589.
2. UK Prospective Diabetes Study (UKPDS) Group: Effect of intensive blood-glucose control with metformin on complications in overweight patients with type 2 diabetes (UKPDS 34). Lancet 1998, 352:854–865.
3. Giugliano D, Standl E, Vilsboll T, Betteridge J, Bonadonna R, Campbell I, Schernthaner G, Staels B, Trichopoulou A, Farinaro E: Is the current therapeutic armamentarium in diabetes enough to control the epidemic and its consequences? What are the current shortcomings? Acta Diabetol 2009, 46:173–181.
4. Kanai Y, Lee WS, You G, Brown D, Hediger MA: The human kidney low affinity Na+/glucose cotransporter SGLT2. Delineation of the major renal reabsorptive mechanism for D-glucose. J Clin Invest 1994, 93:397–404.
5. Wells RG, Pajor AM, Kanai Y, Turk E, Wright EM, Hediger MA: Cloning of a human kidney cDNA with similarity to the sodium-glucose cotransporter. Am J Physiol 1992, 263:F459–F465.
6. You G, Lee WS, Barros EJ, Kanai Y, Huo T, Khawaja S, Wells R, Nigam S, Hediger M: Molecular characteristics of Na(+)-coupled glucose transporters in adult and embryonic rat kidney. J Biol Chem 1995, 270:29365–29371.
7. Bakris GL, Fonseca VA, Sharma K, Wright EM: Renal sodium-glucose transport: role in diabetes mellitus and potential clinical implications. Kidney Int 2009, 75:1272–1277.
8. Nishimura M, Naito S: Tissue-specific mRNA expression profiles of human ATP-binding cassette and solute carrier transporter superfamilies. Drug Metab Pharmacokinet 2005, 20:452–477.

9. Idris I, Donnelly R: **Sodium-glucose co-transporter-2 inhibitors: an emerging new class of oral antidiabetic drug.** *Diabetes Obes Metab* 2009, **11**:79–88.

10. Wright EM, Turk E: **The sodium/glucose cotransport family SLC5.** *Pflugers Arch* 2004, **447**:510–518.

11. Santer R, Kinner M, Lassen CL, Schneppenheim R, Eggert P, Bald M, Brodehl J, Daschner M, Ehrich J, Kemper M, Li Volti S, Neuhaus T, Skovby F, Swift P, Schaub J, Klaerke D: **Molecular analysis of the SGLT2 gene in patients with renal glucosuria.** *J Am Soc Nephrol* 2003, **14**:2873–2882.

12. Handlon AL: **Sodium glucose co-transporter 2 (SGLT2) inhibitors as potential antidiabetic agents.** *Expert Opin Ther Pat* 2005, **13**:1531–1540.

13. Hussey E, Clark R, Amin D, Kipnes M, O'Connor-Semmes R, O'Driscoll E, Leong L, Murray S, Dobbins R, Layko D, Nunez D: **The single-dose pharmacokinetics and pharmacodynamics of sergliflozin etabonate, a novel inhibitor of glucose reabsorption, in healthy volunteers and subjects with type 2 diabetes mellitus.** *J Clin Pharmacol* 2010, **50**:623–635.

14. Isaji M: **Sodium-glucose cotransporter inhibitors for diabetes.** *Curr Opin Investig Drugs* 2007, **8**:285–292.

15. Komoroski B, Vachharajani N, Feng Y, Li L, Kornhauser D, Pfister M: **Dapagliflozin, a novel, selective SGLT2 inhibitor, improved glycemic control over 2 weeks in patients with type 2 diabetes mellitus.** *Clin Pharmacol Ther* 2009, **85**:513–519.

16. Komoroski B, Vachharajani N, Boulton D, Kornhauser D, Geraldes M, Li L, Pfister M: **Dapagliflozin, a novel SGLT2 inhibitor, induces dose-dependent glucosuria in healthy subjects.** *Clin Pharmacol Ther* 2009, **85**:520–526.

17. Asano T, Ogihara T, Katagiri H, Sakoda H, Ono H, Fujishiro M, Anai M, Kurihara H, Uchijima Y: **Glucose transporter and Na+/glucose cotransporter as molecular targets of anti-diabetic drugs.** *Curr Med Chem* 2004, **11**:2717–2724.

18. Ehrenkranz JR, Lewis NG, Kahn CR, Roth J: **Phlorizin: a review.** *Diabetes Metab Res Rev* 2005, **21**:31–38.

19. Katsuno K, Fujimori Y, Takemura Y, *et al*: **Sergliflozin, a novel selective inhibitor of low-affinity sodium glucose cotransporter (SGLT2), validates the critical role of SGLT2 in renal glucose reabsorption and modulates plasma glucose level.** *J Pharmacol Exp Ther* 2007, **320**:323–330.

20. Fujimori Y, Katsuno K, Nakashima I, Ishikawa-Takemura Y, Fujikura H, Isaji M: **Remogliflozin etabonate, in a novel category of selective low-affinity sodium glucose cotransporter (SGLT2) inhibitors, exhibits antidiabetic efficacy in rodent models.** *J Pharmacol Exp Ther* 2008, **327**:268–276.

21. Harrington WW, Milliken NO, Binz JG, *et al*: **Remogliflozin etabonate, a potent and selective sodium-dependent glucose transporter 2 antagonist, produced sustained metabolic effects in zucker diabetic fatty rats.** *Diabetes* 2008, **58**:529-P.

22. Wright EM, Turk E, Martin MG: **Molecular basis for glucose-galactose malabsorption.** *Cell Biochem Biophys* 2002, **36**:115–121.

23. Sigafoos J, Bowers G, Castellino S, Culp AG, Wagner DS, Reese JM, Humphreys JE, Hussey EK, O'Connor-Semmes RL, Kapur A, Tao W, Dobbins RL, Polli JW: **Assessment of the drug interaction risk for remogliflozin etabonate, a sodium-dependent glucose cotransporter-2 inhibitor: evidence from in vitro, human mass balance, and ketoconazole interaction studies.** *Drug Metab Dispos* 2012, **40**:1–13.

24. Yabe D, Watanabe K, Sugawara K, Kuwata H, Kitamoto Y, Sugizaki K, Fujiwara S, Hishizawa M, Hyo T, Kuwabara K, Yokota K, Iwasaki M, Kitatani N, Kurose T, Inagaki N, Seino Y: **Comparison of incretin immunoassays with or without plasma extraction: Incretin secretion in Japanese patients with type 2 diabetes.** *J Diabetes Investig* 2012, **3**:70–79.

25. Deacon CF, Holst JJ, Sugawara K: **Immunoassays for the incretin hormones GIP and GLP-1.** *Best Pract Res Clin Endocrinol Metab* 2009, **23**(4):425–462. ISSN 1521-690X, 10.1016/j.beem.2009.03.006. [http://www.sciencedirect.com/science/article/pii/S1521690X09000256].

26. O'Connor-Semmes R, Hussey EK, Dobbins RL, Nunez DJ: **Simulation and prediction of long-term clinical efficacy in type 2 diabetes resulting from inhibition of the renal sodium-glucose cotransporter 2 (SGLT2).** *Diabetes* 2008, **57**(2132-PO):A589.

18

Assessing the translatability of In vivo cardiotoxicity mechanisms to In vitro models using causal reasoning

Ahmed E Enayetallah[1,2]*, Dinesh Puppala[1], Daniel Ziemek[3], James E Fischer[1], Sheila Kantesaria[1] and Mathew T Pletcher[1,4]

Abstract

Drug-induced cardiac toxicity has been implicated in 31% of drug withdrawals in the USA. The fact that the risk for cardiac-related adverse events goes undetected in preclinical studies for so many drugs underscores the need for better, more predictive in vitro safety screens to be deployed early in the drug discovery process. Unfortunately, many questions remain about the ability to accurately translate findings from simple cellular systems to the mechanisms that drive toxicity in the complex in vivo environment. In this study, we analyzed translatability of cardiotoxic effects for a diverse set of drugs from rodents to two different cell systems (rat heart tissue-derived cells (H9C2) and primary rat cardiomyocytes (RCM)) based on their transcriptional response. To unravel the altered pathway, we applied a novel computational systems biology approach, the Causal Reasoning Engine (CRE), to infer upstream molecular events causing the observed gene expression changes. By cross-referencing the cardiotoxicity annotations with the pathway analysis, we found evidence of mechanistic convergence towards common molecular mechanisms regardless of the cardiotoxic phenotype. We also experimentally verified two specific molecular hypotheses that translated well from in vivo to in vitro (Kruppel-like factor 4, KLF4 and Transforming growth factor beta 1, TGFB1) supporting the validity of the predictions of the computational pathway analysis. In conclusion, this work demonstrates the use of a novel systems biology approach to predict mechanisms of toxicity such as KLF4 and TGFB1 that translate from in vivo to in vitro. We also show that more complex in vitro models such as primary rat cardiomyocytes may not offer any advantage over simpler models such as immortalized H9C2 cells in terms of translatability to in vivo effects if we consider the right endpoints for the model. Further assessment and validation of the generated molecular hypotheses would greatly enhance our ability to design predictive in vitro cardiotoxicity assays.

Keywords: Causal reasoning, Cardiotoxicity, Translatability, In vitro screening, Preclinical safety

Background

In 2007, the leading cause for drug withdrawal from the market was attributed to cardiotoxicity (31%) [1]. The voluntary withdrawal of the COX-2 selective inhibitor Rofecoxib in 2004 due to increased risk of myocardial infarction and stroke is one of the more prominent examples [2]. Addressing the safety issues early would significantly reduce such costly surprises in the drug discovery process and would also improve the survival of pharmaceutical drugs to the market. Although using animal models to predict late stage safety issues has been the norm in the industry for years, there is increased expectation that progress in utilization of computational toxicology predictive models, specialized in vitro models and a combination of both these models will enhance early de-risking, reduce animal use and enhance compound survival. In addition, the US National Academy of Sciences recently released a toxicity testing framework emphasizing the utilization of high throughput in vitro toxicity assays and computational models to assess the risk and underlying mechanism of toxicities triggered by

---

* Correspondence: Ahmed.Enayetallah@Pfizer.com
[1]Compound Safety Prediction, Pfizer Inc., Groton, CT, USA
[2]Drug Safety Research & Development, Pfizer Inc., Groton, CT, USA
Full list of author information is available at the end of the article

pharmaceutical chemicals and environmental contaminants. This is envisioned to include model systems based on stem cell biology, functional genomics and physiologically based pharmacokinetic (PBPK) modeling [3].

There have been several reports wherein computational models have been utilized for predicting the early safety risks based on potassium voltage-gated channel, subfamily H (HERG) binding [4,5], Absorption, Distribution, Metabolism, Excretion and Toxicity (ADMET) properties [6], Adenosine tri-phosphate Binding Cassette (ABC) transporter substrates [7] and Cytochrome P450 (CYP450) inductions [8]. However, the successful utilization of mechanism-based screening assays has been a challenge despite the plethora of published studies on the known mechanisms of drug-induced cardiac toxicity. These include well studied mechanisms of cardiotoxicity such as oxidative stress, calcium dysregulation, energy metabolism disruption, cell cycle/proliferation and tissue remodeling [9-11].

It is believed that a major factor contributing to the limited success of predicting clinical outcome using preclinical models or predicting in vivo outcome using in vitro models is due to limited understanding of the translatability across model systems and species. Hence, the recent increase of models believed to better reflect the physiological and functional roles of cardiomyocytes such as progenitor cardiomyocytes, human embryonic stem cells (ESC) and inducible pluripotent stem cell (iPS) derived cardiomyocytes [12,13]. Recently, Force and Kolaja reviewed the most commonly used models of cardiomyocytes summarizing their advantages and disadvantages [11]. It should be noted, of course, that this methodology will only reveal mechanisms that result from direct action of a compound on a cardiomyocyte. This in vitro system is inadequate for predicting secondary effects mediated by the interaction of multiple complex organ systems, such a rise in heart rate due to increased epinephrine release.

The primary goal of this study is to evaluate the translatability of cardiotoxicity mechanisms from in vitro to in vivo and to compare the elicited mechanisms in different in vitro models. To achieve this we utilized gene expression microarray experiments from rat toxicity studies (Drugmatrix, Iconix [14,15]) and in vitro experiments in H9C2 (embryonic BD1X rat heart tissue derived cells) and neonatal rat ventricular cardiomyocytes (RCM) using nine known pharmaceutical compounds known to induce cardiotoxicity in vivo.

The gene expression microarray data was analyzed using a novel computational tool called the Causal Reasoning Engine (CRE) [16,17]. CRE interrogates prior biological knowledge to generate testable hypotheses about the molecular upstream causes of the observed gene expression changes. Each such hypothesis summarizes ("explains") a

certain number of gene expression changes (see *KLF4+* example below). Notably, hypotheses usually make statements about predicted *protein* abundance or activity changes, e.g. increased or decreased TGFB1 activity. In our experience, CRE hypotheses tend to robustly identify biological phenomena driving gene expression changes and provide several advantages over other gene expression analysis methods [17]. In particular, for the purpose of this study, CRE provided the advantage of better abstracting biological information from gene expression data obtained across different experimental settings (see *Causal Reasoning Convergence* below).

Following the CRE analysis of all individual compound treatments in vitro and in vivo, we compared the hypotheses and the biological processes they compose to assess the translatability of mechanisms from one model system to the other. Subsequently, we experimentally tested *KLF4* and *TGFB1* activities, two of the central molecular hypotheses predicted by CRE, in response to the cardiotoxic compounds used in the CRE analysis using qPCR and reporter assay. Finally, we discuss the implications of our analysis and suggest potential future experiments.

Methods

Tissue culture

H9C2 cells (derived from embryonic BD1X rat heart tissue) were purchased from ATCC. H9C2 cells were grown DMEM (Gibco# 11965) with 10% FBS as per manufacturer's protocol. Neonatal, ventricular Clonetics® Rat Cardiac Myocytes (P1-3) (RCM)(Catalog # R-CM-561) were purchased from Lonza and were grown in RCGM media with supplements as per manufacturer's protocol.

For ATP depletion assays, H9C2 and RCM's cells were plated in 96 well plates per the manufacturer's protocol for 24 hr prior to treatments. For gene expression experiments, H9C2 and RCM cells were plated in 24 well plates per the manufacturer's protocol for 24 hr prior to adding of treatments.

Chemicals

All the chemicals (Table 1) were purchased from Sigma Aldrich. Stock solutions and working solutions were prepared by dissolving compounds in DMSO.

ATP depletion assays

ATP depletion measurements were done using The CellTiter-Glo® Luminescent Cell Viability Assay from Promega (Catalog # G7570) per the manufacturer's protocol. 100 μl per well of reconstituted ATP depletion reagent was added directly to 96 well plate and incubated for 10 minutes on orbital shaker. Luminescence signal was measured using Envison plate reader.

Table 1 In vitro cytotoxicity phenotype (ATP depletion) and known in vivo cardiac safety liabilities of the test compounds

Drug	ATP depletion IC50 at 48 hrs (μM ± SE)	In vivo 5-day treatment (mg/kg)	Reported ECG abnormalities & arrhythmia	Reported structural cardiotoxicity	Primary pharmacology & indication
Amiodarone	12 ± 1.17	147	Yes	No	Anti-arrhythmic
Amitriptyline	5.7 ± 0.67	160	Yes	Yes	Tricyclic antidepressant
Cyclosporine	2.71 ± 0.92	350	No	Yes	Immunosuppressive
Dexamethasone	>300	1	No	Yes	Glucocorticoid
Dobutamine	22.9 ± 0.83	43	Yes	Yes	β1 agonist, inotropic
Doxorubicin	4.23 ± 0.52	3	Yes	Yes	Cytotoxic Anti-neoplastic
Loratadine	39.5 ± 2.11	2000	Yes	No	Anti-histaminic
Mitoxantrone	1.16 ± 0.47	2	Yes	Yes	Cytotoxic Anti-neoplastic
Terbutaline	>300	130	Yes	Yes	β2 agonist

Microarray gene expression data

RNA was extracted 24 hrs after compound treatment using Qiagen's RNeasy Mini kit (Catalog # 74104) per the manufacturer's protocol. Quality and quantity of RNA was assessed using Nanodrop 2000c (A260/280 ratio) from Thermo Fisher Scientific and Agilent RNA analyzer (RIN scores). RNA (n = 2) was submitted to Genelogic for Affymetrix Genechip profiling using Rat Expression Array 230 2.0 chip. The in vivo rat cardiac tissue gene expression comparisons in response to the same compounds (Table 1) used in the in vitro experiments were obtained from the Drugmatrix toxicogenomic database [14,15]. The gene expression data for the effect of Isoprenaline on mouse cardiac tissue was obtained from the public domain (http://www.ncbi.nlm.nih.gov/geo/query/acc.cgi?acc=GSE18801), from a study published by Galindo et al. [18].

For quality control, RNA degradation plots were generated for each CEL file. To assess potential RNA degradation, 3′/5′ ratios and their associated confidence intervals were evaluated [19]. Two techniques were used to distill the probe results into a small number of representative variables; Multidimensional scaling (MDS) [20] and Principal component analysis (PCA). These two techniques were applied to the data before and after Robust Multi-Array Average (RMA) [20] signal processing. During this processing, only the perfect match (PM) probe data were used; the mismatch (MM) probes were not used. To assess differential expression of genes between groups of interest, a common statistical model was applied independently to each probeset. Gene expression for all sample types was analyzed on the log2 scale. Linear models were used to calculate t-statistics, which were subsequently adjusted using the moderated t-statistic procedure [21]. The Benjamini and Hochberg adjustment procedure [22] based on controlling the False Discovery Rate (FDR) was used.

Causal reasoning engine algorithm

Gene expression changes are analyzed to detect potential upstream regulators as previously described [16,17].

Briefly, the approach relies on a large collection of curated biological statements in the form:

A [increases or decreases] **B**, where **A** and **B** are measurable biological entities.

The biological entities can be of different types (e.g. phosphorylated proteins, transcript levels, biological process and compound exposure) and each statement is tied to accessible, peer-reviewed articles. For this work, we licensed approximately 450,000 causal statements from commercial sources (Ingenuity Systems and Selventa).

Each biological entity in the network and its assumed mode of regulation is a potential *hypothesis* (e.g. *predicted decrease in NFE2L2 activity*). For each hypothesis, we can now compare all possible downstream gene expression changes in the knowledge base with the observed gene expression changes in the experiment. We consider two metrics to quantify the significance of a hypothesis with respect to our experimental data set, namely enrichment and correctness. The *Enrichment* p-value for a hypothesis h quantifies the statistical significance of finding *(#incorrect + #correct)* gene expression changes within the set of all genes downstream of h. The *Correctness* p-value is a measure of significance for the score of a hypothesis h defined as *(#correct - #incorrect)*. The *KLF4+* example below shows a depiction of one significant hypothesis with corresponding downstream transcript changes. Molecular entities implicated by individual hypotheses can be grouped into biological processes to get a more comprehensive picture of predicted changes (see example in Figure 1).

Network modeling of the CRE hypotheses

The analysis results are visualized using the Causal Reasoning Browser, a Java application based on the open-source biological network viewer Cytoscape [23] as previously described [17]. Briefly, in the CRE browser an overview graph allows users to visualize hypotheses and examine their network relationships in the context of the causal relationships obtained from the literature

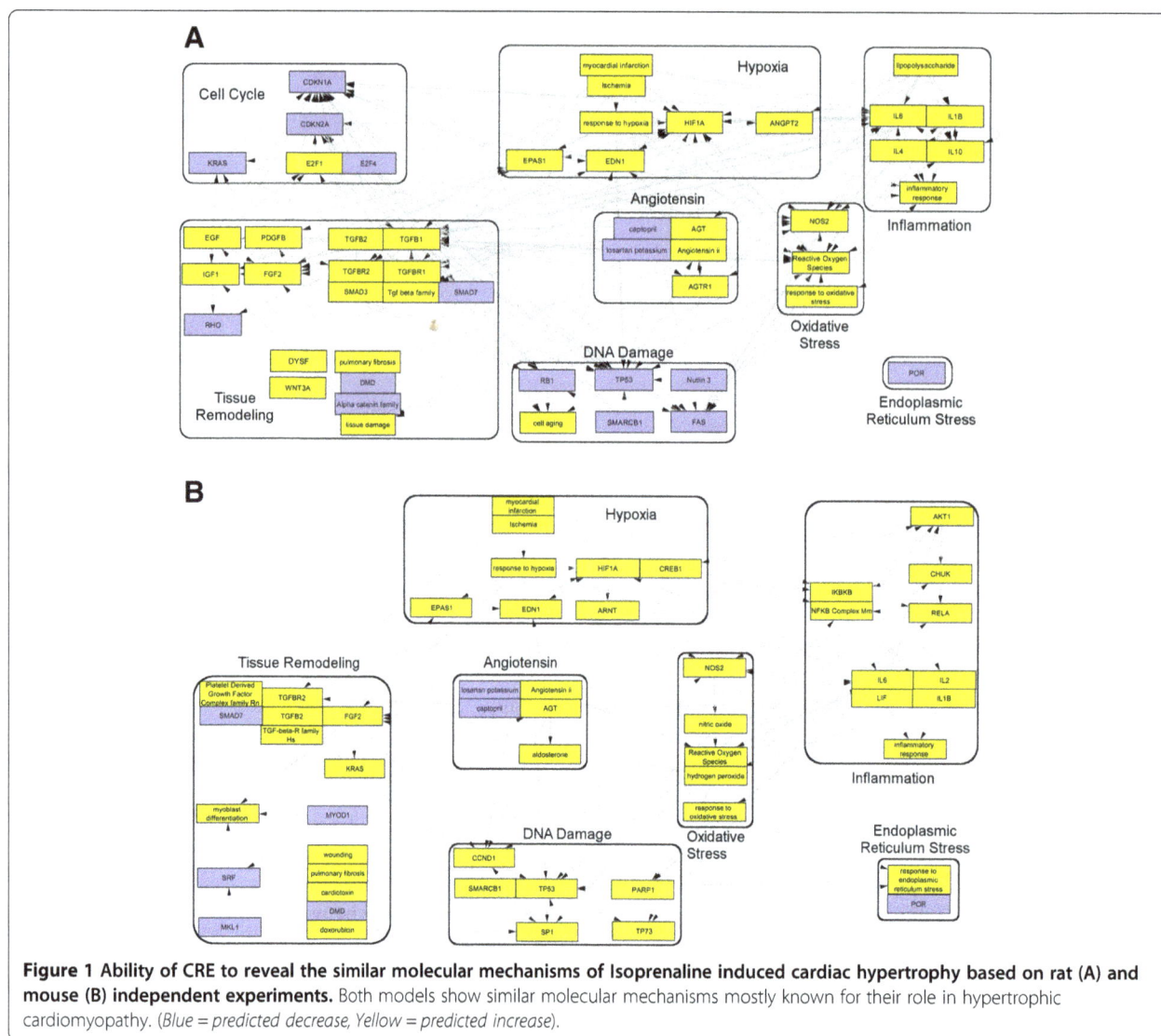

Figure 1 Ability of CRE to reveal the similar molecular mechanisms of Isoprenaline induced cardiac hypertrophy based on rat (A) and mouse (B) independent experiments. Both models show similar molecular mechanisms mostly known for their role in hypertrophic cardiomyopathy. (*Blue = predicted decrease, Yellow = predicted increase*).

based knowledgebase. To facilitate the construction of biological networks from the generated hypotheses, several analytical tools were developed e.g. a clustering tool uses cosine similarity metric and an average linkage method to group related hypotheses together [24].

HEK293 TGFβ reporter assay methods
HEK-293 cell line was obtained from American Type Culture Collection (ATCC; Manassas, VA). HEK-293 cells were grown in Eagles Minimum Essential Medium (ATCC) containing 10% fetal bovine serum and 1% penicillin-streptomycin. Cells were maintained at 37°C, 5% CO2, 95% humidity.

TGFβ *(SMAD2/SMAD3/SMAD4)* Cignal lentiviral construct and transducing reagents were purchased from SABiosciences (Frederick, MD). Cells were plated in 12-well plates at 2.5×10^5 cells per well. Transductions were performed according to manufacturer's directions, using

20 μL of lentiviral particles and 8 μM concentration of Sureentry (SABiosciences) transfection reagent. Stable cell lines were selected using 1 μg/mL puromycin (Sigma, St. Louis, MO). Single cells were isolated from Polyclonal cell lines using a FACS Vantage Cell Sorter (BD, Franklin Lakes, NJ), and expanded.

Transduced cells were plated in 384-well plates at 2000 cells/well. After overnight incubation, cells were induced using 25 ng/ml hTGFβ1 protein (Sigma # T7039) for 1 hour. Cells were then dosed with varying concentrations of test compound at a final 1% DMSO concentration and incubated for 24 hours in a 37° incubator with 5% CO$_2$. Luciferase activity was determined using Steady-Glo Luciferase Assay Reagent to cells. (Promega, Madison, WI). Luminescence was measured on an EnVision 2103 Multilabel Reader (Perkin-Elmer, Waltham, MA). To evaluate inhibitory effects of the test compounds on the TGFB1 reporter, it was necessary to first stimulate

TGFB1 expression. The in vitro reporter cell lines express low basal levels of TGFB1 by design for the original purpose of agonist evaluation. In addition, the Envision plate reader used for detection of the reporter assay luciferase readout is unable detect values lower that zero. Induction of TGFB1 expression with a stimulant allowed us to induce TGFB1 luciferase readout such that we were able run the assay in antagonist mode. This differs from in vivo TGFB1 expression levels, which allow for evaluation of a decrease or increase in expression.

qRT-PCR

Quantitative real time polymerase chain reaction assays were performed in triplicates (n = 3 per treatment group) in rat heart tissue derived immortalized H9C2 cells treated with cardiotoxic and reference compounds using a 384 well format on the ABI 7900HT. Relative quantification values ($\Delta\Delta$Ct) for *Klf4* (p/n 4331182) message were calculated using the ABI SDS 2.3 software comparing compound treatment to DMSO vehicles after normalization to *β-actin* (p/n 4352340E.) The ABI 2X Master Mix (p/n 4370074) was used with standard cycling protocols.

Results

Causal reasoning convergence

One of the proposed advantages in this study is the ability of the causal reasoning approach to abstract similar molecular events from microarray experiments from different sources, models and chips, thus overcoming technical and biological variability that otherwise make the comparison at the gene level challenging. Therefore, we investigated the convergence capability of CRE in detecting expected similar biological events from data generated in different species, gene-chips and different experimental settings (Iconix Drugmatrix database and GEO public data, see Methods). Isoprenaline is a widely studied prototypic compound for hypertrophic cardiomyopathy with documented molecular mechanisms [18] and its effect in rats and mice is compared here. Indeed, comparison of two independently generated gene expression datasets, for Isoprenaline treated mouse heart tissue and from rat heart tissue, reveals very similar causal reasoning biological networks (Figure 1).

The major molecular events (Figure 1) were constructed by selecting the highest ranking hypotheses and their closest significant neighbors followed by elimination of redundant and surrogate hypotheses as previously described [17]. The molecular networks from both rats and mice largely support similar biological events such as increased hypoxia/ischemia, angiotensin signaling, oxidative stress and inflammation, all of which are known mechanisms of cardiac stress response [25-29].

Cardiac liabilities and cytotoxicity of test compounds

We selected a set of test compounds with reported ECG-type abnormalities and/or structural cardiac toxicities and of diverse pharmacology (Table 1). The ATP depletion IC50 concentration at 48 hours in H9C2 cell line was used to determine the microarray experimental concentrations. However, we harvested the cells at 24 hours for RNA extraction and microarray analysis with the rationale of investigating earlier molecular events preceding cell death. All compounds exhibited IC50 in the low micromolar range with the exception of Dexamethasone and Terbutaline.

Examples of in vivo to in vitro causal networks

All in vitro *and* in vivo experiments had a significant number of gene expression changes to drive causal reasoning analysis with the exception of Terbutaline, which did not elicit any gene expression changes in either of the two cell lines used and hence its translatability could not be further investigated. Additional file 1: Table S1 summarizes the significant CRE hypotheses and their statistical values based on the following cutoffs: 3 or more supporting genes, Enrichment and Correctness p-values <0.01 and Rank 35 or less. Figures 2 and 3 depict examples of low and high in vivo to in vitro translatability of molecular responses for Amiodarone and Dexamethasone, respectively.

Outlined in Figure 2 are the major signaling networks differentiating the Amiodarone effect on rat heart (Figure 2A) and primary rat cardiomyocytes (Figure 2B). In vivo, we found a number of hypotheses related to Amiodarone's suggested mechanisms of action through cellular Ca^{++} and potassium modulation [30,31], and reported side effects such as binding to thyroid antagonism and hypothyroidism [32,33]. None of the mechanism related hypotheses were found in vitro. Moreover, all major causal reasoning supported biological networks were significantly different. Inflammation is one of the major signaling networks predicted, albeit with opposite directionality being predicted decreased in vivo and predicted increased in vitro. Suggested downstream effects varied significantly as well, decreased cell cycle in vivo versus apoptosis in vitro and a larger tissue remodeling/structural signal primarily driven by decreased TGFB in vitro. At the hypothesis level very few similarities were found between in vivo cardiac tissue and in vitro primary rat cardiomyoctes, e.g. *Hypoxia-* and *SRF-* hypotheses.

Contrary to Amiodarone, Dexamethasone shows high degree of in vivo to in vitro translatability at both the process and individual hypothesis levels. Figure 3 shows the causal reasoning inferred molecular response to Dexamethasone in rat cardiac tissue (Figure 3A) and Primary rat cardiomyocytes (Figure 3B). Causal reasoning generated a number of individual hypotheses reflective

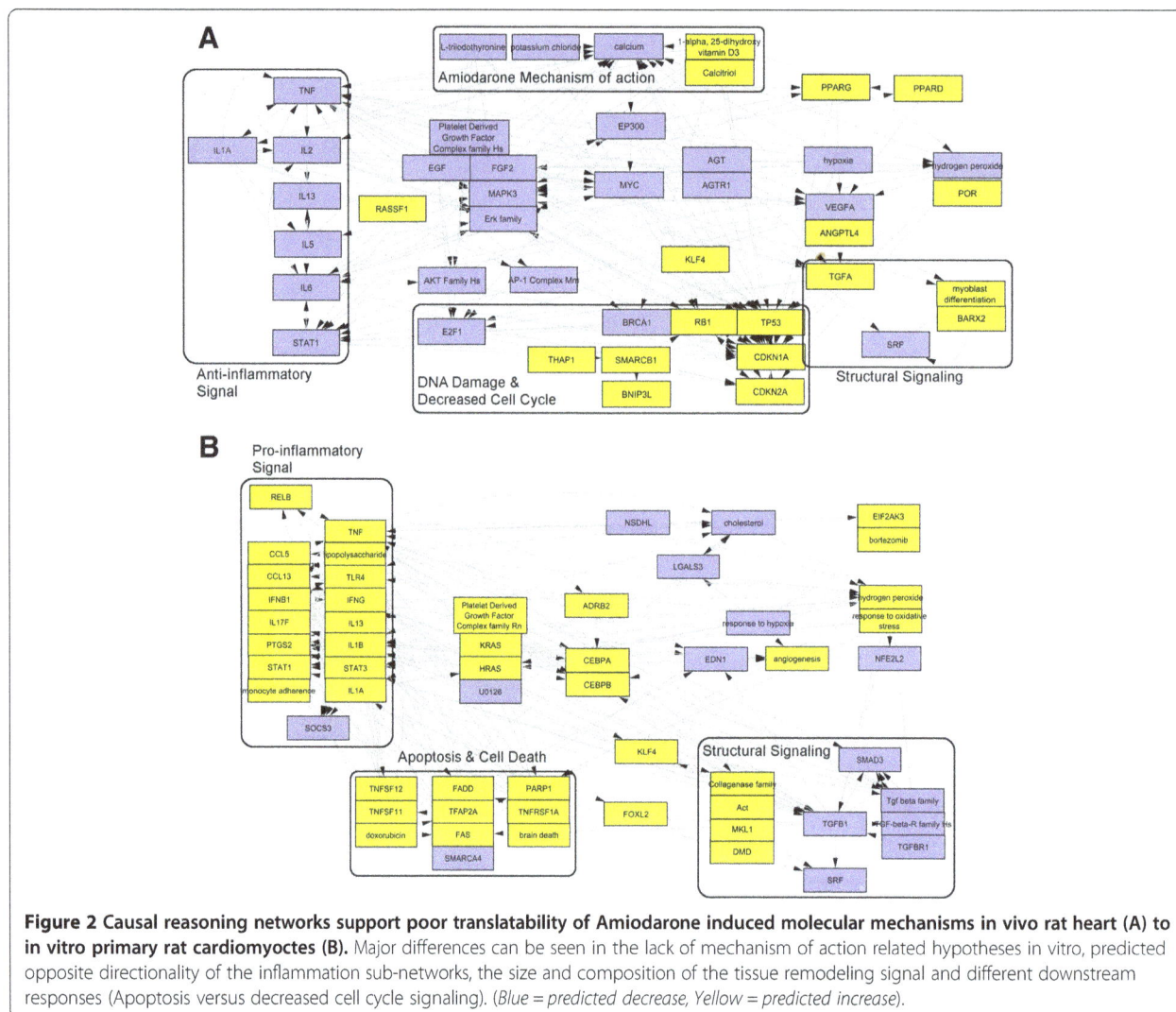

Figure 2 Causal reasoning networks support poor translatability of Amiodarone induced molecular mechanisms in vivo rat heart (A) to in vitro primary rat cardiomyoctes (B). Major differences can be seen in the lack of mechanism of action related hypotheses in vitro, predicted opposite directionality of the inflammation sub-networks, the size and composition of the tissue remodeling signal and different downstream responses (Apoptosis versus decreased cell cycle signaling). (Blue = predicted decrease, Yellow = predicted increase).

of dexamethasone action such as *Dexamethasone+*, *NR3C1+* and *glucocorticoid+*. Known dexamethasone effect is also reflected by supported biological processes such as the anti-inflammatory sub-network both in vivo and in vitro. Dexamethasone is also highly translatable to H9C2 cells as well with a causal network that is highly similar to that of primary rat cardiomyocytes (not shown).

In vivo to in vitro translatability of the major biological processes

The top ranking causal networks from each in vivo or in vitro experiment were summarized at the biological process level in Figure 4. A network was determined to be top ranking if it was supported by a cluster of at least 3 hypotheses and one of which ranks in the top 25 hypotheses as previously described [17]. For every compound at least one process was translatable to at least one of the two cell lines used. Overall, H9C2 cells exhibited larger number of biological networks, perhaps

a reflection of greater sensitivity as compared to both primary rat cardiomyocytes and in vivo cardiac tissue. H9C2 cells also demonstrated a trend of general cell stress/cytotoxicity responses that do not necessarily translate to in vivo events, such as endoplasmic reticulum stress and oxidative stress. However, for every compound there was at least one biological process that translated well from in vivo to H9C2 cells. Some of the biological processes that are supported to translate equally well in H9C2s and RCMs are decreased cell cycle signaling, increased tissue remodeling and increased DNA damage and repair. Hypoxia is one of the mechanisms that is supported to be common in vivo (6 out of 8 compounds) but does not appear to translate consistently well to neither H9C2 cells (2 out of 8 compound) nor RCMs (3 out of 8 compounds). Tissue remodeling biological processes appeared to be the most translatable across all compounds and in both H9C2s and RCMs. However, the tissue remodeling networks makeup was not necessarily homogenous

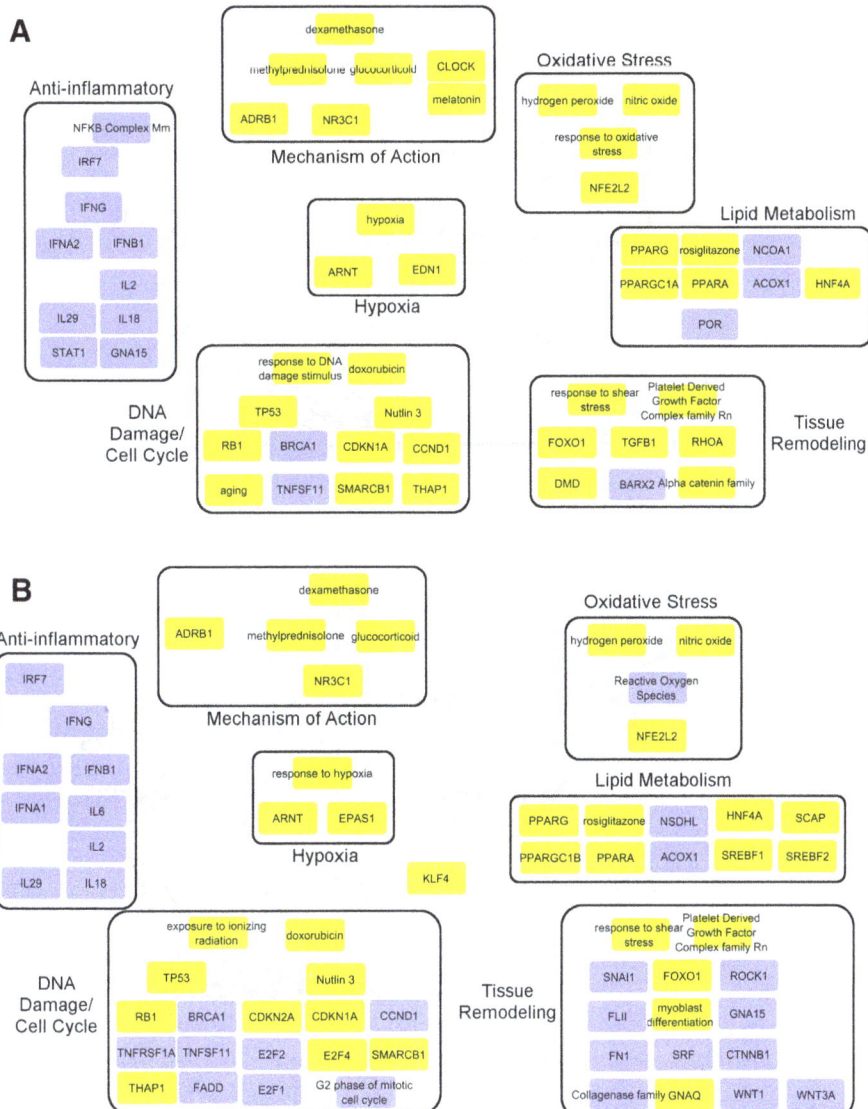

Figure 3 Causal reasoning networks support high translatability of dexamethasone induced molecular mechanisms from in vivo rat heart (A) to in vitro primary rat cardiomyocytes (B). The overview network illustrates hypotheses reflective of the mechanism of action such *Dexamethasone* + and glucocorticoid receptor *NR3C1*+ as well as an anti-inflammatory hypotheses. (*Blue = predicted decrease, Yellow = predicted increase*).

in all treatments with variations in the types of hypotheses as well as the directionality of hypotheses. Examples of tissue remodeling networks included hypotheses of both increased and decreased TGFB signaling, structural protein changes such as Dystrophin (DMD) and Myocardin (MYOCD), and cytoskeleton remodeling proteins such as BARX2 and FLII.

Identifying KLF4 as a potential common hub in cardiotoxicity

KLF4+ was one of the frequent hypotheses in both cell lines and in vivo (See Additional file 2: Figure S1). Additionally, *KLF4*+ was found to be connected to key hypotheses from different toxicity mechanisms such as

IFNG in inflammation, *TGFB1* in tissue remodeling and *TP53* and *CDKN1A* in cell cycle (see example networks in Figures 2 and 3). This suggests a potential role of KLF4 as a central hub in cardiotoxicity. Figure 5 shows an example of a *KLF4*+ hypothesis and the supporting observed gene expression changes. In addition to the CRE prediction of increased KLF4 activity the observed KLF4 gene expression levels from the Affymetrix gene chips showed consistent increase correlating well with the CRE predictions (Figure 6). Finally, subsequent follow-up RT-PCR experiment to measure KLF4 mRNA in H9C2 in response to treatment showed consistent results (Table 2). Doxorubicin was one of the exceptions where there was observed decrease in mRNA on the

	Amiodarone			Amitriptyline			Cyclosporine			Dexamethasone			Dobutamine			Doxorubicin			Loratadine			Mitoxantrone		
	Rat Heart	RCM	H9C2	Rat Heart	RCM	H9C2	Rat Heart	RCM	H9C2	Rat Heart	RCM	H9C2	Rat Heart	RCM	H9C2	Rat Heart	RCM	H9C2	Rat Heart	RCM	H9C2	Rat Heart	RCM	H9C2
Lipid metabolism																								
Endoplasmic reticulum stress																								
Oxidative stress																								
Hypoxia/Ischemia																								
Cell cycle																								
Tissue remodeling																								
Inflammation																								
Apoptosis & cell death																								
DNA damage/repair																								
Energy metabolism																								

Predicted Increase (yellow)   Predicted Decrease (purple)

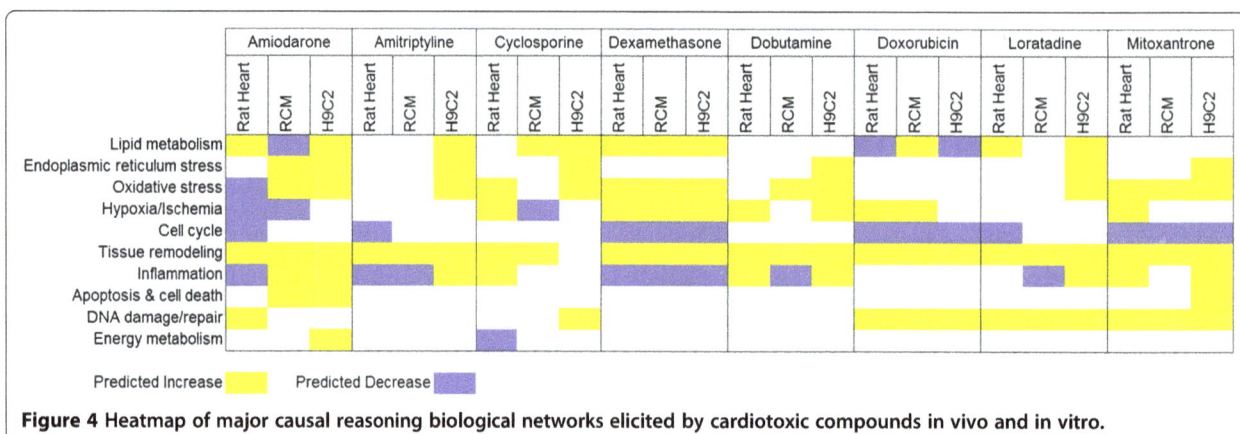

Figure 4 Heatmap of major causal reasoning biological networks elicited by cardiotoxic compounds in vivo and in vitro.

Affymetrix gene chip despite of predicted *KLF4+* hypothesis. However, repeating the experiment with a lower Doxorubicin concentration that corresponds to the IC20 resulted in 2.52 fold increase in *KLF4* mRNA perhaps suggests the CRE prediction was for a molecular event at an earlier time point.

Potential role of TGFB1 in cardiotoxicity and TGFB1 reporter assay

TGFB signaling was one of the most frequently perturbed signaling pathway in vivo and in vitro with all tested compounds with the exceptions of Dexamethasone in RCM and Cyclosporine in H9C2 cells. However, the perturbation was in many cases in opposing directions in vivo vs. in vitro (Table 3). Next, we employed a TGFB1 reporter assay to experimentally test the predicted effect of compounds on TGFB1 activity in vitro. Compound treatment following stimulation with TGFB1 demonstrates the inhibitory effect of the compounds in dose dependant manner consistent with the CRE predictions (Figure 7). In absence of TGFB1 stimulation none of the tested compounds had a stimulatory effect (data not shown).

Discussion

Gene expression changes of nine compounds known to induce cardiotoxicity were profiled in rat cardiomyocytes, rat embryonic heart tissue-derived H9C2 cells, and heart tissue from treated rats. There was, as expected, significant variation between drugs and test systems at the individual gene level. In this work we applied a recently developed method [16,17] to understand convergence of gene expression changes based on their potential upstream regulators. As described the CRE analysis revealed a convergence of the explained changes around a set of biological pathways. Specifically, pathways associated with tissue remodeling, cell cycle, oxidative stress, and DNA damage were particularly well conserved across cardiotoxic drugs and between in vivo and in vitro test systems. This level of concordance between the in vivo and in vitro systems was encouraging but there were some clear points of disagreement between the experimental systems providing a stark reminder of the limitations of in vitro systems. An example of this difference is the greater diversity of signaling in H9C2 cells compared to rat cardiomyocytes. This may be explained by the immortalized nature of H9C2 cells with active cell cycle compared to the primary rat cardiomyocytes. Another possibility is that H9C2 cells are less similar to cardiomyocytes thus more likely to exhibit non-cardiomyocyte phenotype. Although, the wholesale differences between the Amiodarone in vitro and in vivo transcriptional changes highlights that the overall predictivity of cellular systems can vary from compound

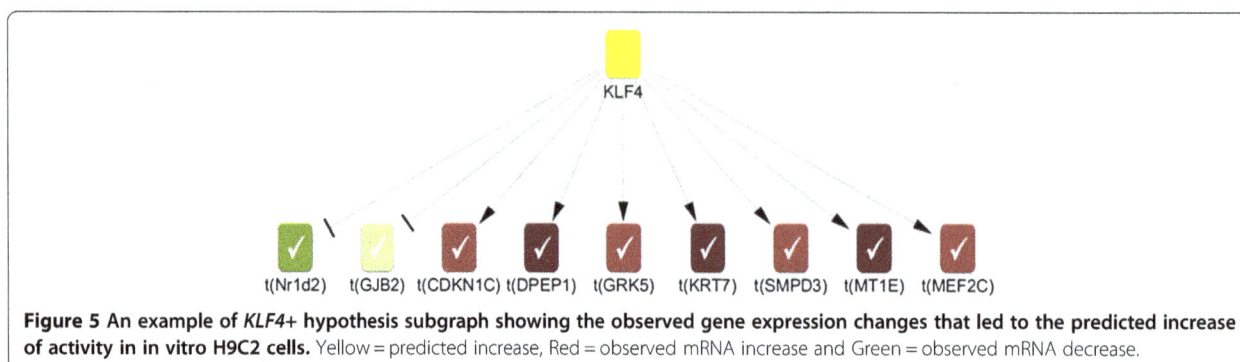

KLF4

t(Nr1d2) t(GJB2) t(CDKN1C) t(DPEP1) t(GRK5) t(KRT7) t(SMPD3) t(MT1E) t(MEF2C)

Figure 5 An example of *KLF4+* hypothesis subgraph showing the observed gene expression changes that led to the predicted increase of activity in in vitro H9C2 cells. Yellow = predicted increase, Red = observed mRNA increase and Green = observed mRNA decrease.

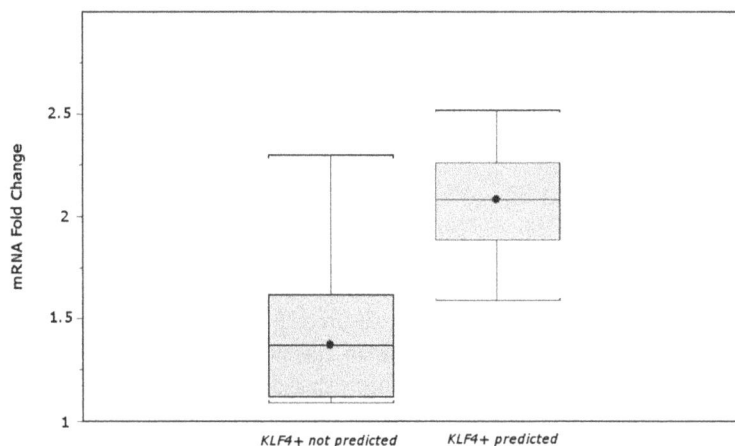

Figure 6 **Box plot shows a trend where predicted *KLF4* hypothesis had a corresponding observed increase in *KLF4* mRNA greater than 1.5 fold on the gene chip for in vitro H9C2 cells.** However, CRE did not predict all significant increases of KLF4 mRNA.

to compound depending on specific expression of drug targets, the opposing TGFB signals observed across the majority of tested drugs points to a more fundamental inability of the in vitro systems to replicate in vivo signaling networks. By better understanding these limitations though, we might still be able to address those instances of successful translations of pathway-level signals of toxicity between in vivo and in vitro systems to quickly and efficiently triage potential therapeutics for their potential to induce adverse events.

The CRE method provided interesting insights in this case and summarized the observed expression changes efficiently for further analysis. However, it is important to note its potential shortcomings. The approach is only as powerful as its underlying knowledgebase of prior biological knowledge. Even a knowledgebase that encompasses all currently known biomedical relationships would not be able to summarize changes that have never been observed before. In our experience [17] the approach usually provides helpful insights as many molecular

Table 2 *KLF4* mRNA fold changes in H9C2 from the gene microarrays and subsequent confirmation using qRT-PCR

	qRT-PCR	Affymetrix
Amiodarone	2.2	1.62
Amitryptiline	2.8	2.3
Cyclosporine	2.1	1.84
Dexamethasone	1.3	2.14
Dobutamine	1.7	1.93
Doxorubicin	−9.7*	−4.92*
Loratadine	2.4	2.1
Mitoxantrone	1.4	2.06

*The decreased levels in Doxorubicin might be a reflection of severe cytotoxicity. However, *KLF4* measurement at a lower dose (IC20 instead of IC50) resulted in 2.52 fold increase.

regulatory processes have been well researched over time. Given a comprehensive knowledgebase results often turn up combinations of upstream regulators that have been observed in a different biological context previously but are novel for the biological problem under study.

Almost as important as the overlap between the in vivo and in vitro outcomes of drug treatment is the notion that the critical biological processes that seem to underlie the drug toxicity can be visualized across various cell types. Much work has been devoted to trying to build an in vitro system that accurately replicates intact organ systems in a dish. These technologies have tended to be expensive, laborious, and low-throughput, thus limiting their utility in any type of routine predictive screening strategy. In addition, these complex culture systems still fail to fully recapitulate the in vivo organ system they seek to model, particularly for long term dosing studies. What this work suggests though is that these types of convoluted cell models might not be necessary for understanding the safety risk of a segment of compounds. When the underlying mechanism of the toxicity is a basic pathway associated with cell health and viability, the specific cell system is of minimal importance. Moving from a primary cardiomyocyte, which recapitulates many important activities of an in vivo cardiac cell; to an immortalized rat heart tissue derived cell line such as H9C2 did not result in the loss of translational power. Likewise, the primary cardiomyocytes were just as likely to show discordance from the in vivo as the immortalized cell line was.

The traditional thinking has been that the reason for the organ specificity of drug toxicity was due to unique innate traits of the particular organ being affected. This thinking has largely driven a desire to have more organ-like in vitro culture systems. The notion that very generic, non-organ specific mechanisms of toxicity might

Table 3 Predicted TGFB signaling in vivo and in cell lines

	Predicted TGFB signaling		
	In vivo	H9C2	RCM
Amiodarone	↑	↓	↓
Amitryptiline	↑	↓	↓
Cyclosporine	↑	↔	↓
Dexamethasone	↑	↑	↔
Dobutamine	↑	↓	↓
Doxorubicin	↑	↑	↓
Loratadine	↑	↓	↓
Mitoxantrone	↑	↓	↓

explain a large portion of organ-specific toxicity runs counter to this thinking and leads to questions of why compounds with these types of liabilities do not show gross, multi-organ toxicities in vivo. It has long been appreciated that differences in distribution and accumulation of medications directly affect their efficacy [34]. The same can be said about toxicity. Cardiotoxicity is not entirely due to the unique "cardiac-ness" of the cells but due to the fact that the heart is the organ that sees the greatest concentration of the compound as a result of a combination of intrinsic and extrinsic expression of transporters and clearance mechanisms. Therefore, in an in vitro system, where one can ensure exposure of the compound to the cell, reproducing an intact organ system is not necessary for visualizing the toxicity risk.

This is not to say that all types of toxicity can be modeled in a generic cell line. There are several types of specific drug-induced toxicities were specific functionalities must be present in a cell system in order to visualize that toxicity. For example, induced pluripotent stem cell derived cardiomyocytes have been extensively characterized (including comparative gene expression profiling) and

evaluated to study cardiac specific end points (such as Beating and Contractility) [35,36]. Utilization of these types of advanced test systems that take advantage of 'cardiac-ness' of these cells might be helpful for certain evaluations. This may be the case for Amiodarone in this study. For instance, drug-induced arrhythmias could be attributed to a very unique feature of cardiomyocytes. Ideally, an in vitro system that predicts this outcome would incorporate a cell that beats so that any alteration in pace or occurrence of rhythmic cell contraction could be directly measured. But even with this example, distilling this very organ-specific toxicity down to the basic molecular mechanism that drives it enables a simple, cell-neutral assay for predicting it, hERG binding and dofetilide competition. As we gain a better appreciation of the mechanisms of toxicity, there will be a reduction in the need for costly primary cell cultures in predictive toxicology.

The mechanisms of toxicity uncovered in this work are not entirely novel. Disregulating cell cycle, inducing DNA damage, and producing oxidative stress has long been appreciated as having a negative effect on cellular health, often leading to obvious cytotoxicity. It is not surprising then that a basic cytotoxicity assay has been shown to have high predictive power for in vivo toxicity regardless of the organ-specific nature of that toxicity [37,38]. This similarity in toxicity across cell lines of different tissue origins can also be seen in our data. Both the primary cardiomyocytes and immortalized skeletal muscle cells showed a clear down regulation of TGFB signaling upon application of cardiotoxicants. We were able to reproduce this data utilizing a reporter system cloned in cell line derived from kidney. Although this response was in opposition to what was observed in vivo, upon moving to the in vitro system, there was a complete conservation of signaling at the pathway level regardless of the tissue type the cell line was meant to

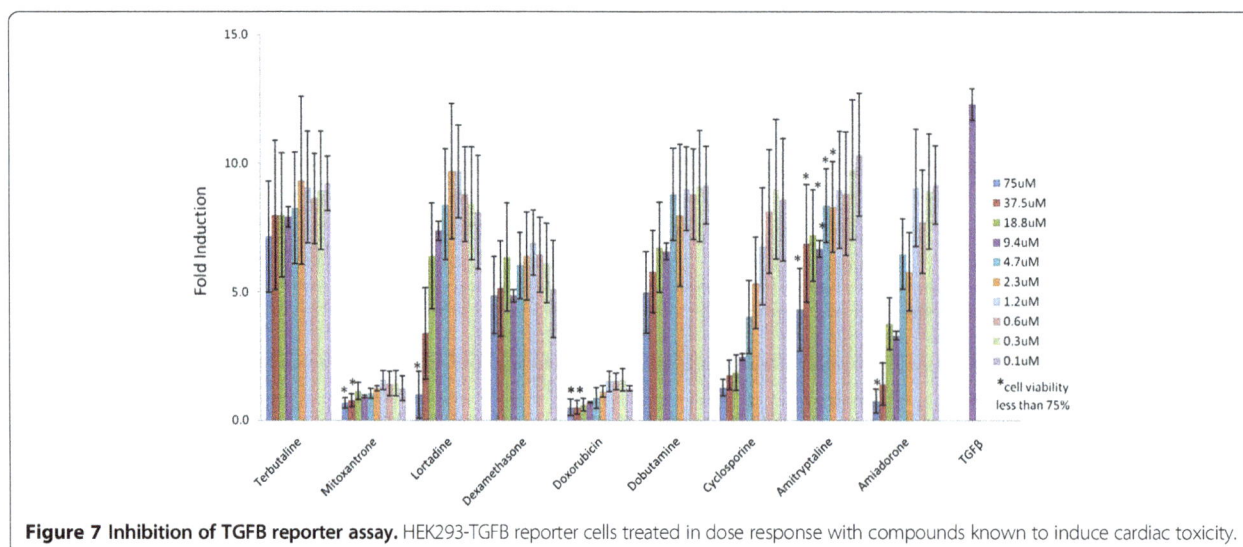

Figure 7 Inhibition of TGFB reporter assay. HEK293-TGFB reporter cells treated in dose response with compounds known to induce cardiac toxicity.

model. Similarly, both primary cardiomyoctes and immortalized H9C2 cells showed predicted increase in KLF4 which we were able to reproduce by measuring KLF4 expression levels using RT-PCR. KLF4 is a hub that mediates the effect of different cell stress signals such as oxidative stress and DNA damage on critical cell functions such as cell proliferation and differentiation [39]. In particular, KLF4 is known to play a role in cardiac function. For example, KLF4 has been shown to mediate cardiac myofibroblast differentiation in response to Angiotensin II stimulation partly through regulating TGFB1 [40]. KLF4 has been also shown to be involved in regulating the cardiac hypertrophic response [41].

The finding concerning TGFB signaling has implications beyond this work. In recognition of the need for more and better in vitro tools for toxicity prediction, many different reporter assays and screening systems have been built and are being marketed for this purpose. The choice of signaling pathways and cellular endpoints used for these products are, for the most part, based not on detailed validation of the tools for their designed purpose. Instead the significance of these endpoints is taken exclusively from literature without fully understanding the impact of moving them to an in vitro detection system. The link between aberrant TGFB signaling and potential adverse events is well established [42-44]. Using a reporter system to measure the potential of a compound to induce that signaling network in vivo is clearly not that straightforward though, based on the finding of this work. Until the translatability of tools like the TGFB reporter system can be validated, caution must be taken in utilizing it and tools like it for predictive screening.

Conclusions

There is a desperate need in modern drug discovery for high-throughput, cost effective assay technologies that are highly predictive of in vivo toxicity. One of the primary concerns in adapting these assays for triaging newly developed compounds is the ability to translate an in vitro signal to an in vivo outcome. This work adds to the growing literature that strongly suggests that an in vivo/in vitro connection can be drawn through the use of basic cellular mechanisms but there are limitations to these predictions that are independent of the relationship between the cell type and the target tissue.

Additional files

Additional file 1: Table S1. Summary of the statistical values used to determine significance of the CRE hypotheses. These include 'Enrichment' and 'Correctness' p-values, number of 'Correctness' genes and the "Rank" of hypotheses based on the on the difference between enriched genes supporting the 'Correctness' and enriched genes not supporting the 'Correctness'.

Additional file 2: Figure S1. Scatter plot analysis for KLF4 transcript levels measured by Affymetrix microarray and RT-PCR. The fold change cut-off (1.3) used for the CRE analysis is indicated by the horizontal and vertical lines.

Competing interests
The authors declare that they have no competing interests.

Financial competing interests
In the past five years have you received reimbursements, fees, funding, or salary from an organization that may in any way gain or lose financially from the publication of this manuscript, either now or in the future? Is such an organization financing this manuscript (including the article-processing charge)? **No**
Do you hold any stocks or shares in an organization that may in any way gain or lose financially from the publication of this manuscript, either now or in the future? **No**
Do you hold or are you currently applying for any patents relating to the content of the manuscript? Have you received reimbursements, fees, funding, or salary from an organization that holds or has applied for patents relating to the content of the manuscript? **No**
Do you have any other financial competing interests? **No**

Non-financial competing interests
Are there any non-financial competing interests (political, personal, religious, ideological, academic, intellectual, commercial or any other) to declare in relation to this manuscript? **No**

Authors' contributions
AEE carried study conception, experimental design, data analysis & interpretation and manuscript writing, DP contributed to experimental design, execution and manuscript writing, DZ contributed Data analysis and manuscript writing, JEF carried experimental execution and manuscript writing, SK contributed to experimental execution and manuscript writing, MTP contributed to study conception, experimental design, interpretation and manuscript writing. All authors read and approved the final manuscript.

Author details
[1]Compound Safety Prediction, Pfizer Inc., Groton, CT, USA. [2]Drug Safety Research & Development, Pfizer Inc., Groton, CT, USA. [3]Computational Sciences CoE, Pfizer Inc., Cambridge, MA, USA. [4]Rare Disease Research Unit, Pfizer Inc., Cambridge, MA, USA.

References
1. Wilke RA, Lin DW, Roden DM, Watkins PB, Flockhart D, Zineh I, Giacomini KM, Krauss RM: Identifying genetic risk factors for serious adverse drug reactions: current progress and challenges. *Nature reviews Drug discovery* 2007, **6**(11):904–916.
2. Topol EJ: Failing the public health–rofecoxib, Merck, and the FDA. *N Engl J Med* 2004, **351**(17):1707–1709.
3. Andersen ME, Krewski D: Toxicity testing in the 21st century: bringing the vision to life. *Toxicol Sci* 2009, **107**(2):324–330.
4. Bhavani S, Nagargadde A, Thawani A, Sridhar V, Chandra N: Substructure-based support vector machine classifiers for prediction of adverse effects in diverse classes of drugs. *J Chem Inf Model* 2006, **46**(6):2478–2486.
5. Gepp MM, Hutter MC: Determination of hERG channel blockers using a decision tree. *Bioorg Med Chem* 2006, **14**(15):5325–5332.
6. Bidault Y: A flexible approach for optimising in silico ADME/Tox characterisation of lead candidates. *Expert Opin Drug Metab Toxicol* 2006, **2**(1):157–168.
7. Demel MA, Schwaha R, Kramer O, Ettmayer P, Haaksma EE, Ecker GF: In silico prediction of substrate properties for ABC-multidrug transporters. *Expert Opin Drug Metab Toxicol* 2008, **4**(9):1167–1180.
8. Hammann F, Gutmann H, Baumann U, Helma C, Drewe J: Classification of cytochrome p(450) activities using machine learning methods. *Mol Pharm* 2009, **6**(6):1920–1926.

9. Octavia Y, Tocchetti CG, Gabrielson KL, Janssens S, Crijns HJ, Moens AL: Doxorubicin-induced cardiomyopathy: from molecular mechanisms to therapeutic strategies. *J Mol Cell Cardiol* 2012, **52**(6):1213–1225.

10. Greineder CF, Kohnstamm S, Ky B: **Heart failure associated with sunitinib: lessons learned from animal models.** *Curr Hypertens Rep* 2011, **13**(6):436–441.

11. Force T, Kolaja KL: **Cardiotoxicity of kinase inhibitors: the prediction and translation of preclinical models to clinical outcomes.** *Nature reviews Drug discovery* 2011, **10**(2):111–126.

12. Braam SR, Tertoolen L, van de Stolpe A, Meyer T, Passier R, Mummery CL: **Prediction of drug-induced cardiotoxicity using human embryonic stem cell-derived cardiomyocytes.** *Stem Cell Res* 2010, **4**(2):107–116.

13. Braam SR, Passier R, Mummery CL: **Cardiomyocytes from human pluripotent stem cells in regenerative medicine and drug discovery.** *Trends Pharmacol Sci* 2009, **30**(10):536–545.

14. Fielden MR, Halbert DN: **Iconix Biosciences, Inc.** *Pharmacogenomics* 2007, **8**(4):401–405.

15. Ganter B, Snyder RD, Halbert DN, Lee MD: **Toxicogenomics in drug discovery and development: mechanistic analysis of compound/class-dependent effects using the DrugMatrix database.** *Pharmacogenomics* 2006, **7**(7):1025–1044.

16. Chindelevitch L, Ziemek D, Enayetallah A, Randhawa R, Sidders B, Brockel C, Huang ES: **Causal reasoning on biological networks: interpreting transcriptional changes.** *Bioinformatics* 2012, **28**(8):1114–1121.

17. Enayetallah AE, Ziemek D, Leininger MT, Randhawa R, Yang J, Manion TB, Mather DE, Zavadoski WJ, Kuhn M, Treadway JL, *et al*: **Modeling the mechanism of action of a DGAT1 inhibitor using a causal reasoning platform.** *PloS one* 2011, **6**(11):e27009.

18. Galindo CL, Skinner MA, Errami M, Olson LD, Watson DA, Li J, McCormick JF, McIver LJ, Kumar NM, Pham TQ, *et al*: **Transcriptional profile of isoproterenol-induced cardiomyopathy and comparison to exercise-induced cardiac hypertrophy and human cardiac failure.** *BMC Physiol* 2009, **9**:23.

19. Archer KJ, Dumur CI, Joel SE, Ramakrishnan V: **Assessing quality of hybridized RNA in Affymetrix GeneChip experiments using mixed-effects models.** *Biostatistics* 2006, **7**(2):198–212.

20. Sammon JW: **A nonlinear mapping for data structure analysis.** *IEEE Trans Comput* 1969, **18**(5):401–409.

21. Smyth GK: **Linear models and empirical bayes methods for assessing differential expression in microarray experiments.** *Stat Appl Genet Mol Biol* 2004, **3**:Article3.

22. Benjamini Y, Hochberg Y: **Controlling the false discovery rate: a practical and powerful approach to multiple testing.** *Journal of the Royal Statistical Society Series B (Methodological)* 1995, **57**(1):289–300.

23. Shannon P, Markiel A, Ozier O, Baliga NS, Wang JT, Ramage D, Amin N, Schwikowski B, Ideker T: **Cytoscape: a software environment for integrated models of biomolecular interaction networks.** *Genome Res* 2003, **13**(11):2498–2504.

24. Jain AK, Dubes RC: *Algorithms for clustering data.* Upper Saddle River: Prentice-Hall, Inc.; 1988.

25. Teekakirikul P, Eminaga S, Toka O, Alcalai R, Wang L, Wakimoto H, Nayor M, Konno T, Gorham JM, Wolf CM, *et al*: **Cardiac fibrosis in mice with hypertrophic cardiomyopathy is mediated by non-myocyte proliferation and requires Tgf-beta.** *J Clin Invest* 2010, **120**(10):3520–3529.

26. Van der Heiden K, Cuhlmann S, le Luong A, Zakkar M, Evans PC: **Role of nuclear factor kappaB in cardiovascular health and disease.** *Clin Sci* 2010, **118**(10):593–605.

27. Aragno M, Mastrocola R, Alloatti G, Vercellinatto I, Bardini P, Geuna S, Catalano MG, Danni O, Boccuzzi G: **Oxidative stress triggers cardiac fibrosis in the heart of diabetic rats.** *Endocrinology* 2008, **149**(1):380–388.

28. Wolkart G, Kaber G, Kojda G, Brunner F: **Role of endogenous hydrogen peroxide in cardiovascular ischaemia/reperfusion function: studies in mouse hearts with catalase-overexpression in the vascular endothelium.** *Pharmacol Res* 2006, **54**(1):50–56.

29. Rona G: **Catecholamine cardiotoxicity.** *J Mol Cell Cardiol* 1985, **17**(4):291–306.

30. Kojima S, Wu ST, Wikman-Coffelt J, Parmley WW: **Acute amiodarone terminates ventricular fibrillation by modifying cellular Ca++ homeostasis in isolated perfused rat hearts.** *J Pharmacol Exp Ther* 1995, **275**(1):254–262.

31. Haworth RA, Goknur AB, Berkoff HA: **Inhibition of ATP-sensitive potassium channels of adult rat heart cells by antiarrhythmic drugs.** *Circulation research* 1989, **65**(4):1157–1160.

32. Goldfine ID, Maddux B, Woeber KA: **Effect of amiodarone on L-triiodothyronine stimulation of [3H] thymidine incorporation into GH3 cells.** *J Endocrinol Invest* 1982, **5**(3):165–168.

33. Jonckheer MH, Blockx P, Broeckaert I, Cornette C, Beckers C: **'Low T3 syndrome' in patients chronically treated with an iodine-containing drug, amiodarone.** *Clin Endocrinol (Oxf)* 1978, **9**(1):27–35.

34. Morgan P, Van Der Graaf PH, Arrowsmith J, Feltner DE, Drummond KS, Wegner CD, Street SD: **Can the flow of medicines be improved? Fundamental pharmacokinetic and pharmacological principles toward improving Phase II survival.** *Drug Discov Today* 2012, **17**(9–10):419–424.

35. Puppala D, Collis LP, Sun SZ, Bonato V, Chen X, Anson B, Pletcher M, Fermini B, Engle SJ: **Comparative gene expression profiling in human-induced pluripotent stem cell–derived cardiocytes and human and cynomolgus heart tissue.** *Toxicol Sci* 2013, **131**(1):292–301.

36. Guo L, Abrams RM, Babiarz JE, Cohen JD, Kameoka S, Sanders MJ, Chiao E, Kolaja KL: **Estimating the risk of drug-induced proarrhythmia using human induced pluripotent stem cell-derived cardiomyocytes.** *Toxicol Sci* 2011, **123**(1):281–289.

37. Lin Z, Will Y: **Evaluation of drugs with specific organ toxicities in organ-specific cell lines.** *Toxicol Sci* 2012, **126**(1):114–127.

38. Benbow JW, Aubrecht J, Banker MJ, Nettleton D, Aleo MD: **Predicting safety toleration of pharmaceutical chemical leads: cytotoxicity correlations to exploratory toxicity studies.** *Toxicol Lett* 2010, **197**(3):175–182.

39. Evans PM, Liu C: **Roles of Krupel-like factor 4 in normal homeostasis, cancer and stem cells.** *Acta Biochim Biophys Sin (Shanghai)* 2008, **40**(7):554–564.

40. Zhang Y, Wang Y, Liu Y, Wang N, Qi Y, Du J: **Kruppel-like factor 4 transcriptionally regulates TGF-beta1 and contributes to cardiac myofibroblast differentiation.** *PloS one* 2013, **8**(4):e63424.

41. Leenders JJ, Pinto YM, Creemers EE: **Tapping the brake on cardiac growth-endogenous repressors of hypertrophic signaling.** *J Mol Cell Cardiol* 2011, **51**(2):156–167.

42. Al-Shabanah OA, Aleisa AM, Hafez MM, Al-Rejaie SS, Al-Yahya AA, Bakheet SA, Al-Harbi MM, Sayed-Ahmed MM: **Desferrioxamine attenuates doxorubicin-induced acute cardiotoxicity through TFG-beta/Smad p53 pathway in rat model.** *Oxid Med Cell Longev* 2012, **2012**:619185.

43. Wang Z, Yao T, Song Z: **Extracellular signal-regulated kinases 1/2 suppression aggravates transforming growth factor-beta1 hepatotoxicity: a potential mechanism for liver injury in methionine-choline deficient-diet-fed mice.** *Exp Biol Med* 2010, **235**(11):1347–1355.

44. Prud'homme GJ: **Pathobiology of transforming growth factor beta in cancer, fibrosis and immunologic disease, and therapeutic considerations.** *Lab Invest* 2007, **87**(11):1077–1091.

19

Coumestrol from the national cancer Institute's natural product library is a novel inhibitor of protein kinase CK2

Shu Liu[†], David Hsieh[†], Yi-Lin Yang, Zhidong Xu, Csaba Peto, David M Jablons and Liang You[*]

Abstract

Background: Casein kinase 2 (CK2) is involved in various cellular events such as proliferation, apoptosis, and the cell cycle. CK2 overexpression is associated with multiple human cancers and may therefore be a promising target for cancer therapy. To identity novel classes of inhibitors for CK2, we screened a natural product library obtained from National Cancer Institute.

Methods: The quantitative luminescent kinase assay ADP-Glo™ was used to screen CK2 inhibitors from the natural product library. The same assay was used to determine cell-free dose-dependent response of CK2 inhibitors and conduct a kinetic study. Docking was performed to predict the binding patterns of selected CK2 inhibitors. Western blot analysis was used to evaluate Akt phosphorylation specific to CK2 and apoptosis effect. The cell viability assay CellTiter-Glo® was used to evaluate the inhibition effects of CK2 inhibitors on cancer cells.

Results: We identified coumestrol as a novel reversible ATP competitive CK2 inhibitor with an IC_{50} value of 228 nM. Coumestrol is a plant-derived compound that belongs to the class of phytoestrogens, natural compounds that mimic the biological activity of estrogens. In our study, coumestrol showed high selectivity among 13 kinases. The hydrogen bonds formed between coumestrol and the amino acids in the ATP binding site were first reviewed by a molecular docking study that suggested a possible interaction of coumestrol with the hinge region of ATP site of CK2. In addition, coumestrol inhibited cancer cell growth partially through down-regulation of CK2-specific Akt phosphorylation. Finally, coumestrol exerted strong inhibition effects on the growth of three cancer cell lines.

Conclusion: Our study shows that coumestrol, a novel ATP competitive and cell permeable CK2 inhibitor with submicromolar IC50, had inhibition effects on the growth of three cancer cell lines and may represent a promising class of CK2 inhibitors.

Keywords: Coumestrol, CK2 inhibitor, Natural product, ATP-competitive

Background

CK2 (previously referred to as casein kinase II) is a serine/threonine protein kinase composed of 2 catalytic subunits (α and/or α') and 2 regulatory subunits (β). The alpha and/or alpha' are linked through two beta subunits to form a stable heterotetrameric structure. CK2 catalyzes the phosphorylation of more than 300 substrates and is itself an evolutionary conserved kinase in eukaryotic cells. Most of the over 300 CK2 substrates have been found to be transcriptional factors (60), effectors of DNA/RNA structure (50) or signalling proteins (more than 80), and a limited number are metabolic enzymes [1]. As such, CK2 plays a critical role on multiple cellular processes, including cell survival [2], apoptosis [3], RNA synthesis [4] and cell transformation [5]. Moreover, CK2 is used by over 40 viruses [1] to phosphorylate the proteins that are essential to their life cycle, including Human Immunodeficiency Virus [6,7], Hepatitis B and C Viruses [8,9], and Human Cytomegalovirus [10].

In addition to its role in viral diseases, CK2 has been reported to be involved in a wide range of neurodegenerative disorders, inflammatory processes, diseases of the

* Correspondence: Liang.you@ucsfmedctr.org

[†]Equal contributors

Thoracic Oncology Laboratory, Department of Surgery, Helen Diller Family Comprehensive Cancer Center, University of California, 2340 Sutter Street, N-221, San Francisco, CA 94115, USA

vascular system, skeletal muscle, and bone, as well as various types of cancer [11], including adenocarcinoma of the colon [12-14], kidney [15], prostate [16,17] and breast [18,19]. The level of CK2 overexpression in colorectal carcinomas was found to range from 38% to 781% when compared to the corresponding non-neoplastic colorectal mucosa in 20 patients [20]. The average kinase CK2 activity from 21 different renal clear cell carcinomas samples was 610 U/mg compared to 318 U/mg U/mg in the corresponding ipsilateral control tissues [15]. In breast cancer, CK2 levels in seven samples showed CK2 activity increased more than 10-fold compared to control [21]. Therefore, regulating CK2 activity may be a promising therapeutic intervention for cancer [22].

In this study, we screened a natural compound library from the National Cancer Institute (NCI) for potential CK2 inhibitors via a cell-free kinase assay. Through this effort, coumestrol was identified as a novel CK2 inhibitor and was further evaluated for its dose-dependent inhibition effect on CK2 kinase activity in a cell-free manner and in three cancer cell lines.

Methods
Cell culture
HeLa, A549 and Jurkat cell lines were purchased from American Type Culture Collection (Manassas, VA). Hela cells were grown in Dulbecco's modified Eagle's medium; A549 and Jurkat cells were cultured in RPMI 1640. Both media were supplemented with 10% fetal bovine serum, 10 units/ml penicillin and 10 μg/ml streptomycin at 37°C and 5% CO_2.

Compound library
The Natural Products Set II (NCI, Bethesda, MD) was used to screen novel CK2 inhibitors. This set of 120 compounds was selected out of 140,000 compounds of the Developmental Therapeutics Program Open Repository Collection. Selection criteria for the compounds were based on origin, purity (>90% by ELSD, major peaks show correct mass ion), structural diversity and availability of compound. Each of the two 96-well polypropylene microtiter plates contains 60 compounds with the outside rows and columns of the plate left empty. Plates are stored at –20°C dry. Each well was deposited in 0.20 μM of compound plus 1 μl of glycerol; adding 19 μl of DMSO to each well can produce 20 μl of a 10 mM solution of each compound.

Cell viability assay
The CellTiter-Glo® luminescent cell viability assay (Promega, Madison, WI) was used to evaluate the cytotoxicity of coumestrol. Cancer cells were seeded in 96-well plates. After 24 hours of attachment to the bottom of the plates, cells were treated by a serial dilution of coumestrol for 72 hours. Then, 50 μl of the CellTiter-Glo reagent was added directly into each well for a 10-minute incubation. The plate was read by GloMax® 96 microplate luminometer (Promega, Madison, WI) after incubation to monitor the luminescence signal generated by the luciferase-catalyzed reaction of luciferin and ATP. A dose–response curve was then plotted as a function of coumestrol concentration used for treatment and luminescence signal.

Kinase assay
The ADP-Glo™ kinase assay (Promega, Madison, WI) was used to screen two plates of Natural Compound Set II for their CK2 inhibition effects or for a kinase selectivity study. The kinase assay was carried out in a 96-well plate in a volume of 25 μl solvent containing 4 μl of 0.1 μg/l Casein kinase 2 (Millipore, Bedford, MA), 5 μl of 1 mM CK2 substrate peptide HRRRDDD-SDDD-NH2 (Millipore, Bedford, MA), 1 μl of serially diluted coumestrol (Fisher Scientific, Pittsburg, PA), and 15 μl of 10 μM ATP (Promega, Madison, WI). Reactions in each well were started immediately by adding ATP and kept going for half an hour under 30°C in a M-36 microincubator (Taitec Co., Tokyo, Japan). After the plate cooled for 5 minutes at room temperature, 25 μl of ADP-Glo reagent was added into each well to stop the reaction and consume the remaining ADP within 40 minutes. At the end, 50 μl of kinase detection reagent was added into the well and incubated for 1 hour to produce a luminescence signal.

Molecular docking
A molecular docking study of screened compounds was performed using Discovery Studio (Accelrys, San Diego, CA). One of the crystal structures of CK2/CX-4945 (PDB ID: 3PE1) was chosen to prepare for the receptor and the binding site because of the low resolution of 1.60 Å. Chain A of the crystal complex was defined as the receptor and the site occupied by CX-4945 was defined as the binding site. Sphere of the binding site was added by the program simultaneously. The high throughput virtual screening protocol LibDock was chosen to perform docking. Compounds to be docked were prepared via the PrepareLigand protocol to give 3D coordinates and confirmation. Number of Hotspots generated by LibDock was set as 100 for each case while the remaining parameters were unchanged. After docking, binding poses of compounds were assessed by LibDock Score and visual inspection to identify the correct poses. CK2/ANP (PDB ID: 3NSZ) was then superimposed with modeled complexes. Protein CK2 in the CK2/ANP complex was deleted to leave the ANP overlayed with predicted poses.

Apoptosis assay
Cells were harvested and stained using an annexin V-FITC apoptosis detection kit according to the manufacturer's

protocol (R&D systems, Minneapolis, MN). Stained cells were analyzed immediately by flow cytometry (FACScan; Becton Dickinson, Franklin Lake, NJ). Early apoptotic cells with exposed phosphatidylserine but intact cell membranes bound to annexin V-FITC, but not to propidium iodide. Cells in necrotic or late apoptotic stages were labeled with both annexin V-FITC and propidium iodide.

RNA interference

Cells were seeded in a 6-well plate as 50,000 cells/well with fresh media without antibiotics 24 h before transfection, with a target of 30–50% confluency at the time of transfection. CK2a siRNA (ON-TARGET plus SMARTpool) and control siRNA were purchased from Thermo Scientific (Waltham, MA, USA). Cells were transfected with 50 nmol/l of siRNA using Lipofectamine

RNAiMAX (Invitrogen, Carlsbad, CA, USA) according to the manufacturer's protocol. Adequate inhibition of the siRNA-mediated knockdown was confirmed by Western blot. The pcDNA3.1-CK2a or control pcDNA3.1-LacZ plasmid vectors were then transfected into the A549 cells (0.5 lg/ml in 24-well plate) using Lipofectamine 2000 transfection reagent (Invitrogen), following the manufacturer's protocol. After siRNA transfection, the plates were incubated for 72 hrs at 37°C before further analysis.

Western blot analysis

After treatment with indicated concentrations of coumestrol or 48 hours, A549 cells were washed with PBS and centrifuged. Cell pellets were lysed with M-PER Mammalian Protein Extraction Reagent (Thermo Scientific) supplied with Complete Protease Inhibitor Cocktails (Roche), and

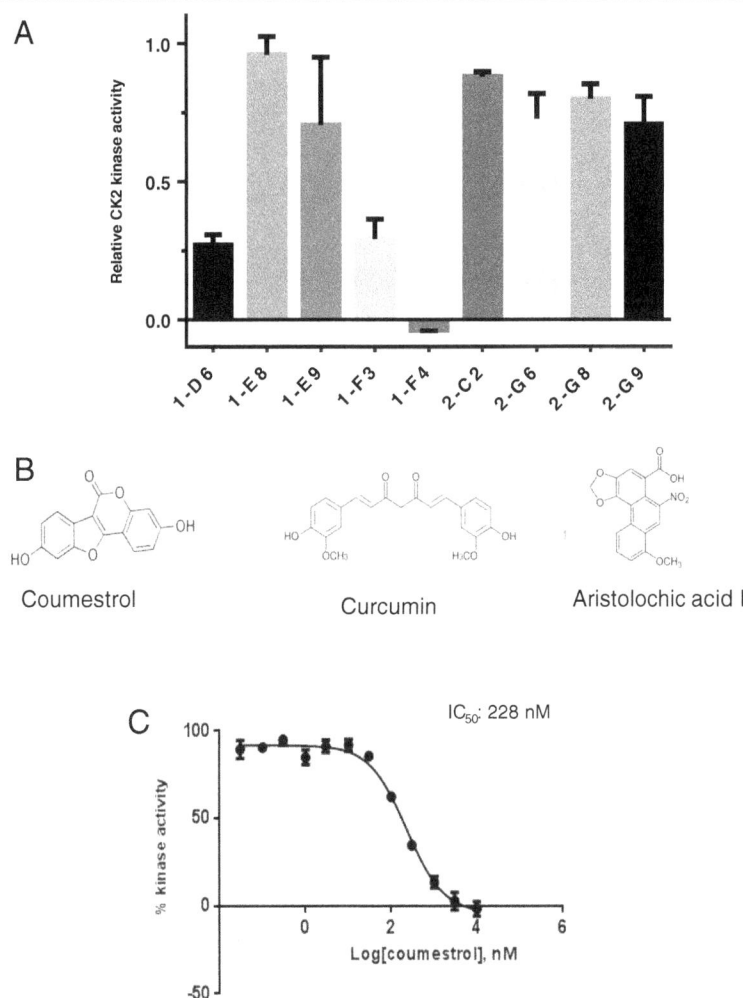

Figure 1 Inhibition effects of representative natural compounds on CK2 kinase activity. A. Natural compounds from NCI plates were screened for their CK2 inhibition activities at 10 μM using a kinase assay. Relative kinase activity of CK2 is shown on the Y axis as a relative number to the control that did not have inhibitor treatment. Compounds 1-F4 (coumestrol), 1-D6 (curcumin) and 1-F3 (aristolochic acid I) showed more than 50% inhibition on kinase activity at 10 μM. Data represents the average of duplicates and bars indicate standard deviation. 1-X represents compounds from NCI plate 13091250 and 2-X represents compounds from NCI plate 13091251. **B.** Chemical structures of coumestrol, curcumin and aristolochic acid I. **C.** IC_{50} of coumestrol.

protein concentration was measured with a colorimetric BCA Protein Assay Kit (Pierce). Total protein samples (50 μg) were separated on 4–20% precast polyacrylamide gels (BioRad) and transferred to PVDF membranes. Membranes were blocked with 5% nonfat milk in Tris Buffered Saline-Tween (TBS-T) and incubated with primary antibodies followed by HRP-conjugated secondary antibodies. Immunoreactive proteins were visualized using SuperSignal West Femto Chemiluminescent Substrate (Thermo Scientific). Primary antibodies used were: rabbit anti-Akt1 (4685; Cell Signaling), rabbit anti-PARP (9542; Cell Signaling), rabbit anti-phospho-Akt1 (S129) (ab133458; Abcam) and mouse anti-β-actin (A2228; Sigma).

Statistical analysis

Data are shown as mean values ± standard deviation (SD). Student's t-test was used to compare cell viability for different treatments. Statistical analysis was carried out using SPSS (version 10.0, Chicago, IL). Significance was defined as $p < 0.05$ with two-sided analysis. The half maximal inhibitory concentration (IC_{50}) values was determined using GraphPad Prism® log (inhibitor) vs. response (variable slope) software (version 6.01, La Jolla, CA).

Results

Screening CK2 inhibitors from a natural compound library

Library screening showed that three compounds had various levels of inhibitory effects on CK2 activity when compared to control samples (DMSO) (Figure 1A). These effects were evaluated in the presence of 10 μM ATP. The three compounds were coumestrol (1-F4; 3,9-Dihydroxy-6-benzofurano [3,2-c]chromenone), curcumin (1-D6; (1E,6E)-1,7-Bis(4-hydroxy-3-methoxy phenyl)-1,6-heptadiene-3, 5-dione) and aristolochic acid I (1-F3; 8-methoxy-6-nitro phenanthro[3,4-d] [1,3] dioxole-5-carboxylic acid (Figure 1B). Although all curcumin and aristolochic acid 1 showed more than 50% inhibition of kinase activity at 10 μM, coumestrol completely inhibited CK2. Therefore, the inhibition effect of coumestrol was further elucidated by kinase assay and a dose-dependent response of coumestrol was plotted to yielded an IC_{50} of 228 nM against CK2 (Figure 1C).

Coumestrol selectively inhibits CK2 kinase activity

To further elucidate the specificity of coumestrol to CK2, we tested a group of 13 kinases representing nine kinase families. We found that coumestrol showed no inhibitory effects on eight kinases: CK1, HER2, MAP2K, MET, AKT2, SRC, PAK1 and mTOR at 10 μM in the presence of 10 μM ATP (Table 1). In contrast, coumestrol inhibited 100% of the kinase activity of CK2, 36% of DYRK1a, 40% of GSK3b and 47% of JAK2. Although coumestrol had a relatively high inhibition of 59% against vascular endothelial growth factor receptor 3 (VEGFR3), this inhibition might be

Table 1 Specificity spectrum of coumestrol

Protein kinase	Kinase activity %
CK2	0
CK1	119
DYRK1a	64
HER2	98
MAP2K	139
MET	101
VEGFR	41
AKT2	164
GSK3b	60
SRC	166
PAK1	129
mTOR	110
JAK2	53

Remaining kinase activity was determined in the presence of 10 μM coumestrol and 10 μM ATP and expressed as a percentage of the control without inhibitor. CK2, Casein kinase 2; CK1, Casein kinase 1; DYRK, Dual-specificity tyrosine-(Y)-phosphorylation regulated kinase; HER2, Human epidermal growth factor receptor 2; c-Met, c-Met receptor tyrosine kinase; VEGFR3, Vascular endothelial growth factor receptor 3; AKT, also known as protein kinase B (PKB); GSK, Glycogen synthase kinase; SRC, src Gene encoded non-receptor tyrosine kinase; PAK1, p21 Protein (Cdc42/Rac)-activated kinase 1; mTOR, Mammalian target of rapamycin; JAK, Janus kinase.

compromised because VEGFR3 is a proven drug target [23]. Overall, our results suggest that coumestrol selectively inhibits kinase activity of CK2 in a cell-free manner.

Coumestrol reversibly inhibits CK2 kinase activity as an ATP competitor

Having shown the affinity and selectivity of coumestrol as a CK2 inhibitor, we next sought to determine the inhibition mode of coumestrol by using a kinetic study. The resulting Linewear-Burk plots showed that coumestrol is an ATP competitor (Figure 2A). A reversibility study was then performed in which coumestrol was pre-incubated with CK2 in a concentration of 100 μg/ml for one hour. A CK2 kinase assay was then done with the final concentration of 100 μM coumestrol. Pre-incubation did not affect the amount of kinase activity (Figure 2B), indicating that coumestrol is a reversible inhibitor toward CK2.

Coumestrol forms hydrogen-bond interactions with the hinge region of the ATP site of CK2

We next examined the binding pattern of coumestrol as an ATP competitor via docking. For this experiment, coumestrol and two other compounds identified from screening—curcumin and aristolochic acid I—were docked into the ATP site, although the inhibition modes of the latter two were not determined. The results suggested that coumestrol forms hydrogen-bond interaction with the hinge region residue Val 116 (Figure 3A). In addition, coumestrol formed another H-bond with Lys68 and a

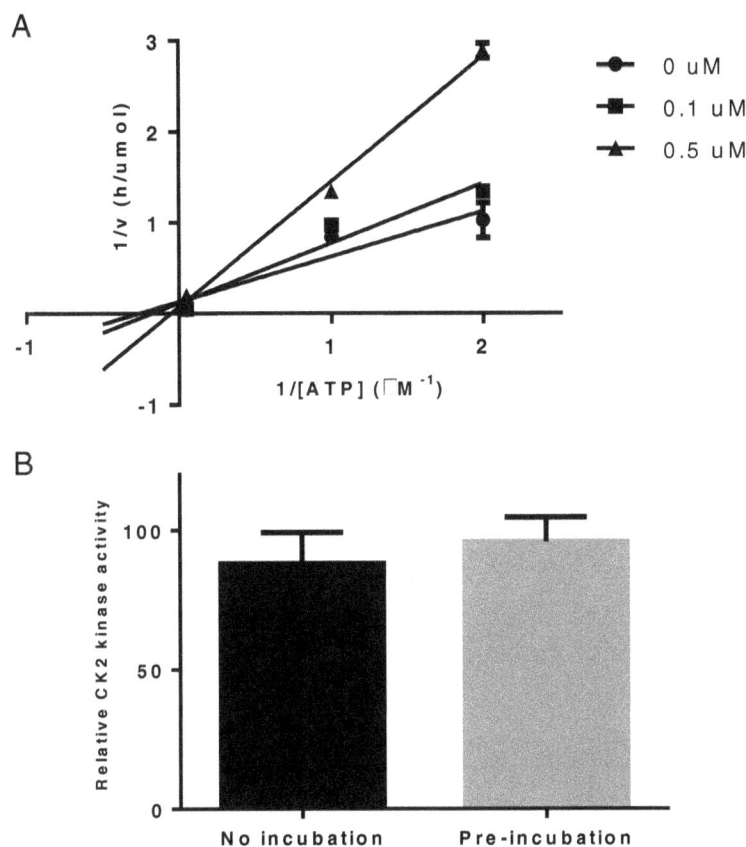

Figure 2 Kinetic analysis and reversibility assay of CK2 inhibition by coumestrol. A. Lineweaver-Burk plots of inhibition of CK2 by coumestrol: ● 0 μM, ■ 0.1 μM, ▲ 0.5 uM. Substrate concentration was fixed at 200 μM. The plots illustrate that coumestrol is an ATP competitive CK2 inhibitor. The data represents means of duplicate experiments. **B**. Reversibility study of coumestrol. Coumestrol was pre-incubated with 100 ug/ml of CK2 for 1 hour and then a kinase assay was performed at a final concentration of coumestrol at 100 uM as described in Methods. CK2 kinase activity is represented as relative CK2 activity to control. Data points represent the average of triplicate experiments and bars indicate standard deviation.

conserved water molecule inside the ATP binding site (Figure 3A). Curcumin and aristolochic acid I were successfully docked into the ATP site as well, suggesting they might be ATP competitors (Figure 3B, 3C). Curcumin established an H-bond with Glu 114 and aristolochic acid I with Val 116. LibDockScores of the three inhibitors correlated with their single concentration inhibition at 10 μM against CK2 (Figure 3D). The docking result for coumestrol provides possible interaction patterns of the compound with CK2. It also suggests that curcumin and aristolochic acid I are potential CK2 inhibitors that regulate kinase activity through competition with ATP; however, proving the inhibition mode would require kinetic studies.

Coumestrol inhibits CK2 kinase activity *cell-free* and downstream Akt phosphorylation in A549 lung cancer cells

Since CK2 showed a dose-dependent response to coumestrol inhibition cell-free, we examined the inhibition effects of

coumestrol on intact cancer cells. A549 lung cancer cells were treated with either 5 μM or 10 μM coumestrol for 48 hours. Interestingly, Akt Ser129, which is phosphorylated by CK2, also showed significantly decreased phosphorylation in A549 cells (Figure 4A). However, total CK2, total Akt and β-actin were comparable. Quantification of expression of pAKT s129 compared to total AKT using different doses of coumestrol in A549 cells showed that coumestrol significantly decreased the expression of pAKT s129 (Figure 4B). Increased cleaved poly ADP-ribose polymerase was also detected in cell lysate treated with 10 uM of coumestrol (Figure 4A), indicating increased caspase-dependent apoptosis of cancer cells after coumestrol treatment. A549 cancer cells were also treated with CK2α siRNA to analyze induced apoptosis. The percentage of apoptotic cells treated with CK2α siRNA was significantly increased, demonstrating a correlation between reduced cell viability and CK2 activity (Figure 4C).

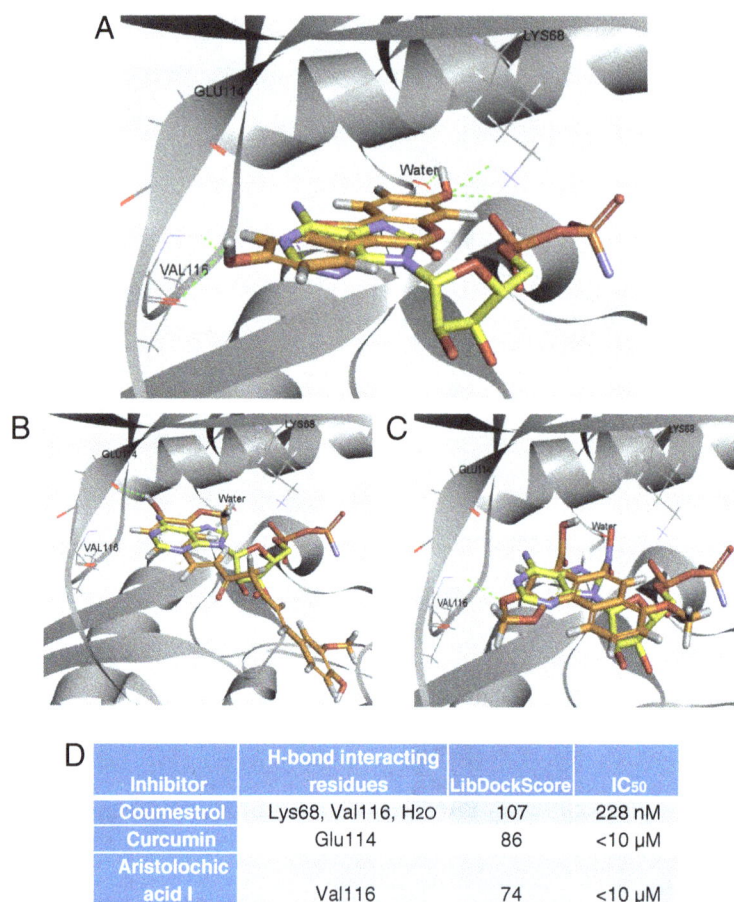

Figure 3 Predicted binding of coumestrol, curcumin and aristolochic acid I in the ATP binding site of CK2. The binding mode of coumestrol (**A**), curcumin (**B**), and aristolochic acid 1 (**C**) in the active site of CK2 was predicted by docking. The three compounds (carbon atoms colored in orange) and an ATP analog, phosphoaminophosphonic acid-adenylate ester (carbon atoms colored in yellow), were overlayed together. The docked pose indicated that hydrogen bonds were formed between coumestrol and CK2. Hydrogen bonds are labeled in green dotted lines. CK2 residues adjacent to coumestrol Glu114, Val116, Lys68, and a conserved water molecule, are shown in line representation along with coumestrol (in A), curcumin (in B), or aristolochic acid 1 (in C) (red represents oxygen, blue represents nitrogen and white represents hydrogen). The rest of the CK2 protein is shown in the flat ribbon. (**D**). Summary of interactions of coumestrol, curcumin and aristolochic acid I with CK2. Residues that make H-bonds, LibDockScore and IC_{50} values of the three inhibitors were listed.

Coumestrol exerts inhibition effects on growth of cancer cells

Finally, we compared the inhibition effects of coumestrol on three cancer cell lines. A549, Jurkat and Hela cells were treated with serially diluted coumestrol for 72 hours, and cell viability was measured via the CellTiter-Glo luminescent cell viability assay. From the dose response curve, IC_{50} values were calculated in A549 (10.3 ±5.9 μM) Jurkat (1.4 uM ± 0.43), and Hela (12.2 ± 5.9 μM) cancer cells (Figure 4D,E,F). The results indicate that coumestrol shows strong inhibition effects towards Jurkat, A549 and Hela cells.

Discussion

Historically, natural products are important starting materials in the lead discovery phase of the drug discovery process and have been a major source for new chemical

entities [24]. More recently, combinatorial chemistry has become an alternative choice. However, the number of lead optimization candidates yielded by combinatorial chemistry has been much less than expected [25]. The underlying reason might be that chemical structures obtained through combinatorial approaches lack essential lead-like properties [24]. Because of these problems, and the fact that CK2 overexpression is associated with multiple human cancers and may therefore be a promising target for cancer therapy, we decided to screen the natural product library obtained from the NCI to identify novel CK2 inhibitors. For this purpose, we used a cell-free kinase assay to screen the libraries. Coumestrol was identified as a promising CK2 inhibitor. Kinetic assays in our study also showed that coumestrol is an ATP competitive and reversible inhibitor toward CK2. The results, combined with those from a kinetic study, led

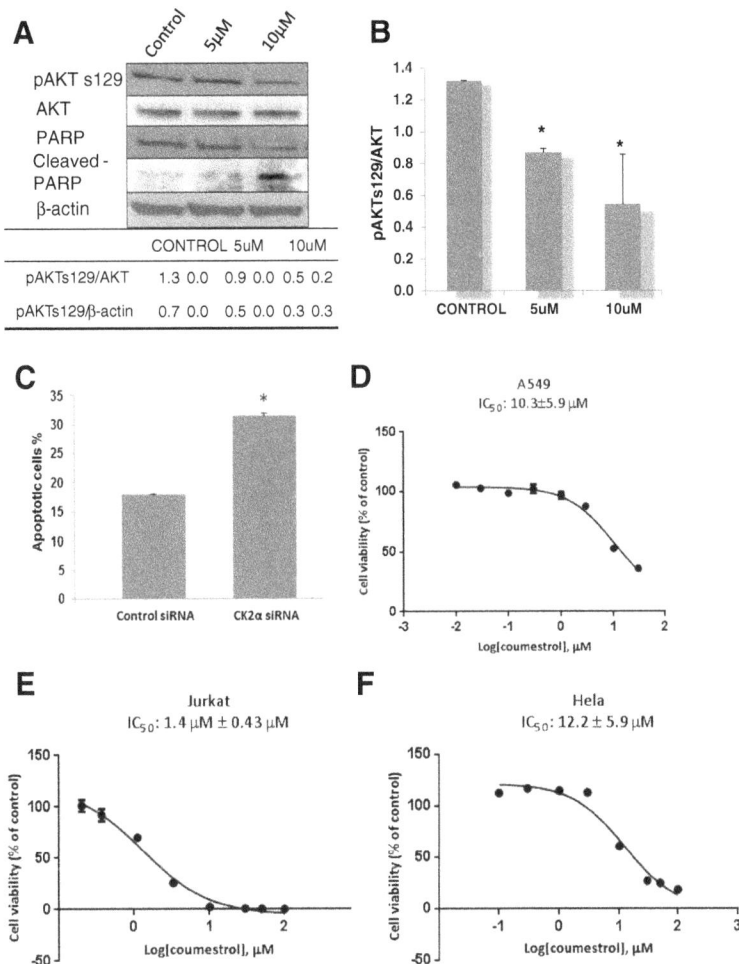

Figure 4 Downstream signalling in A549 lung cancer cells treated with coumestrol and inhibition effects of coumestrol on cellular viability in three cancer cell lines. A. Phosphorylated Akt (Ser129), total Akt, and PARP were measured by western blot analysis. B-actin was used as loading control. Expression of pAKT s129 was quantified using ImageJ software and the mean of relative expression level to β-actin or to total AKT was presented (mean ± SD). **B.** Coumestrol significantly decreased the expression of pAKT s129 in A549 cells (*, $p < 0.05$, Student t-test). **C.** Annexin V analysis of apoptosis induced by CK2α siRNA. A549 cancer cells were treated with 100 nM CK2α siRNA and 100 nM control siRNA for 72 h. **D, E, F.** A549, Jurkat and Hela cells were cultured in the absence and in increasing concentrations of coumestrol (0.1 uM to 100 µM) as indicated. Cellular viability (normalized to DMSO control) was measured after 48 hours using CellTiter-Glo®Luminescent Cell Viability Assay. Data points represent the average of IC_{50} value of coumestrol in triplet experiments and bars indicate SD.

us to identify and validate coumestrol as a novel CK2 kinase inhibitor.

To the best of our knowledge, our study is the first to show that coumestrol is a CK2 kinase inhibitor in both cell-free assay and cancer cells. The cell-free IC_{50} value of coumestrol (0.23 µM) on CK2 kinase activity is comparable to that of several well established CK2 inhibitors, such as 2-Dimethylamino-4,5,6,7-tetrabromo-1H-benzimidazole (DMAT) (0.15 µM), [5-oxo-5, 6-dihydroindolo-(1, 2-a) quinazolin-7-yl] acetic acid (IQA) (0.39 µM), 4,5,6,7-tetrabromo benzotriazole (TBB) (0.50 µM) [22] and 1, 3, 8-trihydroxyanthraquinone (emodin) (0.89 µM) [26].

We also showed that coumestrol triggered apoptosis in cancer cells. Previous studies suggest that CK2 plays an essential role in suppressing apoptosis. Overexpression of CK2 in cancer cells protects cells from etoposide- and diethylstilbestrol-induced apoptosis [27], resulting in suppressed apoptosis mediated through tumor necrotic factor-alpha (TNF-α), TRAIL and Fas L, and augments apoptosis in cells sensitive to these ligands [28]. Treatment of a variety of cancer cells with cell-permeable CK2 inhibitors such as TBB, IQA and DMAT has been shown to induce activation of caspases and then apoptosis [22,29,30]. In our study, coumestrol inhibited Akt/PKB Ser129 phosphorylation in cancer cells. Akt/PKB is activated by CK2 and ensures cell survival via activation of anti-apoptotic pathways, including the NF-κB pathway and suppression of caspase activities [31-33]. Thus, coumestrol induces apoptosis in cancer cells at least partially by inhibiting the Akt/PKB pathway by down regulation of CK2 kinase and then decreased phosphorylation of Akt/PKB Ser129.

Coumestrol belongs to the class of phytoestrogens that includes isoflavones and coumestans. It is the most prevalent derivative of coumestan [34], which can be found in leguminous plants serving as food sources for humans. Coumestrol intake in the Asian population is 10 times greater than that of the non-Asian population [35]. The half-lives of plasma genistein and daidzein, compounds from the same family of coumestrol, were found to be 8.36 and 5.79 hr, respectively, in humans [36]. A pharmacokinetic study of soy-derived phytoestrogens in rats suggested that genestein has a half-life of 4.3 hr, daidzein 2.3 hr and coumestrol 5.5 hr, almost equal to 5.6 hr observed for zearalenone [37].

A specific dietary supplement, selected vegetables (SV), which contains coumestrol, was studied in tumor-bearing mice and in stage IIIB and IV non-small cell lung cancer patients [37]. The study found 53-74% inhibition of tumor growth in mice, but more strikingly, patients in stage IIIB and IV NSCLC who took SV daily for 2–46 months had prolonged survival and attenuation of the normal pattern of progression compared to patients not taking SV [38].

Soy isoflavones, because they are estrogen-like compounds, are thought to have potential side effects on patients with ER-positive breast cancer. The structure of coumestrol is similar to that of estradiol, and coumestrol reportedly can bind to two estrogen receptor subtypes (ERα and ERβ) but with lower binding affinity than that of estradiol [39]. Despite the structural similarities, soy isoflavones bind to ER differently than estrodiol does and are thought to exhibit only beneficial effects of estrogen [40-43]. High consumption of soy foods may reduce the risk of breast cancer [44]. However, whether the use of coumestrol as a cancer treatment may have side effects related to estrogen receptors requires further study.

Coumestrol is a relatively small molecule (MW 268), which provides room for physical/chemical activity modifications. Tumors that overexpress CK2 could be potentially treated with coumestrol or coumestrol derivatives that have better drug-like properties [15,21,45]. Coumestrol and its derivatives can also potentially target several key signaling pathways such as the Akt pathway, a particular example being EGFR mutations [46,47]. Thus, coumestrol may represent a new class of targeted treatments for cancer.

Conclusions

In this study, we showed that coumestrol is a novel ATP competitive and reversible CK2 inhibitor. Coumestrol not only showed inhibition effects on CK2 (IC_{50} 228 nM) cell-free, but also showed the same effects on CK2 *in vitro*. In addition, coumestrol inhibited the growth of three cancer cell lines, indicating its cell-permeable property.

A molecular docking study suggested a possible interaction of coumestrol with the hinge region of ATP site of CK2. Taken together, our findings indicate this compound may represent a promising class of CK2 inhibitors.

Abbreviations
CK2: Casein kinase 2; SD: Standard deviation; VEGFR: Vascular endothelial growth factor receptor; DMAT: 2-Dimethylamino-4,5,6,7-tetrabromo-1H-benzimidazole; IQA: [5-oxo-5, 6-Dihydroindolo-(1, 2-a) quinazolin-7-yl] acetic acid; TBB: 4,5,6,7-Tetrabromo benzotriazole; Emodin: 1, 3, 8-Trihydroxyanthraquinone.

Competing interests
The authors declare that they have no competing interests.

Authors' contributions
SL carried out kinase assay, cell viability assay, molecular docking study, and also drafted the manuscript. DH performed kinase assay and cell viability assay. YLY carried out western blot analysis. ZX carried out the RNA interference, apoptosis and cell line experiments. CP revised the manuscript. SL and LY designed the study and revised the manuscript. All the authors analyzed the results. All authors read and approved the final manuscript.

Acknowledgements
This study was supported by NIH grant R01 CA140654-01A1 (to L.Y.). We are also grateful for support from the Larry Hall and Zygielbaum Memorial Trust and Kazan, McClain, Abrams, Fernandez, Lyons, Greenwood, Harley & Oberman Foundation, Inc., the Estate of Robert Griffiths, the Jeffrey and Karen Peterson Family Foundation, Paul and Michelle Zygielbaum, the Estate of Norman Mancini, and the Barbara Isackson Lung Cancer Research Fund. The funders had no role in study design, data collection and analysis, decision to publish, or preparation of the manuscript. Special thanks to Pamela Derish MA, Scientific Publications Manager, UCSF Department of Surgery for editing the manuscript. The free natural compound library was obtained from National Cancer Institute; we thank them for their generosity and support with drug discovery.

References
1. Meggio F, Pinna LA: One-thousand-and-one substrates of protein kinase CK2? *FASEB J* 2003, **17**(3):349–368.
2. Ahmed K, Gerber DA, Cochet C: Joining the cell survival squad: an emerging role for protein kinase CK2. *Trends Cell Biol* 2002, **12**(5):226–230.
3. Hanif IM, Pervaiz S: Repressing the activity of protein kinase CK2 releases the brakes on mitochondria-mediated apoptosis in cancer cells. *Curr Drug Targets* 2011, **12**(6):902–908.
4. Ghavidel A, Hockman DJ, Schultz MC: A review of progress towards elucidating the role of protein kinase CK2 in polymerase III transcription: regulation of the TATA binding protein. *Mol Cell Biochem* 1999, **191**(1–2):143–148.
5. Ghavidel A, Schultz MC: TATA binding protein-associated CK2 transduces DNA damage signals to the RNA polymerase III transcriptional machinery. *Cell* 2001, **106**(5):575–584.
6. Marin O, Sarno S, Boschetti M, Pagano MA, Meggio F, Ciminale V, D'Agostino DM, Pinna LA: Unique features of HIV-1 Rev protein phosphorylation by protein kinase CK2 ('casein kinase-2'). *FEBS Lett* 2000, **481**(1):63–67.
7. Meggio F, D'Agostino DM, Ciminale V, Chieco-Bianchi L, Pinna LA: Phosphorylation of HIV-1 Rev protein: implication of protein kinase CK2 and pro-directed kinases. *Biochem Biophys Res Commun* 1996, **226**(2):547–554.
8. Enomoto M, Sawano Y, Kosuge S, Yamano Y, Kuroki K, Ohtsuki K: High phosphorylation of HBV core protein by two alpha-type CK2-activated cAMP-dependent protein kinases in vitro. *FEBS Lett* 2006, **580**(3):894–899.
9. Dal Pero F, Di Maira G, Marin O, Bortoletto G, Pinna LA, Alberti A, Ruzzene M, Gerotto M: Heterogeneity of CK2 phosphorylation sites in the NS5A protein of different hepatitis C virus genotypes. *J Hepatol* 2007, **47**(6):768–776.
10. Alvisi G, Jans DA, Guo J, Pinna LA, Ripalti A: A protein kinase CK2 site flanking the nuclear targeting signal enhances nuclear transport of human cytomegalovirus pp UL44. *Traffic* 2005, **6**(11):1002–1013.
11. Guerra B, Issinger OG: Protein kinase CK2 in human diseases. *Curr Med Chem* 2008, **15**(19):1870–1886.

12. Lin KY, Tai C, Hsu JC, Li CF, Fang CL, Lai HC, Hseu YC, Lin YF, Uen YH: Overexpression of nuclear protein kinase CK2 alpha catalytic subunit (CK2alpha) as a poor prognosticator in human colorectal cancer. *PLoS One* 2011, **6**(2):e17193.

13. Zou J, Luo H, Zeng Q, Dong Z, Wu D, Liu L: **Protein kinase CK2alpha is overexpressed in colorectal cancer and modulates cell proliferation and invasion via regulating EMT-related genes.** *J Transl Med* 2011, **9**:97.

14. Homma MK, Li D, Krebs EG, Yuasa Y, Homma Y: **Association and regulation of casein kinase 2 activity by adenomatous polyposis coli protein.** *Proc Natl Acad Sci U S A* 2002, **99**(9):5959–5964.

15. Stalter G, Siemer S, Becht E, Ziegler M, Remberger K, Issinger OG: **Asymmetric expression of protein kinase CK2 subunits in human kidney tumors.** *Biochem Biophys Res Commun* 1994, **202**(1):141–147.

16. Laramas M, Pasquier D, Filhol O, Ringeisen F, Descotes JL, Cochet C: **Nuclear localization of protein kinase CK2 catalytic subunit (CK2alpha) is associated with poor prognostic factors in human prostate cancer.** *Eur J Cancer* 2007, **43**(5):928–934.

17. Yenice S, Davis AT, Goueli SA, Akdas A, Limas C, Ahmed K: **Nuclear casein kinase 2 (CK-2) activity in human normal, benign hyperplastic, and cancerous prostate.** *Prostate* 1994, **24**(1):11–16.

18. Giusiano S, Cochet C, Filhol O, Duchemin-Pelletier E, Secq V, Bonnier P, Carcopino X, Boubli L, Birnbaum D, Garcia S, *et al*: **Protein kinase CK2alpha subunit over-expression correlates with metastatic risk in breast carcinomas: quantitative immunohistochemistry in tissue microarrays.** *Eur J Cancer* 2011, **47**(5):792–801.

19. Eddy SF, Guo S, Demicco EG, Romieu-Mourez R, Landesman-Bollag E, Seldin DC, Sonenshein GE: **Inducible IkappaB kinase/IkappaB kinase epsilon expression is induced by CK2 and promotes aberrant nuclear factor-kappaB activation in breast cancer cells.** *Cancer Res* 2005, **65**(24):11375–11383.

20. Munstermann U, Fritz G, Seitz G, Lu YP, Schneider HR, Issinger OG: **Casein kinase II is elevated in solid human tumours and rapidly proliferating non-neoplastic tissue.** *Eur J Biochem* 1990, **189**(2):251–257.

21. Landesman-Bollag E, Romieu-Mourez R, Song DH, Sonenshein GE, Cardiff RD, Seldin DC: **Protein kinase CK2 in mammary gland tumorigenesis.** *Oncogene* 2001, **20**(25):3247–3257.

22. Sarno S, Pinna LA: **Protein kinase CK2 as a druggable target.** *Mol Biosyst* 2008, **4**(9):889–894.

23. Zhang J, Shan Y, Pan X, He L: **Recent advances in antiangiogenic agents with VEGFR as target.** *Mini Rev Med Chem* 2011, **11**(11):920–946.

24. Feher M, Schmidt JM: **Property distributions: differences between drugs, natural products, and molecules from combinatorial chemistry.** *J Chem Inf Comput Sci* 2003, **43**(1):218–227.

25. Leach AR, Hann MM: **The in silico world of virtual libraries.** *Drug Discov Today* 2000, **5**(8):326–336.

26. Pagano MA, Meggio F, Ruzzene M, Andrzejewska M, Kazimierczuk Z, Pinna LA: **2-Dimethylamino-4,5,6,7-tetrabromo-1H-benzimidazole: a novel powerful and selective inhibitor of protein kinase CK2.** *Biochem Biophys Res Commun* 2004, **321**(4):1040–1044.

27. Guo C, Yu S, Davis AT, Wang H, Green JE, Ahmed K: **A potential role of nuclear matrix-associated protein kinase CK2 in protection against drug-induced apoptosis in cancer cells.** *J Biol Chem* 2001, **276**(8):5992–5999.

28. Ahmad KA, Harris NH, Johnson AD, Lindvall HC, Wang G, Ahmed K: **Protein kinase CK2 modulates apoptosis induced by resveratrol and epigallocatechin-3-gallate in prostate cancer cells.** *Mol Cancer Ther* 2007, **6**(3):1006–1012.

29. Ruzzene M, Penzo D, Pinna LA: **Protein kinase CK2 inhibitor 4,5,6,7-tetrabromobenzotriazole (TBB) induces apoptosis and caspase-dependent degradation of haematopoietic lineage cell-specific protein 1 (HS1) in Jurkat cells.** *Biochem J* 2002, **364**(Pt 1):41–47.

30. Yde CW, Frogne T, Lykkesfeldt AE, Fichtner I, Issinger OG, Stenvang J: **Induction of cell death in antiestrogen resistant human breast cancer cells by the protein kinase CK2 inhibitor DMAT.** *Cancer Lett* 2007, **256**(2):229–237.

31. Di Maira G, Salvi M, Arrigoni G, Marin O, Sarno S, Brustolon F, Pinna LA, Ruzzene M: **Protein kinase CK2 phosphorylates and upregulates Akt/PKB.** *Cell Death Differ* 2005, **12**(6):668–677.

32. Duncan JS, Litchfield DW: **Too much of a good thing: the role of protein kinase CK2 in tumorigenesis and prospects for therapeutic inhibition of CK2.** *Biochim Biophys Acta* 2008, **1784**(1):33–47.

33. Ponce DP, Maturana JL, Cabello P, Yefi R, Niechi I, Silva E, Armisen R, Galindo M, Antonelli M, Tapia JC: **Phosphorylation of AKT/PKB by CK2 is

34. Kirihata Y, Kawarabayashi T, Imanishi S, Sugimoto M, Kume S: **Coumestrol decreases intestinal alkaline phosphatase activity in post-delivery mice but does not affect vitamin D receptor and calcium channels in post-delivery and neonatal mice.** *J Reprod Dev* 2008, **54**(1):35–41.

35. Greendale GA, Huang MH, Leung K, Crawford SL, Gold EB, Wight R, Waetjen E, Karlamangla AS: **Dietary phytoestrogen intakes and cognitive function during the menopausal transition: results from the Study of Women's Health Across the Nation Phytoestrogen Study.** *Menopause* 2012, **19**(8):894–903.

36. Watanabe S, Yamaguchi M, Sobue T, Takahashi T, Miura T, Arai Y, Mazur W, Wahala K, Adlercreutz H: **Pharmacokinetics of soybean isoflavones in plasma, urine and feces of men after ingestion of 60 g baked soybean powder (kinako).** *J Nutr* 1998, **128**(10):1710–1715.

37. Mallis LM, Sarkahian AB, Harris HA, Zhang MY, McConnell OJ: **Determination of rat oral bioavailability of soy-derived phytoestrogens using an automated on-column extraction procedure and electrospray tandem mass spectrometry.** *J Chromatogr B Analyt Technol Biomed Life Sci* 2003, **796**(1):71–86.

38. Sun AS, Yeh HC, Wang LH, Huang YP, Maeda H, Pivazyan A, Hsu C, Lewis ER, Bruckner HW, Fasy TM: **Pilot study of a specific dietary supplement in tumor-bearing mice and in stage IIIB and IV non-small cell lung cancer patients.** *Nutr Cancer* 2001, **39**(1):85–95.

39. Kuiper GG, Lemmen JG, Carlsson B, Corton JC, Safe SH, van der Saag PT, van der Burg B, Gustafsson JA: **Interaction of estrogenic chemicals and phytoestrogens with estrogen receptor beta.** *Endocrinology* 1998, **139**(10):4252–4263.

40. Jordan VC, Morrow M: **Tamoxifen, raloxifene, and the prevention of breast cancer.** *Endocr Rev* 1999, **20**(3):253–278.

41. Brzozowski AM, Pike AC, Dauter Z, Hubbard RE, Bonn T, Engstrom O, Ohman L, Greene GL, Gustafsson JA, Carlquist M: **Molecular basis of agonism and antagonism in the oestrogen receptor.** *Nature* 1997, **389**(6652):753–758.

42. Pike AC, Brzozowski AM, Hubbard RE, Bonn T, Thorsell AG, Engstrom O, Ljunggren J, Gustafsson JA, Carlquist M: **Structure of the ligand-binding domain of oestrogen receptor beta in the presence of a partial agonist and a full antagonist.** *EMBO J* 1999, **18**(17):4608–4618.

43. Cummings SR, Eckert S, Krueger KA, Grady D, Powles TJ, Cauley JA, Norton L, Nickelsen T, Bjarnason NH, Morrow M, *et al*: **The effect of raloxifene on risk of breast cancer in postmenopausal women: results from the MORE randomized trial, multiple outcomes of raloxifene evaluation.** *JAMA* 1999, **281**(23):2189–2197.

44. Zheng W, Dai Q, Custer LJ, Shu XO, Wen WQ, Jin F, Franke AA: **Urinary excretion of isoflavonoids and the risk of breast cancer.** *Cancer Epidemiol Biomarkers Prev* 1999, **8**(1):35–40.

45. Masliah E, Iimoto DS, Mallory M, Albright T, Hansen L, Saitoh T: **Casein kinase II alteration precedes tau accumulation in tangle formation.** *Am J Pathol* 1992, **140**(2):263–268.

46. Tapia JC, Torres VA, Rodriguez DA, Leyton L, Quest AF: **Casein kinase 2 (CK2) increases survivin expression via enhanced beta-catenin-T cell factor/lymphoid enhancer binding factor-dependent transcription.** *Proc Natl Acad Sci U S A* 2006, **103**(41):15079–15084.

47. Siddiqui-Jain A, Drygin D, Streiner N, Chua P, Pierre F, O'Brien SE, Bliesath J, Omori M, Huser N, Ho C, *et al*: **CX-4945, an orally bioavailable selective inhibitor of protein kinase CK2, inhibits prosurvival and angiogenic signaling and exhibits antitumor efficacy.** *Cancer Res* 2010, **70**(24):10288–10298.

necessary for the AKT-dependent up-regulation of beta-catenin transcriptional activity. *J Cell Physiol* 2011, **226**(7):1953–1959.

20

Anakinra pharmacokinetics in children and adolescents with systemic-onset juvenile idiopathic arthritis and autoinflammatory syndromes

Saik Urien[1,2]*, Christophe Bardin[3], Brigitte Bader-Meunier[2,4], Richard Mouy[4], Sandrine Compeyrot-Lacassagne[4], Franz Foissac[1,2], Benoît Florkin[4], Carine Wouters[4], Bénédicte Neven[2,4], Jean-Marc Treluyer[1,2,3]† and Pierre Quartier[2,4]†

Abstract

Background: Anakinra pharmacokinetics and pharmacodynamics were investigated in children and adolescents treated for systemic-onset juvenile idiopathic arthritis (SJIA) and autoinflammatory syndromes.

Methods: Anakinra was given subcutaneously at doses between 2 and 10 mg/kg (maximum 100 mg) per day. Anakinra concentrations were recorded in patients, as well as C-reactive protein (CRP) levels, on different occasions. The data were fitted to a pharmacokinetic-pharmacodynamic model via a population approach using Monolix.

Results: A total of 87 children and adolescents, 8 months to 21 years old, were available for pharmacokinetic evaluation. A one compartment model with linear absorption and elimination described the pharmacokinetics. Taking into account bodyweight to explain variations in apparent clearance (CL/F) and distribution volume (V/F) significantly reduced the associated between-subject and between-occasion variabilities. The final estimates were 6.24 L/h/70 kg and 65.2 L/70 kg for CL/F and V/F respectively. A mixture pharmacodynamic model described the CRP level change during anakinra treatment for the SJIA patients with 2 subpopulations, patients with high baseline and large CRP decrease and patients with low baseline and small CRP decrease followed by a re-increase in CRP levels. There was no significant effect of the combined anti-inflammatory treatment. The proportion of patients for which the development of a resistance to treatment was significant was 62% and the corresponding time was approximately 60 days.

Conclusions: Based on effects in SJIA, a prospective dosage adjustment was proposed based on a 0.4 mg/L Css target in order to obtain a CRP decrease to 10 mg/L or below.

Background

Anakinra, a recombinant nonglycosylated homolog of human IL-1 receptor antagonist, competitively inhibits the binding of IL-1α and IL-1β to the IL-1 receptor and thus inhibits the effects of this pro-inflammatory cytokine. Il-1 blockade using selective IL-1β blockade (canakinumab) or IL-1 α and β blockade (anakinra, rilonacept) has proven efficacy in cryopyrin-associated periodic syndromes (CAPS) [1] and more recently in systemic-onset juvenile idiopathic arthritis (SJIA) [2-5]. In patients with CAPS, anakinra has been shown to induce clinical remission in most cases, decrease the inflammatory markers including C-reactive protein (CRP) and improve patient's quality of life on the long term [1,6]. In the first randomized placebo-controlled trial published with anakinra in SJAI, the number of active joints, CRP and the physician global disease activity assessment using a visual analalog scale (VAS) were significantly decreased in the anakinra group compared to the

---

* Correspondence: saik.urien@cch.aphp.fr
†Equal contributors
[1]CIC-0901 Inserm Necker-Cochin (Assistance Publique-Hopitaux de Paris), Paris EA-3620, France
[2]Université Paris Descartes Sorbonne Paris Cité et Institut IMAGINE, Paris, France
Full list of author information is available at the end of the article

placebo group at one month. However, some patients eventually experienced a disease flare and the authors hypothesised that suboptimal anakinra dosage might be partly responsible for a lack of sustained efficacy, in low-weight children [3].

The aim of the present study was to investigate anakinra pharmacokinetics in children and young adult patients with SJIA and autoinflammatory conditions. The effects of anakinra on CRP was also modelled in relation to the anakinra pharmacokinetics in children with SJIA.

Methods

Patients

Following IRB (CPP Paris V) approval and patients and/or parents (for children) written informed consent, pharmacokinetic data were obtained from a phase IIB trial testing anakinra in SJIA patients (ANAJIS)(5) and from patients subsequently treated for diverse autoinflammatory conditions. In ANAJIS trial all the patients received anakinra once-a-day at the dose of 2 mg/kg subcutaneously, maximum 100 mg. In patients with autoinflammatory syndromes treated afterwards, anakinra was given at doses ranging between 2 and 10 mg/kg daily (the highest doses were in low-weight CAPS patients who had failed to respond to lower doses). In the patients who took part to ANAJIS trial, CRP was recorded at each visit and retained for the pharmacodynamic modeling.

Anakinra plasma determination

Anakinra plasma determinations were performed on blood taken at one or repeated occasions depending on the study group. Whole blood samples were collected into tubes containing heparin. Plasma was separated immediatly after sampling and frozen at −20°C. Concentrations of anakinra in plasma samples were determined using the antibody (Ab) ELISA purchased from R&D Systems (Minneapolis, Minnesota, USA). Briefly, samples and quality controls were diluted with buffered animal serum and added to a microtiter plate which have been pre-coated with a monoclonal antibody specific for IL-1ra. An enzyme-linked polyclonal antibody specific for IL-1ra (horseadish peroxydase) was added to the wells. Following a wash, a substrate solution was added for color development. Reaction was stopped with sulfuric acid. Optical density was determined using a microplate reader set to 450 nm. Anakinra concentration were calculated for each sample by log-log curve fitting of the plate standards dilutions. The lower limit of quantification (LOQ) for anakinra concentrations in plasma samples was 40 ng/mL.

Pharmacokinetic modelling

Pharmacokinetic data was ascribed to an open one-or two-compartment models with linear absorption. Zero-order absorption and absorption with transit compartments

models, as well as the possibility of non-linear elimination, were also considered.

Pharmacodynamic modelling

The CRP levels as a function of time and drug treatment were ascribed to a indirect response model. In this model, anakinra is thought to inhibit the response production rate, $k_{TR}*R0$ (transit time rate constant multiplied by response at baseline). The model equation was then

$$dR/dt = k_{TR} * R_0 * [1–C/(C_{50} + C)] – k_{TR} * R \qquad (1)$$

where R, C_{50} and C stand for the pharmacodynamic response, 50% inhibitor concentration and drug concentration. When the drug treatment starts, the system is at equilibrium (stable disease) what is defined by the baseline parameter, $R = R_0$.

Some individual time-courses showed that there was a loss of drug effect during the treatment time. To take this into account, an empirical resistance function was as a function of time was defined

$$Resis = exp(–k_{RESI}t)$$

where k_{RESI} is a time rate constant of resistance appearance. Then the response model becomes

$$dR/dt = k_{TR} * R_0 * [1–Resis\ C/(C_{50} + C)] – k_{TR} * R$$
$$(2)$$

Therefore, using a mixture model, the patients were ascribed to either equation (1) or (2). The CRP levels were analysed in the 22 SJIA patients from the ANAJIS trial.

Population pharmacokinetic and pharmacodynamic analysis

Pharmacokinetic and pharmacodynamic data were analysed using the nonlinear mixed effect modelling software program Monolix version 3.2 (http://www.lixoft.com/) [7]. Pharmacodynamic data were obtained from the 22 ANAJIS trial patients: the CRP concentrations were log_{10}–transformed to take into account the wide range of observed data during the analysis. The data were analysed sequentially; the pharmacokinetic estimates were fixed for the pharmacodynamic analysis. Parameters were estimated by computing the maximum likelihood estimator of the parameters without any approximation of the model (no linearization) using the stochastic approximation expectation maximization (SAEM) algorithm combined to a MCMC (Markov Chain Monte Carlo) procedure. The number of MCMC chains was allowed to vary in order to obtain a nice and reliable convergence of the SAEM algorithm. Additive and proportional error models were used to describe the residual variability (ε) for the pharmacokinetic and pharmacodynamic data respectively, and the between-subject or between occasion variabilities (η or φ) were generally ascribed to an exponential model, except specific indication. The likelihood ratio test (LRT) including the log-likelihood, the Akaike information criterion (AIC) and the bayesian information criterion (BIC) was used to test different hypotheses regarding the final model, covariate effect on structural parameter(s), residual variability model (proportional versus proportional plus additive error model), structure of the variance-covariance matrix for the BSV parameters. The normalised prediction distribution errors (NPDE) metrics [8] were used used as a main diagnostic tool to evaluate the final model and were directly computed by Monolix. Diagnostic graphics and other statistics were obtained by using RfN (http://wfn.sourceforge.net/) with the R program [9].

Results

Population pharmacokinetic modeling

A total of 87 children (32 girls, 52 boys) with 148 anakinra concentrations were available for pharmacokinetic evaluation, four concentrations were observed below the limit of quantification (BLQ) and coded as left censored data for the analysis. The distribution of sampling times can be observed in Figure 1.

The 22 SJIA patients were 2.26 – 16.8 years old (median 7.6) weighing 10 – 83 kg (median 21). The other patients were 0.73 – 21 years old (median 8) weighing 4.3 – 60 kg (median 21). These included 20 patients with CAPS (14 with the chronic, inflammatory, neurologic, cutaneous and articular (CINCA) syndrome / neonatal onset multisystem inflammatory disease (NOMID) and 6 with Muckle-Wells syndrome),

mevalonate kinase deficiency (n = 3), TNF-receptor associated periodic syndromes (n = 2), familial mediterranean fever (n = 1) and patients with genetically undetermined autoinflammatory conditions.

A one-compartment with linear absorption and elimination model adequately described the data. Other candidate models included one-compartment with non-linear elimination and two-compartment models. The parameters of the model were Ka, V/F and CL/F, respectively the absorption rate, the apparent volume of distribution and clearance, F being the unknown bioavailability. The statistical model included a between-subject variability for CL/F, η_{CL}, and a between-occasion variability for V/F, $\gamma_{V/F}$. The residual variability was described as an additive component.

The only covariates that influenced the pharmacokinetic parameters were age and bodyweight (BW). CL/F and V/F were then related to BW using an allometric function with estimated power exponents. This decreased the CL/F and V/F variabilities from 0.41 to 0.28 and from 1.34 to 0.475 and the AIC and BIC criteria by more than 15 units. This BW effect finally removed the effect of age. No other covariate effect could be identified, gender or combined use of corticoids or anti-inflammatory drugs, AINS. The final models for CL/F and V/F were then

$$CL/F = 0.847 \times BW^{0.47}$$
$$V/F = 2.581 \times BW^{0.76}$$

Figure 1 depicts anakinra observed time-courses and the median and 5th/95th percentiles of the model predictions. Table 1 summarises the final population pharmacokinetic estimates. As shown, all parameters were well estimated with low relative standard errors.

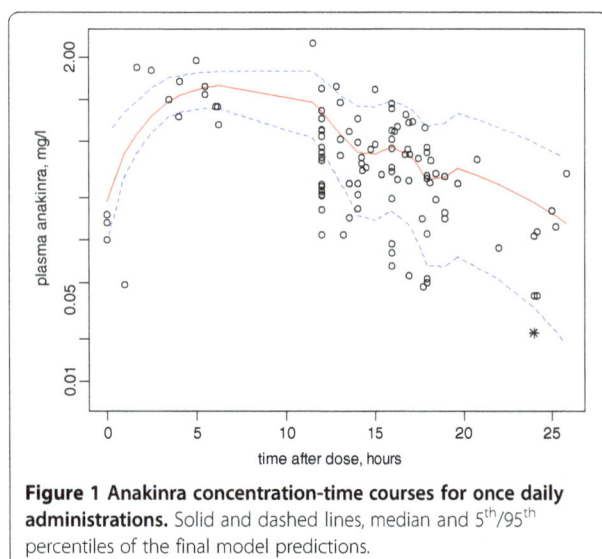

Figure 1 Anakinra concentration-time courses for once daily administrations. Solid and dashed lines, median and 5th/95th percentiles of the final model predictions.

Table 1 Parameter estimates of the final anakinra population pharmacokinetic model in 87 pediatric patients

Parameter	Estimate	Relative standard error (%)
CL/F (L h^{-1} 70 kg^{-1})	6.24	8
β_{CL}, TV(CL)·(BW/70)$^{\beta CL}$	0.47	14
V/F (L)	65.2	12
β_V, TV(V)·(BW/70)$^{\beta V}$	0.76	16
Ka (h^{-1})	0.38	19
$\eta_{CL/F}$	0.28	15
$\gamma_{V/F}$	0.47	17
ε, mg/L	0.072	10

Key: *CL/F*, apparent elimination clearance; *V/F*, apparent volume of distribution; *Ka*, absorption rate constant; *F*, unknown bioavailability; *TV()*, typical value for the mean covariate value; *β*, covariate effect parameter; *η*, between-subject variability; *γ*, between occasion variability; *ε*, constant residual variability; *BW*, bodyweight (CL/F and V/F estimates are normalized to a 70 kg BW).

Pharmacodynamic modeling

An indirect response model assuming that the production rate of the inflammatory process is inhibited by anakinra concentrations described well the CRP time-courses in the 22 ANAJIS trial patients (195 observations were available). The C_{50} parameter was related to the mean steady-state anakinra concentration (Css), allowing the determination of the corresponding dosage to obtain for example 90% of the maximal effect ($C_{90} \sim 10 \times C_{50}$), i.e., dose rate (mg/h) = CL/F*C_{90}. A mixture model with 2 subpopulations, patients with high baseline and large CRP decrease and patients with low baseline and small CRP decrease followed by a slow re-increase in baseline levels (delayed "resistance" to treatment), was finally retained. The corresponding observed baselines (median [range]), 120 [44, 230] and 43 [2.5, 152] mg/L, were significantly different (p = 0.02, Kruskal-Wallis test). However it was impossible to estimate a clear cut-off value between the 2 groups, probably because of the small sample size. There was no significant effect of the combined anti-inflammatory treatment. The proportion of patients for which the development of a "resistance" to treatment was significant was 62% and the corresponding time was approximately 60 days. Table 2 summarizes the results and Figure 2 depicts the CRP observed time-courses and the median and 5th/95th percentiles of the model predictions.

Evaluation and validation

Figures 1 and 2 show that the average prediction matches the observed concentrations or CRP time courses and that the variability is reasonably estimated. Moreover, the NPDE residuals corresponding to these modellings also

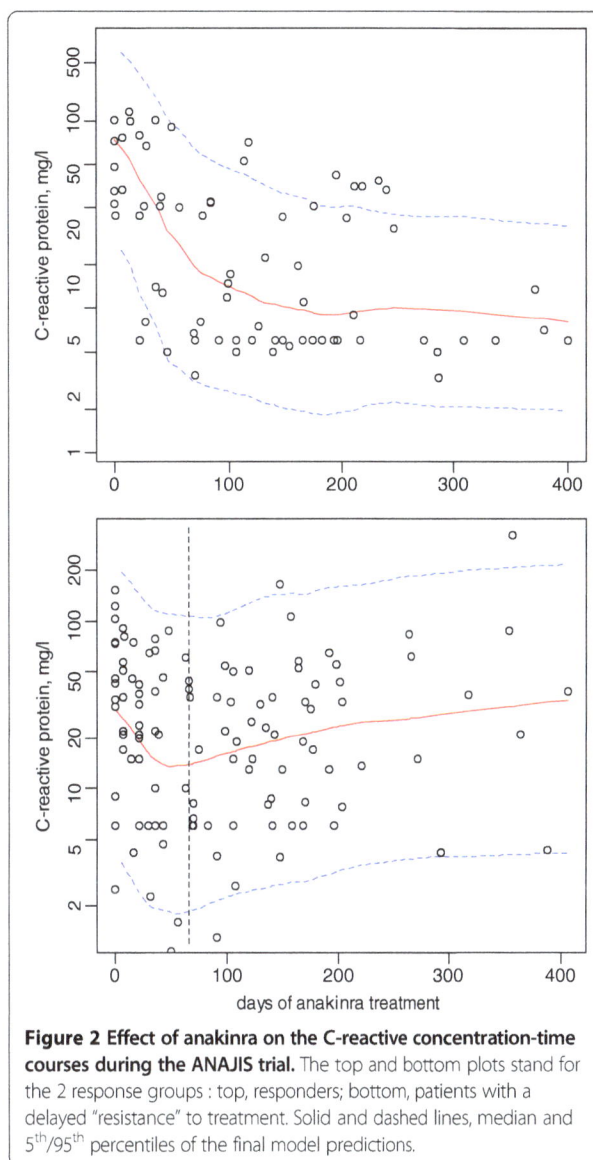

Figure 2 Effect of anakinra on the C-reactive concentration-time courses during the ANAJIS trial. The top and bottom plots stand for the 2 response groups : top, responders; bottom, patients with a delayed "resistance" to treatment. Solid and dashed lines, median and 5th/95th percentiles of the final model predictions.

Table 2 Parameter estimates of the anakinra effect on c-reactive protein concentrations in 22 SJIA patients (RESP = responders and RESI = patients with onset of "resistance" to treatment)

Parameter	Estimate	Relative standard error (%)
Baseline (mg/L)		
RESP	141	27
RESI	37.9	29
k_{TR} (day^{-1})	0.042	27
C_{50} (mg/L)	0.03	37
k_{RESI} (day^{-1})	0.0048	0.0018
Proportion of RESP	0.37	31
$\eta_{BASELINE.RESI}$	0.79	24
η_{KTR}	081	25
ε, mg/L (*)	0.39	6

Key: *Baseline*, CRP level before treatment; k_{TR}, transit time rate constant; C_{50}, anakinra concentration that induces a 50% decrease of CRP level; k_{RESI}, time rate constant of resistance appearance; η, between-subject variability; ε, constant residual variability, *log-additive model.

validated these population models, the mean and variance were not significantly different from 0 and 1 and the distribution did not differ from normality.

Dosage simulations

Figure 3 shows the model-predicted CRP time-courses for different Css values. Clearly, the target Css is 0.4 mg/L in order to obtain a CRP decrease to 10 mg/L or below. Accordingly, the anakinra dosage as a function of bodyweight can be deduced as shown in Figure 4.

Discussion

This is the first pharmacokinetic study of anakinra in children. In pediatric patients with SJIA and diverse autoinflammatory conditions, the pharmacokinetics of anakinra following sub-cutaneous administration was

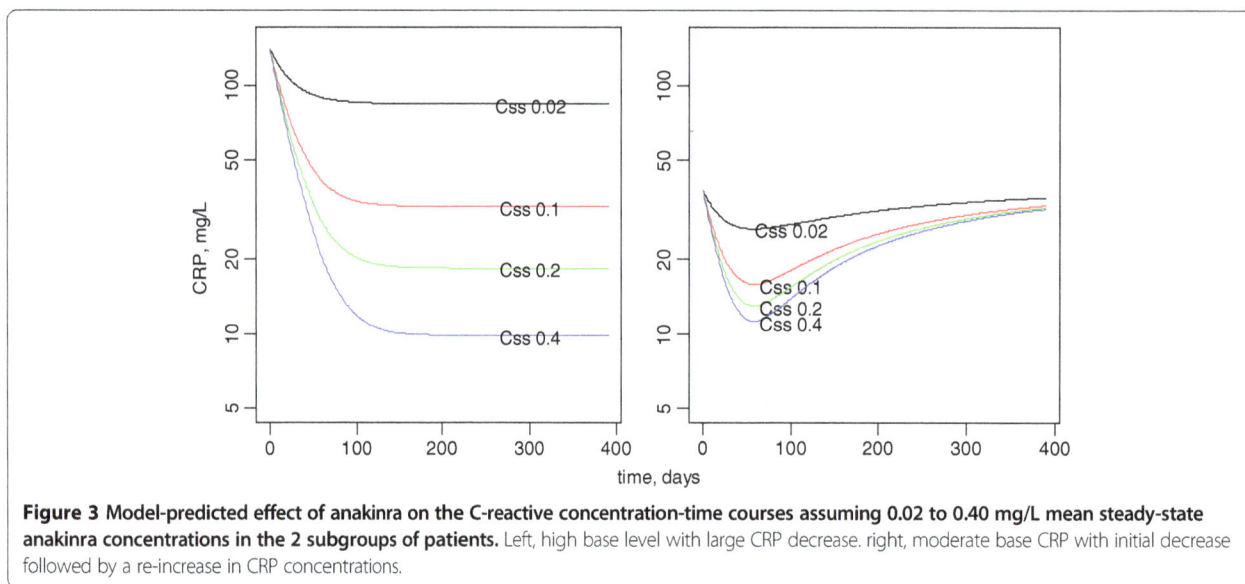

Figure 3 Model-predicted effect of anakinra on the C-reactive concentration-time courses assuming 0.02 to 0.40 mg/L mean steady-state anakinra concentrations in the 2 subgroups of patients. Left, high base level with large CRP decrease. right, moderate base CRP with initial decrease followed by a re-increase in CRP concentrations.

satisfactorily described by a one compartment model with 1st order absorption. Bodyweight was identified as the sole significant covariate that could finally explain a significant part of the variability and this BW effect was modeled via an allometric scaling of CL/F and V/F. The allometric power values are typically 1 and 0.75 for BW effect on V and CL respectively [10]. Because our estimates were not so close to these theoretical values and

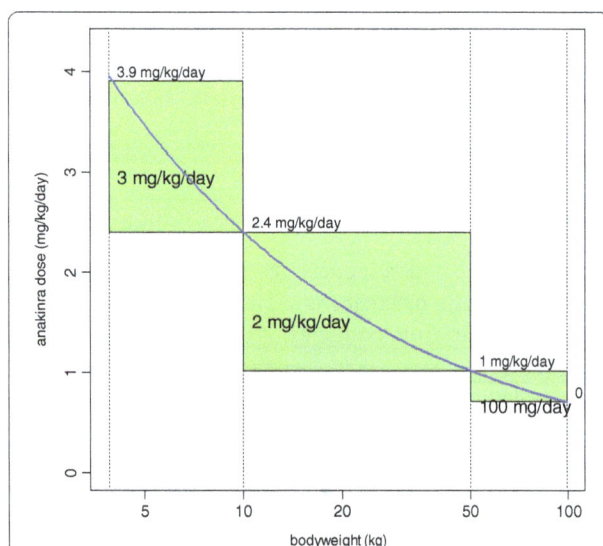

Figure 4 Daily dose of anakinra (mg/kg, thick curve) as a function of bodyweight in order to reach the mean anakinra steady-state concentration of 0.4 mg/L. The 0.4 mg/L target corresponds to a maximal effect on the CRP biological marker of inflammation. Bold text in rectangles defines possible mean dosage recommendation for 3 bodyweight ranges. Text on top side stands for the maximal dosage in the corresponding bodyweight range.

because anakinra is a 153 amino acids peptide chain and somewhat different from standard drugs, the estimated power effects were retained in the final pharmacokinetic model. The improvement of the predictive performance of the model (observed vs. predicted data, not shown) as well as a decrease in the CL/F and V/F variabilities validated this model.

Assuming that anakinra inhibits the production of the inflammatory marker CRP via an "Emax" model allowed a satisfactory description of the CRP time-course during anakinra treatment in SJIA patients. As seen in Figure 2, this was monitored and modelled up to approximately 400 days of treatment. The C_{50} estimate was low (0.03 mg/L) and nearly all the observed concentrations were above this limit. According to the predicted time-course effects of different mean Css values (Figure 3), a Css value of 0.4 mg/L was retained to obtain the maximal effect. The dosages per 24 h that produce this 0.4 mg/L Css are depicted in Figure 4. Therefore, the actual dosage of 2 mg/kg/day in SJIA patients was appropriate in the 10 – 50 kg BW range children, but not in low weight or early age children, BW < 10 kg, for which the efficient mean dose would be 3 mg/kg/day. Also, the oldest chilgren, > 50 kg BW, could have received a flat dose of 100 mg/day, similar to the adult dosage.

Conclusions

Bodyweight significantly influenced the pharmacokinetics of anakinra. An allometric BW scaling of apparent clearance and distribution volume was sufficient to describe the variation of anakinra pharmacokinetics in these 87 pediatric patients weighing from 4 to 80 kg and

9 months to 21 years old. The effect on the C-reactive protein was adequately described by a turn-over model and allowed to derive some concentration-dose guidelines for SJIA disease.

Competing interests

The authors declare that they have no competing interests.

Authors' contributions

SU, JMT and PQ wrotre the paper; SU and FF performed the modelling and analysis of the data; PQ, JMT, BBM, CB designed the research; CB was responsible for the drug assay; BBM, RM, SCL, BF, CW, BN, PQ conducted the research; SU, PQ and JMT had primary responsibility for the final content. All authors read and approved the final content.

Acknowledgements

We acknowledge Agnès Mogenet, MD (CIC Hopital Necker), Solimda Sotou-Bere and Yamina Boulahdaj, clinical research assistants, and the nurses for their time and dedication to this study. We also acknowledge the young patients and their families who participated to these trials.

Author details

[1]CIC-0901 Inserm Necker-Cochin (Assistance Publique-Hopitaux de Paris), Paris EA-3620, France. [2]Université Paris Descartes Sorbonne Paris Cité et Institut IMAGINE, Paris, France. [3]Pharmacologie, Hôpital Cochin, Assistance Publique-Hopitaux de Paris, Paris, France. [4]Unité d'Immuno-Hématologie et Rhumatologie pédiatriques, Hôpital Necker-Enfants Malades, Assistance Publique-Hopitaux de Paris, Paris, France.

References

1. Lachmann HJ, Quartier P, So A, Hawkins PN: **The emerging role of interleukin-1β in autoinflammatory diseases.** *Arthritis Rheum* 2011, **63**:314–324.
2. Ruperto N, Brunner HI, Quartier P, Constantin T, Wulffraat N, Horneff G, Brik R, McCann L, Kasapcopur O, Rutkowska-Sak L, Schneider R, Berkun Y, Calvo I, Erguven M, Goffin L, Hofer M, Kallinich T, Oliveira SK, Uziel Y, Viola S, Nistala K, Wouters C, Cimaz R, Ferrandiz MA, Flato B, Gamir ML, Kone-Paut I, Grom A, Magnusson B, Ozen S, Sztajnbok F, Lheritier K, Abrams K, Kim D, Martini A, Lovell DJ: **Two randomized trials of canakinumab in systemic juvenile idiopathic arthritis.** *N Engl J Med* 2012, **367**:2396–2406.
3. Quartier P, Allantaz F, Cimaz R, Pillet P, Messiaen C, Bardin C, Bossuyt X, Boutten A, Bienvenu J, Duquesne A, Richer O, Chaussabel D, Mogenet A, Banchereau J, Treluyer J-M, Landais P, Pascual V: **A multicentre, randomised, double-blind, placebo-controlled trial with the interleukin-1 receptor antagonist anakinra in patients with systemic-onset juvenile idiopathic arthritis (ANAJIS trial).** *Ann Rheum Dis* 2011, **70**:747–754.
4. Lequerré T, Quartier P, Rosellini D, Alaoui F, De Bandt M, Mejjad O, Kone-Paut I, Michel M, Dernis E, Khellaf M, Limal N, Job-Deslandre C, Fautrel B, Le Loët X, Sibilia J: **Interleukin-1 receptor antagonist (anakinra) treatment in patients with systemic-onset juvenile idiopathic arthritis or adult onset Still disease: preliminary experience in France.** *Ann Rheum Dis* 2008, **67**:302–308.
5. Pascual V, Allantaz F, Arce E, Punaro M, Banchereau J: **Role of interleukin-1 (IL-1) in the pathogenesis of systemic onset juvenile idiopathic arthritis and clinical response to IL-1 blockade.** *J Exp Med* 2005, **201**:1479–1486.
6. Neven B, Marvillet I, Terrada C, Ferster A, Boddaert N, Couloignier V, Pinto G, Pagnier A, Bodemer C, Bodaghi B, Tardieu M, Prieur AM, Quartier P: **Long-term efficacy of the interleukin-1 receptor antagonist anakinra in ten patients with neonatal-onset multisystem inflammatory disease/chronic infantile neurologic, cutaneous, articular syndrome.** *Arthritis Rheum* 2010, **62**:258–267.
7. Lavielle M, Mentré F: **Estimation of population pharmacokinetic parameters of saquinavir in HIV patients with the MONOLIX software.** *J Pharmacokinet Pharmacodyn* 2007, **34**:229–249.
8. Comets E, Brendel K, Mentré F: **Computing normalised prediction distribution errors to evaluate nonlinear mixed-effect models: the npde add-on package for R.** *Comput Methods Programs Biomed* 2008, **90**:154–166.
9. Ihaka R, Gentleman R: **R: A Language for Data Analysis and Graphics.** *Journal of Computational and Graphical Statistics* 1996, **5**:299–314.
10. Anderson BJ, Holford NHG: **Mechanism-based concepts of size and maturity in pharmacokinetics.** *Annu Rev Pharmacol Toxicol* 2008, **48**:303–332.

21

Active post-marketing surveillance of the intralesional administration of human recombinant epidermal growth factor in diabetic foot ulcers

Isis B Yera-Alos[1]*, Liuba Alonso-Carbonell[1], Carmen M Valenzuela-Silva[2], Angela D Tuero-Iglesias[2], Martha Moreira-Martínez[3], Ivonne Marrero-Rodríguez[4], Ernesto López-Mola[2] and Pedro A López-Saura[2]

Abstract

Background: After several exploratory and confirmatory clinical trials, the intralesional administration of human recombinant epidermal growth factor (hrEGF) has been approved for the treatment of advanced diabetic foot ulcers (DFU). The aim of this work was to evaluate the effectiveness and safety of this procedure in medical practice.

Methods: A prospective, post-marketing active pharmacosurveillance was conducted in 41 hospitals and 19 primary care polyclinics. Patients with DFU received hrEGF, 25 or 75 µg, intralesionally 3 times per week until complete granulation of the ulcer or 8 weeks maximum, adjuvant to standard wound care. Outcomes measured were complete granulation, amputations, and adverse events (AE) during treatment; complete lesion re-epithelization and relapses in follow-up (median: 1.2; maximum 4.2 years).

Results: The study included 1788 patients with 1835 DFU (81% Wagner's grades 3 or 4; 43% ischemic) treated from May 2007 to April 2010. Complete granulation was observed in 76% of the ulcers in 5 weeks (median). Ulcer non-ischemic etiology (OR: 3.6; 95% CI: 2.8-4.7) and age (1.02; 1.01-1.03, for each younger year) were the main variables with influence on this outcome. During treatment, 220 (12%) amputations (171 major) were required in 214 patients, mostly in ischemic or Wagner's grade 3 to 5 ulcers. Re-epithelization was documented in 61% of the 1659 followed-up cases; 5% relapsed per year. AE (4171) were reported in 47% of the subjects. Mild or moderate local pain and burning sensation, shivering and chills, were 87% of the events. Serious events, not related to treatment, occurred in 1.7% of the patients.

Conclusions: The favorable benefit/risk balance, confirms the beneficial clinical profile of intralesional hrEGF in the treatment of DFUs.

Keywords: Diabetic foot ulcer, Epidermal growth factor, Pharmacoepidemiology

Background

Pharmacovigilance and post-marketing studies are key elements to monitor the safety and effectiveness of approved drugs. They are excellent scenarios to confirm and extend the safety profile and efficacy data acquired in previous clinical trials.

Products for the treatment of diabetic foot ulcers (DFU) available in the market have been scarcely effective in advanced and/or ischemic lesions [1]. Necrotic tissue, sepsis, inflammation and wound proteases impair the effective distribution of the active pharmaceutical ingredients when they are administered in topically [2].

A new procedure has been recently developed for the treatment of these advanced DFU based on the intralesional infiltration of recombinant, human epidermal growth factor (rhEGF) as a lyophilized formulation under the brand name Heberprot-P®. The rationale of this procedure has been published and reviewed recently [2,3].

* Correspondence: isis.yera@cigb.edu.cu
[1]Center for the Development of Pharmacoepidemiology, Havana, Cuba
Full list of author information is available at the end of the article

Exploratory [4-6] and confirmatory [7] clinical trials have been successfully completed with this product in patients suffering from advanced DFUs with potential amputation risk (reviewed in ref. 3). These trials demonstrated that the intralesional administration of rhEGF accelerates the wound healing process. The generation of useful granulation tissue on the ulcer bed facilitated its closure by either second intention or a skin graft. The product's safety profile was acceptable and the benefit-risk analysis of its use yielded a largely favorable balance. These results granted the approval by the Cuban Regulatory Authority (CECMED).

In April 2007 this treatment was included in the country's Basic Drugs List and its use was extended to all Angiology services, firstly in the secondary healthcare level (hospitals) and subsequently in the primary level (polyclinics).

At the same time, postmarketing active surveillance was initiated in order to evaluate the effectiveness and safety of the drug in the current medical practice. This article reports the first results of this surveillance.

Methods
Design and participants
A multicenter, prospective, intensive, post-marketing surveillance was conducted on patients treated from May 2007 to April 2010; follow-up extended to December 2011. The study was coordinated by the Center for the Development of Pharmacoepidemiology (CDF) from the Cuban Ministry of Health and its national network. There were 41 participating hospitals from the 15 Cuban provinces and 19 polyclinics from 7 provinces.

Patients, more than 18 years-old, suffering from 1 cm^2 or larger DFUs were prescribed with rhEGF and included. The indication comprised Wagner's [8] grades 3 and 4 DFU, but some patients with grades 1, 2, and 5 were included, under off-label use according to the physicians' decision. Patients with diabetic coma, uncontrolled heart, renal or liver disease, history or suspicion of malignancy, pregnancy or breastfeeding were not treated. Prescription was part of the patient's regular care, not induced by the present work. The protocol was approved by the CDF Institutional Review Board. The confidentiality of the patients' personal data was preserved.

Lesion etiology was classified as ischemic or not. When the ankle/brachial index (ABI) was available, patients with values below 0.75 were considered ischemic, following the same criterion used in the clinical trials. Otherwise, clinical signs of ischemia such as absence of pulses (femoral-popliteal, tibial or distal), intermittent claudication, pain, local atrophy, coldness, and hair loss were taken into account for this classification.

Since it was not feasible to standardize the ulcer size measurement among so many clinical sites, lesion extension-location was considered in three categories:

(i) simple, if the ulcer covered only one region of the foot (toes, dorsum, sole, internal edge, external edge, except calcaneus); (ii) complex, if the extension of the ulcer comprised several regions but not the heel, and (iii) calcaneal if this region was involved.

Intervention
The treatment was as in-patients, although ambulatory care was allowed if the subject could attend the treatment visits. The standard care included the patient's metabolic control, lesion area sanitation and systematic cures, sharp debridement of the necrotic or infected tissue with minor amputation of the affected zones if necessary, and moist gauze dressing. Wide spectrum antimicrobial drugs were prescribed in patients exhibiting local clinical signs of infection. Pressure off-loading of the affected zones was recommended as well.

The product (Heberprot-P®, Heber Biotec, Havana) is lyophilized, containing 75 or 25 μg of rhEGF per vial, to be dissolved with 5 ml of water for injection. In every visit this volume was distributed throughout the lesion in 0.5–1 ml injections. The solution was injected first into the dermo-epidermal junction at equidistant points all over the lesion contours and then downward into the wound bottom to ensure a uniform distribution. The needle was changed for each puncture. The product label indicates injections 3 times per week (tpw) on alternate days. However, in some cases the physicians decided to modify the schedule to daily, twice or once per week. A treatment cycle continued until complete granulation was achieved, lesion closed by autografting or 8 weeks maximum.

The rhEGF dose (25 μg or 75 μg) was selected according to the label (25 μg in ulcers smaller than 20 cm^2 and non-ischemic), but the choice was also determined by each physician's criteria, his/her experience with this product, and the availability of either drug presentation in the healthcare unit at a certain moment.

Outcomes and measurement methods
The main effectiveness variable was lesion complete granulation, evaluated by direct visual inspection. It was defined as productive material, able to mediate the complete lesion closure by second intention or an autologous skin graft. Macroscopically, it was characterized by the presence of reddish, diffused, dispersed and lustrous miliary granular formations that bleed easily after manipulation.

Secondary outcomes were time-to-complete granulation, need for amputation and its type during treatment. During the follow-up period wound closure (complete re-epithelization), relapses, and patient's survival were evaluated.

The variables used to evaluate safety were the adverse events (AE) during the treatment period, considering the type of event, organ and system affected [9], its seriousness and causality relation with the treatment. The latter was done according to the World Health Organization (WHO) algorithm [10] only for serious adverse events (SAE) by the provincial pharmaco-epidemiologists and a consulting multidisciplinary team created *ad hoc* for this purpose. SAE reported were included in the Cuban Pharmacosurveillance System Database, which guarantees the absence of duplicated data when processing reports received from different sources.

Information was gathered by the physicians in case report forms (CRF) which covered the in-patient treatment period. Patients' final outcome was collected in a further follow-up visit, done by the hospital or municipality pharmaco-epidemiology staff, scheduled annually. Emphasis was placed on the training of the personnel in all aspects related to the drug safety evaluation.

Deaths during treatment were further investigated by review of the clinical records and, if necropsy was performed, its report. Causes of death were taken from the death certificates, coded according to the International Classification of Disease-10.

The occurrence of any type of cancer was actively investigated through: (i) direct interview to the patient in the follow-up visits; (ii) cross-search in the National Cancer Registry (NCR), or (iii) findings in the National Mortality Registry. The latter cross search was also useful for the identification and confirmation of follow-up period deceases.

Statistical analyses

One patient could be treated more than once for the same or a different lesion at different moments. Then the experimental unit considered was the treatment cycle, since each of them generated one CRF. Short term AE were evaluated on this basis. The lesion was the unit taken into account for the analyses of granulation, amputations, healing, and relapses. Survival and long term AE were done on patient basis.

The statistical treatment of the data was conducted with the PASW 18.0 software. Measures of central tendency and dispersion such as mean, median, standard deviation (SD), 95% CI, quartile range (QR), minimal and maximal values, were calculated to describe quantitative variables. Graphical normality analysis (QQPlot) and Kolmogorov-Smirnov test for goodness of fit were applied. The chi-square values were calculated to evaluate dependency among qualitative variables. Time variables were estimated using Kaplan-Meier plots and compared with the log-rank test. Logistic or Cox regression models were adjusted to assess the influence of control variables on the outcomes. For the variable-association analyses only the results from the first treatment cycle on each patient were taken into account to avoid considering non-independent observations. Safety related variables were subjected to descriptive

statistics. A Bayesian approach was used for the benefit-risk ratio analysis.

Results

Characteristics of the subjects

CRFs were available from 1788 subjects bearing 1835 DFU. This population represents approximately 80% of all the DFU patients treated with rhEGF in the study period, according to weekly reports received at CDF. Of them, 1676 (93.7%), were seen in hospitals and 112 (6.3%) in polyclinics. Most of the patients (1729; 96.7%) received one treatment cycle; 56 (3.1%) were given two cycles; four of them simultaneously on two different lesions and 3 (0.2%) had three cycles. Therefore the whole patient population received 1851 treatment cycles with rhEGF.

The main demographic characteristics are shown in Table 1. Females, white colored, and diabetes type 2 were predominant. Patients older than 75 years were 248 (14%). The main co-morbidities were hypertension, ischemic cardiopathy, previous DFU, and amputations. Ulcers were mostly advanced (82% Wagner's grades 3–5). Ischemic lesions were 34% diagnosed clinically and 9% by ABI. Simple lesions (mainly on the toes) were the most frequent.

Treatment compliance

There were some treatment schedule deviations according to doctors' decisions: 267 Wagner's grade 1, 2, or 5 ulcers (15% of all lesions) were treated as off-label indications; 281 ischemic lesions (36%) were treated with the 25 μg dose; 50 lesions were treated with both doses, considered as 75 μg for the analyses; the three tpw schedule was not followed strictly (see next paragraph); 48 treatment cycles comprised more than 24 injections.

The 75 μg dose was given more frequently to Wagner's grades 3–5 ulcers (61%) than to less severe cases (53%) and to patients with ischemia (64%) than without it (54%). The thrice weekly regime was the most frequently used. However, some cases were treated daily (9%) or less than three tpw (14%). The median number of infiltrations was 10 (range 1–47). The median total exposure to rhEGF was 500 μg (range 25–3825).

Interruptions occurred in 462 treatment cycles (25%). The causes were: voluntary abandon in 200 (10.8%) cases; worsening of the lesion in 207 (11.2%); local hypergranulation in 16 (0.9%), and other AE in 39 (2.1%).

Granulation

Complete granulation was achieved in 76% of the ulcers at the end of treatment (Table 2). This favorable response was more likely to occur in patients without clinical manifestations of ischemia. The other variables with significant enhancing influence on the granulation outcome in bivariate analyses were age ≤ 75 years better than older (78% vs.

Table 1 Clinical and demographical characteristics of the patients or ulcers

Characteristics		Results (N = 1788 patients)
Age (years): median ± QR (minimum; maximum)		65.0 ± 14.0 (19; 98)
Gender: masculine/feminine (% feminine)		825/963 (53.9%)
Ethnic groups (24 missing)	White	1132 (63.3%)
	Black	289 (16.2%)
	Mixed	333 (18.6%)
	Chinese	10 (0.6%)
Diabetes mellitus: type 1/type 2 (% type 2) (47 missing)		379/1362 (76.2%)
Smokers (6 missing)		368 (20.6%)
Arterial hypertension (4 missing)		1085 (60.7%)
Ischemic cardiopathy (9 missing)		411 (23.0%)
Antecedents of foot ulcers		662 (37.0%)
Antecedents of amputations		420 (23.5%)
		N = 1835 ulcers
Etiology of the ulcer (1 missing)	Ischemic	790 (43.1%)
	Non ischemic	1044 (56.9%)
Location-extension of the lesion (118 missing)	Simple	1140 (62.1%)
	Complex	354 (19.3%)
	Calcaneal	223 (12.2%)
Wagner's classification (83 missing)	Grade 1	26 (1.4%)
	Grade 2	228 (12.4%)
	Grade 3	981 (53.5%)
	Grade 4	504 (27.5%)
	Grade 5	13 (0.7%)

59%), non-smoker (77% vs. 68%), three tpw schedule better than <3 tpw (78% vs. 65%), non-calcaneus location (77% vs. 66%), non-history of hypertension (79% vs. 73%), non-history of ischemic cardiopathy (78% vs. 66%), and the 25 µg dose (81% vs. 72%). In a multivariate, logistic regression model granulation response was favored by non-ischemia (OR: 3.6; 95% CI: 2.8-4.7), non-smoking (1.3; 1.01–1.8), age (1.02; 1.01–1.03, for each younger year), three tpw schedule (1.9; 1.4–2.7), and the 25 µg dose (1.6; 1.2–2.0). The healthcare level, gender, ethnic group, and Wagner's classification were not significantly related to the granulation outcome. The time-to-complete granulation differed significantly between non-ischemic and ischemic lesions (log-rank test; p < 0.001).

Amputations

At the end of treatment 214 patients required 220 amputations (12%) (Table 2); 23 of them were disarticulations, 26 transmetatarsal and 171 major amputations (9.3% of the lesions). Ischemic ulcers caused more amputations. Most of the amputations (85%) were in cases

with Wagner's 3–5 ulcers. Calcaneus location of the ulcers was also an unfavorable factor for the amputation outcome (18.5% vs. 11.0% in non-calcaneus ulcers). Smoking habit (17% vs. 11% in non-smokers) and history of previous amputation (15% vs. 11%) conditioned a higher amputation rate too.

Adverse events

A total of 4171 AE were reported (70 different types) in 46% (856/1851) of the treatment cycles in 838 subjects (47%). The AE occurring in more than 1% of the patients and the maximal number of repetitions of the event in any subject are summarized in Table 3. Pain and burning sensation at the administration site, shivering and chills account for 87% of all the AE reported. Their frequency decreased as the treatment continued: from more than 14% in the first application to less than 2% after 40 days. More than 85% of the events were mild or moderate and easily manageable. Except for local infection, all common AE were more frequent with the 75 µg dose. The rate of local infection as an AE (4%) was not dependent on the baseline infection status of the ulcer (Table 4).

The 31 SAE reported are shown in Table 5. Two of them (ketoacidosis and gastroenterocolitis) were unrelated to the treatment. The other 29 were classified as conditional or possible, since there was a temporal relation with treatment but there are alternative explanations to the clinical findings. Local infection accounted for 32% of the SAE and cardiovascular syndromes for 14 SAE. Thirteen of the latter patients had antecedent of cardiovascular disease (hypertension, ischemic cardiopathy, or arrhythmia).

The benefit/risk ratio is presented in Figure 1. The odds for benefit were larger than for risk (Bayes Factor = 5.4; difference between probabilities: 61%; 95% CI: 59%–64%).

Follow-up: wound closure

Post-treatment follow-up information was obtained from 1620 subjects (91%) with 1659 ulcers, at least once during the 4 years after the end of treatment. The follow-up period (median: 1.2; maximum 4.2 years) comprised 2270.6 years-person. The baseline and demographic characteristics of the followed-up subjects do not differ from the whole patient population (data not shown). Complete ulcer re-epithelization was achieved in 55% of all the lesions ("intention-to-treat" evaluation), 61% of those evaluated (Table 2). In a logistic regression model significant positive influence on this outcome was shown by: non-ischemic etiology (OR: 2.1; 95% CI: 1.6–2.6), age (1.012; 1.002–1.022, for each younger year), and not-history of amputation before treatment (1.7; 1.3–2.1). Relapses occurred in 5% person-years, regardless of the ulcer etiology or other characteristics (Table 2).

Table 2 Lesion response to treatment according to pathogeny

	Ischemic	Non-ischemic	Total
Complete granulation	486/790	905/1044	1392/1835
%	61.5	86.7	75.9
(95% CI)	(58.1; 64.9)	(84.6; 88.7)	(73.9; 77.8)
Weeks to complete granulation median (95% CI)	6 (5.6; 6.3)	4 (3.8; 4.2)	5 (4.8; 5.2)
Healing	371/742	641/916	1012/1659
Evaluated ("per protocol") %	50.0	69.9	61.0
(95% CI)	(48.1; 54.9)	(66.9; 73.3)	(58.2; 62.9)
Included ("intention-to-treat") %	47.0	61.4	55.1
(95% CI)	(43.4; 50.4)	(58.4; 64.4)	(52.9; 57.4)
Relapses: (years-person of follow- up)	26/333 (561)	49/584 (927)	75/917 (1488)
Rate per year (95% CI)	4.6 (2.9; 6.4)	5.3 (3.8; 6.7)	5.0 (3.9; 6.2)
Amputations during treatment	180/790	40/1044	220/1835
%	22.8	3.8	12.0
(95% CI)	(19.9; 25.7)	(2.7; 5.0)	(10.5; 13.5)

Survival and long-term safety

During treatment or follow-up 352 patients (20%) died. Table 6 lists the causes of death. The most frequent were cardiovascular disorders (41.8%); among them acute myocardial infarct and ischemic cardiopathy. Diabetes itself and its complications (renal disease and others) represented 17%, and tumors caused 8% of the deceases. A Cox-regression yielded that the variables with significant unfavorable influence on survival were (HR; 95% CI): ischemic etiology (1.4; 1.1–1.8), history of ischemic cardiopathy (1.3; 1.01–1.6), and older age (1.03; 1.01–1.04 per year increment), whereas ulcer healing showed a significant protective effect (0.25; 0.19–0.31). Amputation after treatment had an inverse lineal correlation with healing. Figure 2 illustrates the effects of healing, etiology, and amputation on survival through the corresponding Kaplan-Meier plots.

Table 3 Frequent adverse events (> 1.0%)

Type of event	Treatment cycles N = 1851		Maximum number of repetitions
	N	%	
Pain at the administration site	402	21.7	24
Shivering	368	19.9	23
Burning sensation at the administration site	297	16.0	17
Chills	171	9.2	16
Local infection	70	3.8	4
Fever	42	2.3	7
Ulcer worsening*	30	1.6	2
Vomits	25	1.4	10

*:Reported by the doctors as adverse events. In fact, worsening of the ulcer as a therapeutic failure occurred in 209 cycles (11.3%).

During the follow-up 42 subjects were identified with neoplasia, not diagnosed before treatment. None of them was on the rhEGF treated region. Locations were: breast (11), colon (5), prostate (4), uterus (4), bladder (2), lung (3), peritoneum (2), and skin basal cell, rectum, endometrium, stomach, fibrosarcoma, pancreas, kidney, pharynx, spinal column, mouth, and not specified, one each. Cancer was not related to the extent of exposure to rhEGF treatment: all these patients had received one treatment cycles; the average exposure was 535 μg of rhEGF (range: 75–2100 μg).

Discussion

The postmarketing surveillance covered all the Angiology wards that manage DFU in Cuba and some primary care units that have incorporated this drug as part of the diabetic patients integral care program. The demographic and baseline characteristics of the subjects parallel those of people with DFU that took part in the clinical trials with this procedure [3-7]: predominantly diabetes type 2, median age 65 years, approximately equal gender distribution, high proportions of hypertension, ischemic cardiopathy, and previous ulcers, as well as the ethnic distribution

Table 4 Local infection as an adverse event vs. baseline

		Occurrence of local infection as adverse event		Total
		Yes	No	
Local infection as baseline	Yes	52	1270	1322
	No	15	358	373
Total		67	1628	1695

Information on baseline infection was missing in one subject with local infection as adverse event and in 90 subjects without it. The OR was 0.98; 95% CI: 0.54–1.76.

Table 5 Serious adverse events

Motive for seriousness	Events	N	%*
Caused death	Acute myocardial infarct	5	
	Sudden cardiac death	2	
	Acute pulmonary edema	2	
	Ventricular fibrillation	1	
	Uncompensated heart insufficiency	1	
	Ischemic stroke	1	
	Acute respiratory failure	1	
	Acute gastroenterocolitis	1	
	Diabetic ketoacidosis-septic shock	1	
	Subtotal	15	0.8%
Endangered life	Acute pulmonary edema	2	
	Loss of consciousness	2	
	Local infection	1	
	Glottic spasm	1	
	Faintness	1	
	Subtotal	7	0.4%
Prolonged hospitalization	Local infection	4	0.2%
Produced disability	Local infection	5	0.3%
TOTAL		31	1.7%

*Percent calculated from 1851 treatment cycles.

of the Cuban population [11]. Co-morbidities such as hypercholesterolemia, arterial hypertension and ischemic cardiopathy have been reported in other settings [12] too. Nearly half of the subjects had ischemic ulcers, mostly Wagner's grades 3–4, which singularizes the application of intralesional hrEGF from other procedures that are mainly indicated in less advanced

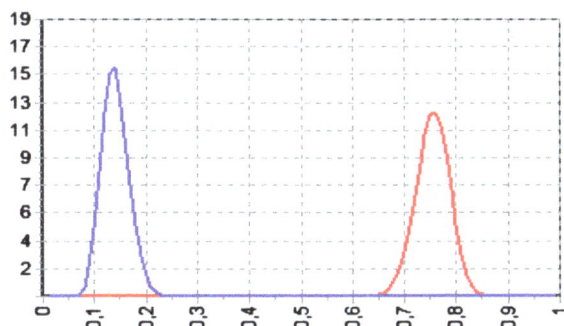

Figure 1 Risk-benefit analysis. Given $p(x \mid benefit)$ by the probability distribution function for benefit (complete granulation) and $p(x \mid risk)$ by the probability distribution function for risk (moderate and severe adverse events or amputation) then the Bayes Factor (B_{br}) is: $B_{br} = \frac{p(x\mid benefit)}{p(x\mid risk)}$ representing a summary of the evidence provided by the data in favor of benefit (red), as opposed to risk (blue). A value larger than 1 means a favorable benefit-risk ratio. In this case: Bayes factor = 5.4; difference between probabilities: 61% (95% CI: 59%–64%).

lesions [13]. Calcaneus ulcers were not excluded, which is also an unfavorable condition [14].

Some deviations from the labeled pattern of hrEGF application were seen, which were due to doctors' preference, according to their judgment of the patient's evolution. In some cases, ambulatory patients could not attend all the visits. The dose deviations were also determined, eventually, by product availability at a given moment. The off-label use of medicaments, particularly biologics, is not a seldom practice in many settings as part of the common medical practice [15,16].

Treatment interruptions were mainly due to failure that determined amputation mostly in ischemic, Wagner's 3–5 lesions. Very few were because of patients' intolerance (AE or voluntary abandonments). Hypergranulation is noteworthy since it is due to the same mechanism of healing enhancement. It was easily controlled by tissue excess removal and there is no information of related sequels, such as hypertrophic scars or keloids.

The results of the previous clinical trials with intralesional hrEGF (79.4% granulation in 296 patients; 95% CI: 74.8–84.0%) were confirmed in this study. The re-epithelization rate found falls within the pooled analysis of the clinical trials too: 59.2%; 95% CI: 53.4– 64.5% [3]. Granulation response showed good predictive value for final healing in this series [17]. The relapse rate (5% year-persons) is better than reported [18,19]. For example, Boulton et al. [20] refer an estimate of 50–70% for the UK and 34% after one year follow-up in other series. The fact that postmarketing data confirm the results of the clinical trials is an important feature that endorses the use of intralesional rhEGF in medical practice for the treatment of advanced DFU. Topical EGF [21,22] or other growth factors [23,24] have been reported in smaller and/or less advanced ulcers. However, there is scarce information on their effectiveness in regular medical practice or have not fulfilled the expectations raised from clinical trials [25].

The main variables with influence on the treatment effectiveness, both for granulation and re-epithelization, were ischemia and age, which are well-known adverse prognosis factor for ulcer healing [26]. However, the granulation and healing rates attained indicate that the effect of the product is evident in ischemic patients too. Ischemia was considered when ABI < 0.75 or clinically. The ABI cutoff for ischemia varies among different guidelines, from 0.7 [27,28] to 0.9 [29]. Consequently, 40 subjects (85% granulation; 80% re-epithelization) classified as non-ischemic in this work would fall into a "mild" ischemia category (with scarce clinical expose) according to other thresholds. This supports the notion that the product is also effective in patients with impaired blood supply.

Although this work did not include a non-treated control group to measure the impact of the treatment on amputation rate, other independent investigations in additional

Table 6 Causes of death in diabetic foot ulcer patients treated with intralesional hrEGF

Cause	Number	Percent of all deaths	Rate (per 100 person-years)
Cardiovascular disorders	145	41.2%	6.38%
Acute myocardial infarct	37	10.5%	1.63%
Stroke and its sequels	33	9.4%	1.45%
Ischemic cardiopathy	29	8.2%	1.28%
Cardiac failure	18	5.1%	0.79%
Hypertensive cardiac disease	9	2.6%	0.40%
Other: peripheral angiopathy (5); acute pulmonary edema (4); cardiac arrhythmias (4); cardiac arrest and cardiogenic shock (3); generalized atherosclerosis; non specified (2); abdominal aorta aneurism rupture (1)	19	5.4%	0.84%
Other complications of diabetes	60	17.0%	2.64%
Diabetic coma	6	1.7%	0.26%
Diabetes mellitus with renal complications	30	8.5%	1.32%
Diabetes mellitus with other complications	13	3.7%	0.57%
Diabetic foot	11	3.1%	0.48%
Respiratory disorders	53	15.1%	2.33%
Pneumonia and bronchopneumonia	49	13.9%	2.16%
Acute respiratory insufficiency	4	1.1%	0.18%
Neoplasia: breast (8); prostate (3); colon (4); bladder (2); lung (3); peritoneum (2); pancreas (1); kidney (1); pharynx (1); spinal column (1); mouth (1); tumor of unknown behavior, encephalus, supratentorial (1)	28	8.0%	1.23%
Peripheral venous thrombosis and thromboembolism	12	3.4%	0.53%
Amputations and other surgical complications	12	3.4%	0.53%
Other causes: sepsis (8); upper digestive bleeding (4); gastroenteritis (2); liver cirrhosis (2); rheumatoid arthritis (1); viral encephalitis (not specified) (1); multiorgan failure (1); alcoholic hepatitis (1); prostate hyperplasia (1); accidents and traumatisms (2); sudden death (1)	24	6.8%	1.06%
Unknown	18	5.1%	
Total	352		15.50%

(From the national death certificate database).

patient series have made such comparisons. González-Acosta et al. found a major amputation rate reduction from 26.7% to 8.3% when intralesional rhEGF was added to conventional standard care [30]. García-Herrera et al. report a 43.1% to 8.1% major amputation rate reduction [31]. These data are consistent with the 9.2% major amputation rate found in the present work.

The most frequently observed AE such as pain and burning sensation at the injection site, shivering, chills, and local infection coincide with the reported intralesional hrEGF safety profile [3-7].

Local infection is one of the most fearsome AE because it frequently leads to amputation. Approximately 60% of amputations are preceded by infected ulcers [32]. Local infection was classified with "possible" causality relationship with the treatment. This is difficult to evaluate since most of these ulcers were infected at baseline. This diagnosis was defined by signs such as edema, ulcer border redness, and secretion. Heberprot P* labeling says that these signs

should be cleared (antibiotics, debridement) before the product is applied. Even though, a negative culture is never obtained. It is unlikely that the injection procedure contributes to spread any subclinical infection as shown by the fact that the occurrence of this AE was not associated to the baseline infection of the ulcer.

There is not enough information to relate cardiovascular AE and deaths to the treatment, since the patients have frequent antecedents of cardiovascular diseases. The relationship of diabetes and cardiovascular diseases is well known, moreover if DFU is present [33,34]. In data from the national death certificate database and the Annual Health Report [35] for 2007–2010, the death rates due to these causes in people with diabetes among the three main causes of death in the certificate double that of the general population. This death profile agrees with the literature for DFU patients [36,37].

A particular concern on the use of growth factors is the possibility of development or stimulation of a pre-

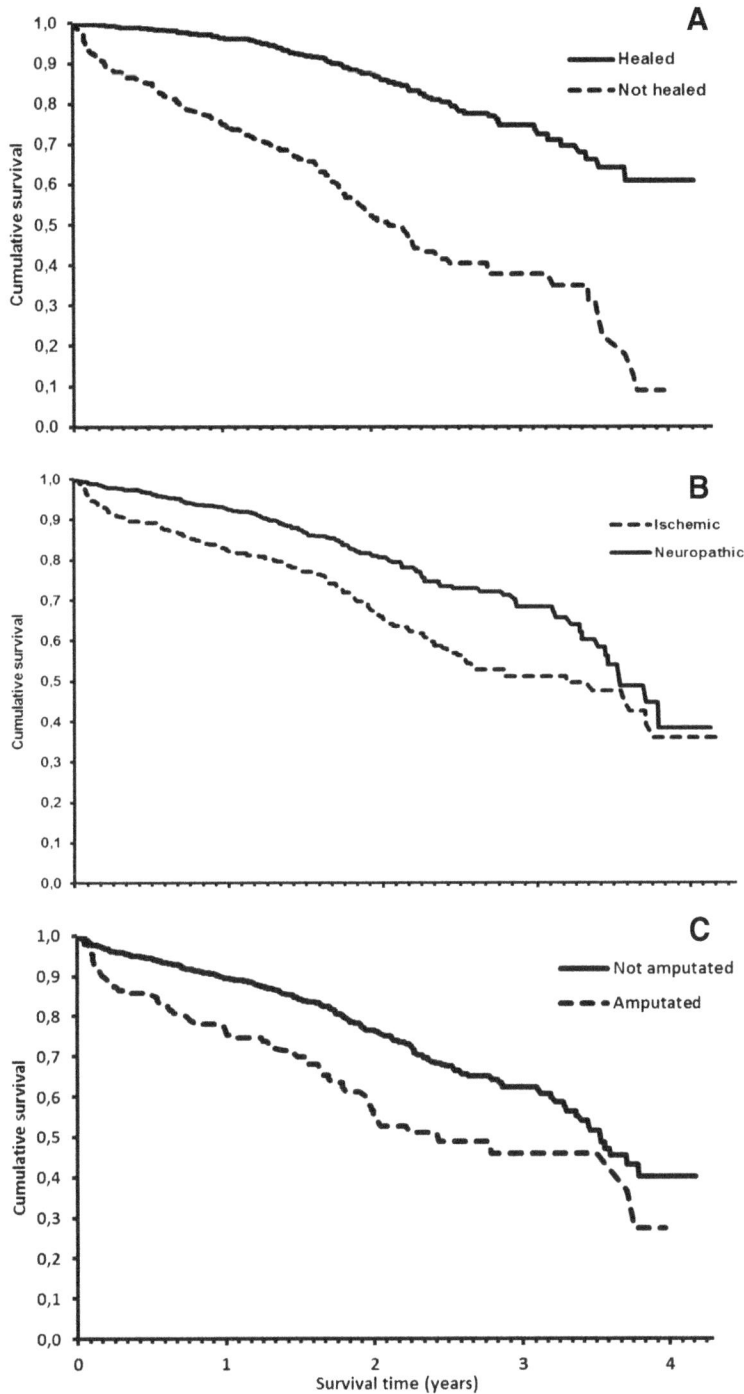

Figure 2 Kaplan-Meier curves for survival time according to A) whether the ulcer healed or not; B) ulcer etiology or C) whether the affected limb was amputated or not.

existing malignancy. Contrary to PDGF, EGF cannot initiate malignant transformation [38] and results with EGF in experimental models have not demonstrated tumor promotion consistently [3,39]. Diabetes is a known cancer risk boosting condition [40-43]. The data do not support any cancer promotion by rhEGF treatment.

Giovannucci et al. discuss the possible mechanisms of the diabetes-cancer association, either by common risk factors or specific mechanisms in diabetes metabolism and management [44]. This aspect has to be further investigated and followed in the product risk-management program.

Conclusions

In summary this postmarketing, prospective study is consistent with earlier findings from exploratory and confirmatory clinical trials, while extending the data to a larger clinical setting. The positive findings, related to the clinical evolution of the patients treated at secondary and primary Cuban healthcare levels, suggest a relevant role of this drug in the treatment of DFUs. Further clinical research and post-marketing information from other countries should enrich the evidence shown in this paper.

Appendix
(Cuban Group for the Introduction of Heberprot P in Diabetic Foot Ulcers)

Patient recruitment, treatment and follow-up.

Health Unit, Province (number of treatment cycles performed), investigators: "Camilo Cienfuegos" Hospital, Sancti Spíritus (211): Regla Soto-Águila (province coordinator), Pablo Sánchez Pentón, Irelio Borroto Carpio, Reidel Veloso, Yanet Hernández, Ana Tavio Reyes, Mayilé Gómez, Liliam Moreno Perera; "Gustavo Aldereguía Lima" Hospital, Cienfuegos (154): Ivonne Marrero Rodríguez, Belkis Calaña González Posada, Ivette García, Mabel Medina, Nancy Ramírez, Sahily González Acosta, Yadira Alonso, Javier Borrego; "Abel Santamaría" Hospital, Pinar del Río (128): Martha Moreira Martínez, Aida Hernández, Antonio Díaz Díaz, Agustina Gómez García Yanet Crespo, Etty Chirolde, Laureano Peña Bazant Pérez Jose Ortega Baez, Ana Lidia Hernández Méndez; "Arnaldo Milián" Hospital, Villa Clara (101): Teresita Fleito Castex, Felicia García, Seco, Angel Alfaro, Cecilio González Benavidez; "Lucía Iñiguez" Hospital, Holguín (99): Armando González, Eneida Caraballosa, Esther Peña, Isel Sánchez Mirna Enel Pérez Muñoz; "Carlos M. de Céspedes" Hospital, Granma (95): Francisco Vázquez, José Ortega, Juan Planas Brooks, Juan Carrazona, Eberto Caravana; "Antonio Luaces Iraola" Hospital, Ciego de Ávila (87): José Hernández Cañete, Mislene Álvarez Hernández, Xiomara Herrera, Jorge Herrera Zamora; "Manuel Ascunce" Hospital, Camagüey (84): Ariel Hernández Varela, Yanor Agüero, Fidel Rivero Fernández, Raúl Romay Boitrago, Jorge Luis Valdez, Nicolás Socarras, Pedro Vejerano, Ramón Bentrogo, Misleidis González Cedeño, Nelina Morales, Odalis Escalante; "José R. López Tabranes" Hospital, Matanzas (77): Edel Fleitas Pérez, Leydis Hernández Rodríguez, Jaqueline Ramos Serpa, Martha Jiménez, Arístides García Herrera, Elizabeth Cao, Isis de la Caridad Abreu Jiménez, Daymar Bom Pérez, Yadira García; "Agostinho Neto" Hospital, Guantánamo (72): Zulema Mena, Georgina Grave de Peralta, Vladimir Sarrión; "Ernesto Guevara" Hospital, Las Tunas (58): Dianelis González, Zulema Elliot Pérez, José Luis Solis, José Luis Rivero Miranda, José Pablo Ponce; "Ambrosio Grillo" Hospital, Santiago de Cuba (57): Emilio Goulet, Lisandra Betancourt, Alina Echevarría, Jorge Lockhant; "Enrique

Cabrera" Hospital, Havana (44): Heriberto Artaza Sans, Sandra González Pelegrí, Angela Blanco Díaz, Natalia Poll Marrón, Evaristo Vargas Machirán, Eduardo Atencio Soriol, Pedro Goicochea Díaz; "Julio Arestegui" Hospital, Matanzas (37): Leitter Pérez, Juan Díaz; "Julio Trigo" Hospital, Havana (36): Reinaldo Martínez Garrido; "Saturnino Lora" Hospital, Santiago de Cuba (36): Natacha Sancho Sueto, Arelis Frómeta, David Díaz, Hever Viguera, Mayelin Sabourit; "Amalia Simoni" Hospital, Camagüey (35): Alberto Álvarez Varona, Jorge Gómez , Gustavo Pérez Hechevarría, Denny González, Victor Alfonso; "Guillermo Domínguez" Hospital, Las Tunas (29): Wilber Velázquez Chacón; "Calixto García" Hospital, Havana (26): Osmel Castillo, Aimeé Rodríguez Hernández, María Campos, Remberto García, Joaquín David Liziaga Vázquez, Julio César Nuñez Vázquez; "Joaquín Castillo" Hospital, Santiago de Cuba (26): Bencay Joa Liranza; Octavio de la Concepción Hospital, Guantánamo (26): Arturo Pons; "Celia Sánchez" Hospital, Granma (24): Odelaisys Hernández Saborit, Sergio Fernández; "Victoria de Girón" Polyclinic, Santiago de Cuba (23): Carlos Calderón, Orlando San Pedro; "Carlos Font" Hospital, Holguín (22): Tamara Pérez; "Roberto Rodríguez" Hospital, Ciego de Ávila (22): Elier del Castillo, Jorge Morales Florat; "Alcides Pino" Polyclinic, Holguín (20): María Antonia Rodríguez, Tania García; "Mártires de Mayarí" Hospital, Holguín (19): Isabel Carrasco, Eneida Caraballosa; Military Hospital, Holguín (18): Pedro Matos García, Olides Cobas Díaz, Daniel Rodríguez Curí; "Diez de Octubre" Hospital, Havana (17): Deysi Acosta Lapera, Héctor Chivas, Manuel Hernández Rivero; National Institute for Angiology and Vascular Surgery, Havana (17): José Fernández Montequín , Calixto Valdez Pérez, José Llanes Barrios, Williams Savingne Gutierrez, Neobalis Franco Pérez, Daniel Reynaldo Concepción; "Comandante Manuel Fajardo" Accommodation, Havana (13): Reyna Lourdes Morejón Vega; "Manuel Fajardo" Hospital, Havana (12): Milagros Romero Gamboa, Máximo Sander López, "Orlando Pantoja" Hospital, Santiago de Cuba (12): Raúl Mesa; "Máximo Gómez" Polyclinic, Granma (12): Rafaela Rondón; "Ciro Redondo" Hospital, Artemisa (11): Odelaysis Hernández Saborí; "Aleida Fernández" Hospital, Mayabeque (11): Pedro González, Vicente Vega Mederos; "Comandante Pinares" Hospital, Artemisa (8): José Ortega Baez; "Martha Abreu" Polyclinic, Villa Clara (8): Juan Miguel García Velázquez; "XXX Anniversary" Polyclinic, Villa Clara (7): Juan Miguel García Velázquez; "Edor Reyes" Polyclinic, Granma (6): Salvador Oliva; "Roberto Fleites" Polyclinic, Villa Clara (6): Juan Miguel García Velázquez; "Miguel Enriquez" Hospital, Havana (5): Luis Olivera Baez, Justa Peñalver; "Santa Cruz del Sur" Hospital, Camagüey (5): Luis Gustavo Cisneros; Banes Hospital, Holguín (4): Antonio Ricardo García; "XXX Aniversario" Hospital, Villa Clara (4): Juan Miguel García Velázquez; Camilo Cienfuegos Polyclinic, Havana (3): Carmen Luisa Ramos; "Manuel A

Varona" Polyclinic, Camagüey (3): Esteban Lopez; "Tamara Bunke" Polyclinic, Holguín (3): Luis Aguilar; "Gustavo Aldereguía" Hospital, Holguín (2): Manuel Balán; "Juan Bruno Zayas" Hospital, Santiago de Cuba (2): Rolando Castillo; "San Luis" Polyclinic, Pinar del Río (2): Aida Rosa Hernández; "XX Anniversary" Polyclinic, Villa Clara (2): Juan Miguel García Velázquez; "19 de Abril" Polyclinic, Havana (2): Reyna Lourdes Morejón Vega; "Wajay" Polyclinic, Havana (2): Angela Blanco Díaz; "Colón" Hospital, Matanzas (1): Alejandro Piedra-Fita Tejeda; "Mario Muñoz" Hospital, Matanzas (1): Maylin Torres; "Ramón Pando Ferrer" Polyclinic, Villa Clara (1): Juan Miguel García Velázquez; "Santa Clara" Polyclinic, Villa Clara (1): Juan Miguel García Velázquez; "Isabel Rubio" Polyclinic, Pinar del Río (1): Aida Rosa Hernández; "Raúl Sanchez" Polyclinic, Pinar del Río (1). Aida Rosa Hernández.

Monitoring, data management, and analyses.

Center for the Development of Pharmacoepidemiology: Isis Belkis Yera Alós, Liuba Carbonell Alonso, Julián Pérez Peña, Francisco Debesa García, Alina Alvarez Crespo, Ismary Alfonso Orta, Giset Jiménez López, Jenny Ávila Pérez, Ana García Milián, Aleida Díaz Hernández; National Pharmacoepidemiology Network: Yumara Díaz Castro (Pinar del Río), Gustavo Rodríguez (Artemisa–Mayabeque), Deborah Rodríguez Piñeiro (Havana), Adis Martín (Havana), Lia Mónica Bravo (Havana), Loida Báez (Havana), Armando Morri (Havana), Leydis Santos Muñoz (Matanzas), Miraida Baute (Cienfuegos), Luis Orlando Rico Martell (Ciego de Ávila), Orlando René Águila González (Villa Clara), Betania Rodríguez (Sancti Spíritus), Natacha Caballero (Camagüey), Soraida García (Las Tunas), Maria Elena Fernández Tablada (Holguín), Gloria Zaldivar (Holguín), Zayda Herrera López (Holguín), Yeraldis Ramírez Calzadilla (Granma), Sheila Tamayo (Santiago de Cuba), Yudeisi Trabanca Beltrán (Guantánamo); Center for Genetic Engineering and Biotechnology: Ernesto López Mola, Angela Tuero Iglesias, Carmen Valenzuela Silva, Jorge Berlanga Acosta, Miriela Gil Mena, Ricardo Silva Rodríguez, Marianela García Siverio, Francisco Hernández Bernal, Elizeth García Iglesias, Leovaldo Álvarez Falcón, María Dolores Castro Santana, Rafael Ibargollín Ulloa, Luis Herrera Martínez, Pedro Antonio López Saura.

Abbreviations
ABI: Ankle/brachial pressure index; AE: Adverse event; CDF: Center for the development of pharmacoepidemiology; CECMED: State center for the control of medicaments, diagnostics and medical devices; CRF: Case report form; DFU: Diabetic foot ulcer; NCR: National cancer registry; rhEGF: Recombinant human epidermal growth factor; SAE: Serious adverse event; Tpw: Times per week.

Competing interests
Authors IBYA, CMVS, ADTI, ELM, and PALS. are employees of the Center for Genetic Engineering and Biotechnology (CIGB), where rhEGF is produced and sponsored the clinical trials and postmarketing study where the data were taken from. The postmarketing study was also financed by the Ministry of Public Health of Cuba. IBYA had no conflict of interest when the study was done. The rest of the authors have no conflict of interests.

Authors' contributions
IBYA wrote the manuscript and participated in the protocol design, interpretation of the results, and final report writing; LAC took part in protocol design, data collection, and monitoring; CMVS made all the statistical analyses of this work, the interpretation of the results, and final report writing; ADTI participated in the statistical analyses; MMM and IMR were the site principal investigators that included more subjects and were part of the work steering committee; ELM took part in study design and organization; PALS collaborated in this manuscript writing and reviewing and contributed in protocol designs, analyses and interpretation of the results, and final report writing.

Acknowledgements
The authors appreciate the contribution of the Medicine Students from all Cuban Medical Universities that helped to locate the patients for the follow-up visits; the National Statistics Direction and the National Cancer Registry of the Ministry of Public Health of Cuba provided information from the mortality and cancer databases, respectively; Dr. Carlos Duarte from the Biomedical Research Direction, CIGB, for his review of the manuscript.

Author details
[1]Center for the Development of Pharmacoepidemiology, Havana, Cuba. [2]Center for Genetic Engineering and Biotechnology, Havana, Cuba. [3]"Abel Santamaría" Hospital, Pinar del Río, Cuba. [4]"Gustavo Aldereguía" Hospital, Cienfuegos, Cuba.

References
1. Armstrong DG, Cohen K, Courric S, Bharara M, Marston W: **Diabetic foot ulcers and vascular insufficiency: our population has changed, but our methods have not.** *J Diabetes Sci Technol* 2011, 5:1591–1595.
2. Berlanga J: **Diabetic lower extremity wounds: the rationale for growth factors-based infiltration treatment.** *Int Wound J* 2011, 8:612–620.
3. López-Saura PA, Berlanga-Acosta J, Fernández-Montequín JI, Valenzuela-Silva C, González-Díaz O, Savigne W, Morejon-Vega L, Del Río-Martín A, Herrera-Martínez L, López-Mola E, Acevedo-Castro B: **Intralesional human recombinant epidermal growth factor for the treatment of advanced diabetic foot ulcer: from proof of concept to confirmation of the efficacy and safety of the procedure.** In *Global perspective on diabetic foot ulcerations.* Edited by Dihn T. Rijeka: InTech Europe; 2011:217–238. http://www.intechopen.com/articles/show/title/intralesional-human-recombinant-epidermal-growth-factor-for-the-treatment-of-advanced-diabetic-foot-.
4. Berlanga J, Savigne W, Valdez C, Franco N, Alba JS, Del Rio A, López-Saura P, Guillén G, Lopez E, Herrera L, Férnandez-Montequín J: **Epidermal growth factor intra-lesional can prevent amputation in diabetic patients with advanced foot wounds.** *Int Wound J* 2006, 3:232–239.
5. Fernández-Montequín JI, Infante-Cristiá E, Valenzuela-Silva C, Franco-Pérez N, Savigne-Gutierrez W, Artaza-Sanz H, Morejón-Vega L, González-Benavides C, Eliseo-Musenden O, García-Iglesias E, Berlanga-Acosta J, Silva-Rodríguez R, Betancourt BY, López-Saura PA, Cuban Citoprot-P Study Group: **Intralesional injections of Citoprot P® (recombinant human epidermal growth factor) in advanced diabetic foot ulcers with risk of amputation.** *Int Wound J* 2007, 4:333–343.
6. Fernández-Montequín JI, Betancourt BY, Leyva-Gonzalez G, López Mola E, Galán-Naranjo K, Ramírez-Navas M, Bermúdez-Rojas S, Rosales F, García-Iglesias E, Berlanga-Acosta J, Silva-Rodriguez R, Garcia-Siverio M, Herrera Martinez L: **Intralesional administration of epidermal growth factor-based formulation (Heberprot-P) in advanced diabetic foot ulcer: treatment up to complete wound closure.** *Int Wound J* 2009, 6:67–72.
7. Fernández-Montequín JI, Valenzuela-Silva CM, González-Díaz O, Savigne W, Sancho-Soutelo N, Rivero-Fernández F, Sánchez-Penton P, Morejón-Vega L, Artaza-Sanz H, García-Herrera A, González-Benavides C, Hernández-Cañete CM, Vázquez-Proenza A, Berlanga-Acosta J, López-Saura PA, for the Cuban Diabetic Foot Study Group: **Intralesional injections of recombinant human epidermal growth factor promote granulation and healing in advanced diabetic foot ulcers. Multicenter, randomized, placebo-controlled, double blind study.** *Int Wound J* 2009, 6:432–443.

8. Armstrong DG, Lavry LA, Harkless LB: **Validation of a diabetic wound classification system: the contribution of depth, infection, and ischemia to risk of amputation.** *Diabetes Care* 1998, **21**:855–859.

9. The Uppsala Monitoring Centre, WHO Collaborating Centre for International Drug Monitoring: *WHO Adverse reaction terminology 2008.* Uppsala: UMC; 2008. Available from http://www.umc-products.com/DynPage.aspx?id=73589&mn1=1107&mn2=1664.

10. Edwards RI, Biriell C: **Harmonisation in pharmacovigilance.** *Drug Saf* 1994, **10**:93–102.

11. National Report of the Population and Housing Census of Cuba 2002: La Habana: Bureau for Statistics; 2002. Available from: http://www.cubagob.cu/otras_info/censo/tablas_html/ii_3.htm; accessed on 06/23/2012.

12. Prompers L, Huijberts M, Apelqvist J, Jude E, Piaggesi A, Bakker K, Edmonds M, Holstein P, Jirkovska A, Mauricio D, Ragnarson Tennvall G, Reike H, Spraul M, Uccioli L, Urbancic V, Van Acker K, Van Baal J, Van Merode F, Schaper N: **High prevalence of ischaemia, infection and serious comorbidity in patients with diabetic foot disease in Europe. Baseline results from the Eurodiale study.** *Diabetologia* 2007, **50**:18–25.

13. Fang RC, Galiano RD: **A review of becaplermin gel in the treatment of diabetic neuropathic foot ulcers.** *Biologics* 2008, **2**:1–12.

14. Chipchase SY, Treece KA, Pound N, Game FL, Jeffcoate WJ: **Heel ulcers don't heal in diabetes. Or do they?** *Diabet Med* 2005, **22**:1258–1262.

15. Smith DI, Swamy PM, Heffernan MP: **Off-label uses of biologics in dermatology: Interferon and intravenous immunoglobulin (Part 1 of 2).** *J Am Acad Dermatol* 2007, **56**(Suppl 1):e1–e54.

16. Graves JE, Nunle K, Heffernan MP: **Off-label uses of biologics in dermatology: rituximab, omalizumab, infliximab, etanercept, adalimumab, efalizumab, and alefacept (Part 2 of 2).** *J Am Acad Dermatol* 2007, **56**(Suppl 1):e55–e79.

17. Valenzuela-Silva CM, Tuero-Iglesias AD, García-Iglesias E, González-Díaz O, Del Río-Martín A, Year-Alos IB, Fernández-Montequín JI, López-Saura PA: **Granulation response and partial wound closure predict healing in clinical trials on advanced diabetes foot ulcers treated with recombinant, human epidermal growth factor.** *Diabetes Care* 2013, **36**:210–215.

18. Matricali GA, Deroo K, Dereymaeker G: **Outcome and recurrence rate of diabetic foot ulcers treated by a total contact cast: short-term follow-up.** *Foot Ankle Int* 2003, **24**:680–684.

19. Frigg A, Pagenstert G, Schäfer D, Valderrabano V, Hintermann B: **Recurrence and prevention of diabetic foot ulcers after total contact casting.** *Foot Ankle Int* 2007, **28**:64–69.

20. Boulton AJM, Vileikyte L, Ragnarson-Tennvall G, Apelqvist J: **The global burden of diabetic foot disease.** *Lancet* 2005, **366**:1719–1724.

21. Tsang MW, Wong WK, Hung CS, Lai KM, Tang W, Cheung EYN, Kam G, Leung L, Chan CW, Chu CM, Lam EKH: **Human epidermal growth. Factor enhances healing of diabetic foot ulcers.** *Diabetes Care* 2003, **26**:1851–1856.

22. Viswanathan V, Pendsey S: **A phase III study to evaluate the safety and efficacy of recombinant human epidermal growth factor (REGEN-D™ 150) in healing diabetic foot ulcers.** *Wounds* 2006, **18**:186–196.

23. Wieman TJ, Smiell JM, Su Y: **Efficacy and safety of a topical gel formulation of recombinant human platelet-derived growth factor- B (becaplermin) in patients with chronic neuropathic diabetic ulcers. A phase III randomized placebo-controlled double-blind study.** *Diabetes Care* 1998, **21**:822–827.

24. Uchi H, Igarashi A, Urabe K, Koga T, Nakayama J, Kawamori R, Tamaki K, Hirakata H, Ohura T, Furue M: **Clinical efficacy of basic fibroblast growth factor (bFGF) for diabetic ulcer.** *Eur J Dermatol* 2009, **19**:461–468.

25. Papanas N, Maltezos E, Benefit-Risk: **Assessment of becaplermin in the treatment of diabetic foot ulcers.** *Drug Saf* 2010, **33**:455–461.

26. Prompers L, Schaper N, Apelqvist J, Edmonds M, Jude E, Mauricio D, Uccioli L, Urbancic V, Bakker K, Holstein P, Jirkovska A, Piaggesi A, Ragnarson-Tennvall G, Reike H, Spraul M, Van Acker K, Van Baal J, Van Merode F, Ferreira I, Huijberts M: **Prediction of outcome in individuals with diabetic foot ulcers: focus on the differences between individuals with and without peripheral arterial disease. The EURODIALE Study.** *Diabetologia* 2008, **51**:747–755.

27. Frykberg RG, Zgonis T, Armstrong DG, Driver VR, Giurini JM, Kravitz SR, Landsman AS, Lavery LA, Moore JC, Schuberth JM, Wukich DK, Andersen C, Vanore JV: **Diabetic foot disorders: a clinical practice guideline (2006 revision).** *J Foot Ankle Surg* 2006, **45**(Suppl 5):S1–S66.

28. Verdú J, Marinel-lo J, Armans E, Carreño P, March JR, Soldevilla J: *National conference for consensus on low extremity ulcers.* Spain: EdikaMed S.L; 2009 (in Spanish).

29. Snyder RJ, Kirsner RS, Warriner RA 3rd, Lavery LA, Hanft JR, Sheehan P: **Consensus recommendations on advancing the standard of care for treating neuropathic foot ulcers in patients with diabetes.** *Ostomy Wound Manage* 2010, **56**(4 Suppl):S1–S24.

30. González-Acosta S, Calaña-González-Posada B, Marrero-Rodríguez I, López-Fernández R: **Clinical evolution of diabetic foot treatment with Heberprot-P or with the conventional method.** *Rev Cubana Angiología y Cirugía Vascular* 2011, **11**(2):11. (in Spanish). Available from http://bvs.sld.cu/revistas/ang/vol_11_2_11/ang07211.htm.

31. García Herrera AL, Rodríguez Fernández R, Ruiz VM, Rodríguez Hernández L, Acosta Cabadilla L, Febles Sanabria R, Pancorbo Sandoval C, Cantero Calderón S, Vázquez Díaz O, Moliner Cartaya M: **Reduction in the amputation rate with Heberprot P in the local treatment of diabetic foot.** *Spanish Journal of Surgical Research* 2011, **XIV**:21–26 (in Spanish).

32. Lipsky BA: **Medical treatment of diabetic foot infections.** *Clin Infect Dis* 2004, **39**(Suppl 2):S104–S114.

33. Iversen MM, Tell GS, Riise T, Hanestad BR, Østbye T, Graue M, Midthjell K: **History of foot ulcer increases mortality among individuals with diabetes: ten-year follow-up of the Nord-Trøndelag health study, Norway.** *Diabetes Care* 2009, **32**:2193–2199.

34. Wannamethee SG, Shaper AG, Whincup PH, Lennon L, Sattar N: **Impact of diabetes on cardiovascular disease risk and all-cause mortality in older men: influence of age at onset, diabetes duration, and established and novel risk factors.** *Arch Intern Med* 2011, **171**:404–410.

35. Ministry of Public Health: *Cuban health yearbook 2011.* La Habana; 2012. Available from: http://files.sld.cu/bvscuba/files/2012/05/anuario-2011-e.pdf.

36. Brownrigg JRW, Davey J, Holt PJ, Davis WA, Thompson MM, Ray KK, Hinchliffe RJ: **The association of ulceration of the foot with cardiovascular and all-cause mortality in patients with diabetes: a meta-analysis.** *Diabetologia* 2012, **55**:2906–2912.

37. Campbell PT, Newton CC, Patel AV, Jacobs EJ, Gapstur SM: **Diabetes and cause-specific mortality in a prospective cohort of one million U.S. adults.** *Diabetes Care* 2012, **35**:1835–1844.

38. Berlanga-Acosta J, Gavilondo-Cowley J, García del Barco-Herrera D, Martín-Machado J, Guillen-Nieto G: **Epidermal Growth Factor (EGF) and Platelet-Derived Growth Factor (PDGF) as tissue healing agents: clarifying concerns about their possible role in malignant transformation and tumor progression.** *J Carcinogene Mutagene* 2011, **2**:1.

39. Berlanga-Acosta J, Gavilondo-Cowley J, López-Saura P, González-López T, Castro-Santana MD, López-Mola E, Guillén-Nieto G, Herrera-Martinez L: **Epidermal Growth Factor (EGF) in clinical practice–a review of its biological actions, clinical indications and safety implications.** *Int Wound J* 2009, **6**:331–346.

40. Barone BB, Yeh HC, Snyder CF, Peairs KS, Stein KB, Derr RL, Wolff AC, Brancati FL: **Postoperative mortality in cancer patients with preexisting diabetes.** *Diabetes Care* 2010, **33**:931–939.

41. Hense HW, Kajüter H, Wellmann J, Batzler WU: **Cancer incidence in type 2 diabetes patients -first results from a feasibility study of the D2C cohort.** *Diabetol Metabol Syndrome* 2011, **3**:15.

42. Varlotto JM, Recht A, Flickinger JC, Medford-Davis LN, Dyer AM, DeCamp MM: **Factors associated with local and distant recurrence and survival in patients with resected non-small cell lung cancer.** *Cancer* 2009, **115**:1059–1069.

43. Onitilo AA, Engel JM, Glurich I, Stankowski RV, Williams GM, Doi SA: **Diabetes and cancer I: risk, survival, and implications for screening.** *Cancer Causes Control* 2012, **23**:967–981.

44. Giovannucci E, Harlan DM, Archer MC, Bergenstal RM, Gapstur SM, Habel LA, Pollak M, Regensteiner JG, Yee D: **Diabetes and cancer. A consensus report.** *Diabetes Care* 2010, **33**:1674–1685.

22

Efficacy of RNA polymerase II inhibitors in targeting dormant leukaemia cells

Monica Pallis[1,4*], Francis Burrows[2], Abigail Whittall[3], Nicholas Boddy[3], Claire Seedhouse[3] and Nigel Russell[1,3]

Abstract

Background: Dormant cells are characterised by low RNA synthesis. In contrast, cancer cells can be addicted to high RNA synthesis, including synthesis of survival molecules. We hypothesised that dormant cancer cells, already low in RNA, might be sensitive to apoptosis induced by RNA Polymerase II (RP2) inhibitors that further reduce RNA synthesis.

Methods: We cultured leukaemia cells continuously *in vitro* in the presence of an mTOR inhibitor to model dormancy. Apoptosis, damage, RNA content and reducing capacity were evaluated. We treated dormancy-enriched cells for 48 hours with the nucleoside analogues ara-C, 5-azacytidine and clofarabine, the topoisomerase targeting agents daunorubicin, etoposide and irinotecan and three multikinase inhibitors with activity against RP2 - flavopiridol, roscovitine and TG02, and we measured growth inhibition and apoptosis. We describe use of the parameter $2 \times IC_{50}$ to measure residual cell targeting. RNA synthesis was measured with 5-ethynyl uridine. Drug-induced apoptosis was measured flow cytometrically in primary cells from patients with acute myeloid leukaemia using a CD34/CD71/annexinV gating strategy to identify dormant apoptotic cells.

Results: Culture of the KG1a cell line continuously in the presence of an mTOR inhibitor induced features of dormancy including low RNA content, low metabolism and low basal ROS formation in the absence of a DNA damage response or apoptosis. All agents were more effective against the unmanipulated than the dormancy-enriched cells, emphasising the chemoresistant nature of dormant cells. However, the percentage of cell reduction by RP2 inhibitors at $2 \times IC_{50}$ was significantly greater than that of other agents. RP2 inhibitors strongly inhibited RNA synthesis compared with other drugs. We also showed that RP2 inhibitors induce apoptosis in proliferating and dormancy-enriched KG1a cells and in the CD71[neg] CD34[pos] subset of primary acute myeloid leukaemia cells.

Conclusion: We suggest that RP2 inhibitors may be a useful class of agent for targeting dormant leukaemia cells.

Keywords: Leukemia, Dormancy, RNA polymerase II inhibitors

Background

Relapse in cancer patients after therapy is due to the continued presence of a subset of cells which is likely to have evaded the effects of treatment by lying dormant [1,2]. Dormant cells are characterised by low levels of RNA, consistent with their lack of proliferation and need to conserve energy [3]. However, cancer cells may be dependent on ("addicted to") survival gene expression [4,5] and thus be primed for death if the survival genes are down-regulated [6]. Hence we hypothesised that dormant cancer cells, in which RNA levels are already low, may be sensitive to agents that target the transcriptional machinery. Transcriptional cyclin dependent kinases, i.e. CDK9 and CDK7, are permissive for transcription through modulation of the essential RNA elongation factor RNA Polymerase II (RP2). RP2 serine 5 phosphorylation by CDK7 normally occurs early in the initiation of transcription, whereas RP2 serine 2 phosphorylation by CDK9 predominates later, during elongation and termination [7]. Inhibition of RP2, although ultimately fatal to all cells, can allow for a therapeutic window by selectively affecting molecules essential to cancer cell survival. Foremost candidates for this role are those molecules with a short message and protein

* Correspondence: monica.pallis@nottingham.ac.uk
[1]Nottingham University Hospitals, Nottingham, UK
[4]Academic Haematology, Clinical Sciences Building, Nottingham University Hospitals City Campus, Nottingham NG5 1PB, UK
Full list of author information is available at the end of the article

half-life [4,8]. An emerging group of multi-kinase inhibitors such as flavopiridol, roscovitine and TG02 inhibit transcriptional CDKs and thus RP2 activation in cells from patients with haematological malignancies [9-15].

A large amount of material is needed to study mechanisms of drug targeting and resistance, but dormant cancer cells are rare. Thus *in vitro* models of the dormant subpopulation would be valuable. In contrast to primary samples, leukaemia cell lines are plentiful and highly proliferative, so we sought a suitable method of inducing dormancy in these cells.

MTOR is a critical mediator of cell cycle progression [16,17]. In normal cells, mTOR integrates nutrient and growth factor signals such that factor deprivation inhibits mTOR, allowing the cell to conserve resources, quiesce and survive. This paper first addresses the chemosensitivity of the KG1a cell line, which retains long-term viability and is undamaged by mTOR inhibition. We show that these cells, which have a CD34$^+$CD38$^-$, p-glycoprotein$^+$ phenotype characteristic of leukaemic progenitor cells [18], are enriched for features of dormancy by mTOR inactivation. We treat unmanipulated and dormancy-enriched cells with the nucleoside analogues ara-C, 5-azacytidine and clofarabine, the topoisomerase targeting agents daunorubicin, etoposide and irinotecan and three multikinase inhibitors with activity against RP2 - flavopiridol, roscovitine and TG02. We report our findings and extend them to primary leukaemia samples.

Methods
Materials
Phenotyping antibodies and isotype controls were obtained from BD Biosciences. TG02-citrate was synthesised by Tragara Pharmaceuticals. Other drugs and reagents were obtained from Sigma unless otherwise stated.

Cells and rapamycin pre-treatment
The KG1a myeloid leukaemia cell line was obtained from the European Collection of Animal Cell Cultures (Salisbury, UK) and was maintained in RPMI 1640 medium with 10% foetal calf serum (FCS; First Link, Birmingham, UK) and 2 mM L-glutamine. All experiments were performed with cell lines in log phase. Continued testing to authenticate the cells was performed by genetic fingerprinting towards the final passage of each batch thawed and through repeated assays of CD34, CD38 and p-glycoprotein status. The cells were pre-treated with rapamycin (LC labs) for 2–9 days before addition of chemotherapy drugs.

Ethics statement
Blood or bone marrow samples were obtained after written informed consent from AML patients. Use of these samples was approved by the Nottingham 1 Ethics Committee (reference 06/Q2403/16) and the Nottingham University Hospitals NHS Trust. Frozen, banked samples were used.

Drug treatment in cell lines
Unmanipulated and rapamycin-pre-treated KG1a cells were pelleted and re-suspended in 96 well plates at 2×10^5 cells per ml for 48 hours with and without drugs. Cytosine arabinoside (Ara-C), flavopiridol, irinotecan and daunorubicin stock solutions were made in water. Clofarabine stock was made in PBS. 5-azacytidine, etoposide, roscovitine (LC labs) and TG02 were dissolved in DMSO as was the RP2 inhibitor 5,6-dicholoro-1-β-D-ribofuranoslybenzimidazole (DRB). DMSO diluent controls were used for etoposide and roscovitine (because the final DMSO concentration was greater than 1 in 10,000). Drug dilutions were made in culture medium.

Determination of RNA status and RNA synthesis
For flow cytometry, the method of Schmid was used using 7-amino actinomycin D (7-AAD) to label DNA and pyronin Y to label RNA [19]. RNA was also measured on unselected cells by spectrophotometry. RNA synthesis was measured flow cytometrically using the method of Jao and Salic [20]: 5-ethynyl uridine (EU, Invitrogen) incorporation (20 μM, 1 hour) was followed by detection with Alexa 488 azide (Invitrogen). A non-specific fluorescence control tube, missing out the EU incorporation step, was set up for each condition, and the result subtracted from the test fluorescence value before calculating the percentage of untreated control fluorescence for each drug.

To determine modulation of RP2S2, treated and untreated cells were fixed and permeabilized using the Leucoperm kit (AbD Serotec) and were incubated with antibodies to RP2S2 (Abcam #5095,) then with a FITC conjugated second layer.

Determination of reactive oxygen species (ROS)
Cells were incubated with the (non-fluorescent) 15 μM 2′,7′-Dichlorofluorescin diacetate (DCFDA) in triplicate for 25 minutes at 37°C and at 4°C, placed on ice and the fluorescent oxidation product dichlorofluorescin (DCF) was measured immediately by flow cytometry. Baseline (4°C) values were subtracted from test (37°C) values.

Determination of metabolism
Cellular metabolism was measured using the reduction of 2,3-bis(2-methoxy-4-nitro5-sulfophenyl)-5-{(phenylamino) carbonyl}-2H-tetrazolium hydroxide (XTT, Roche) [21]. Cells were plated at 2×10^5/ml and cultured for 48 hours, with XTT for the final 6 hours. Relative absorbance was

calculated after adjustment for final cell concentration (measured by haemocytometer).

Immunocytochemistry

Gamma-H2A.X foci were identified and counted using the H score system as previously described [22].

Determination of cell viability and apoptosis in cell lines

Toxicity was measured using the XTT assay kit according to manufacturer's instructions (Roche). Apoptosis was measured flow cytometrically using the Trevigen Annexin V kit (R & D) according to manufacturers' instructions.

Dormancy and apoptosis of primary AML cells

Primary cells were cultured in triplicate at 1×10^6/ml in fibronectin coated wells of a flat-bottomed plate in serum-free medium supplemented with cytokines. (A previous publication [23] has further details). Drugs were added after 2–3 hours. After 14–18 hours of further culture, cells were harvested and stained with CD34PerCP and CD45-APCCy7, and with CD71PE or isotype controls. Following two rinses in PBS, the cells were counterstained with Annexin V FITC in the buffer provided (R&D Systems). CD71 expression was measured in cells gated tightly on forward and side scatter, with secondary gating on CD45 and side scatter to exclude lymphocytes. A third gate was set on CD34/low side scatter and a fourth gate on annexin V low positive cells. To ensure at most a 15% co-efficient of variation, cultures with a low number of cells after this four-part gating, i.e. less than 50 positive events, were excluded (explained in detail elsewhere [24]).

Statistical analysis

Univariate analysis of variance main effects modelling was used for comparing multiple treatments, and significant findings were further analysed in 2 way comparisons using paired T-tests, carried out using the Statistical Package for Social Sciences, version 16 (SPSS, Chicago, IL, USA).

Results

mTOR inhibition induces the principal features of dormant cells

Given that inhibition of the mTOR pathway is experimentally proven to maintain the *in vivo* dormancy and transplantability of haematopoietic and leukaemic cells [25-28], we experimented with the possibility of inhibiting growth in a leukaemic cell line with the mTOR inhibitor rapamycin. In preliminary studies, we cultured KG1a cells with 50-500 nM rapamycin and found similar percentage growth inhibition across the dose range (data not shown), such that 100 nM was

chosen for further study. We now show that continuous culture of KG1a cells in 100 nM rapamycin for up to 11 days induced no detectable apoptosis, whereas serum withdrawal, the common method for inducing cells to exit the cell cycle, induced a statistically significant induction of Annexin V within 48 hours, and most cells were dead within a week (Figure 1A,B). Sublethal damage in the rapamycin-treated cells might sensitise them to chemotherapeutic drugs, but we determined that no measurable γH2A.X damage foci were induced by rapamycin (Figure 1C).

We have already previously shown that rapamycin inhibits phosphorylation of the mTOR targets 4E-BP1 and P70S6K in KG1a cells [29]. In a series of experiments performed after 48 hours' incubation with rapamycin we found that, despite cell growth being slowed rather than totally arrested by rapamycin, the cells acquired key properties of dormant cells. There was a decrease in RNA, measured as a 3.5fold increase in Pyronin Y^{low} cells, from 13.6 to 48.6% cells and a decrease in total RNA per cell of 54% (Figure 2A). This is an especially important finding, as Pyronin Y^{low} cells are enriched for dormancy rather than terminal differentiation as demonstrated by their engraftment capacity in both normal haematopoietic cells and tumour initiating cells [30,31]. We also observed a corresponding decrease in cell size (Figure 2C) [3]. We noted that formazan production from XTT, an indicator of mitochondrial metabolism, was reduced by 34% in dormancy- enriched cells (Figure 2D). We also noted a 32% ROS decrease in dormancy-enriched cells (Figure 2E).

Superiority of transcriptional CDK/RP2 inhibitors in targeting dormancy-enriched cells

As nucleoside analogues and topoisomerase inhibitors are the mainstay of AML therapy, we examined the toxicity of these drug classes as well as that of RP2 inhibitors against unmanipulated and dormancy-enriched KG1a cells. We derived dose response curves for the topoisomerase- targeting agents daunorubicin, etoposide and irinotecan, nucleoside analogues ara-C, 5-azacytidine and clofarabine and the transcriptional CDK/RP2 inhibitors flavopiridol, roscovitine and TG02 in proliferating and dormancy-enriched KG1a cells. We also used the specific RNA polymerase 2 inhibitor 5,6-dicholoro-1-β-D-ribofuranoslybenzimidazole (DRB) as positive control for RP2 targeting [4,32]. Figure 3A demonstrates that dose response curves from dormancy-enriched cells have a greater tendency than those from unmanipulated cells to flatten out and there are more residual cells under the flattened part of the curve. We therefore asked a novel question: namely, how can we measure the difficulty for a drug to target further cells after the initial IC_{50} has been passed? For this measure,

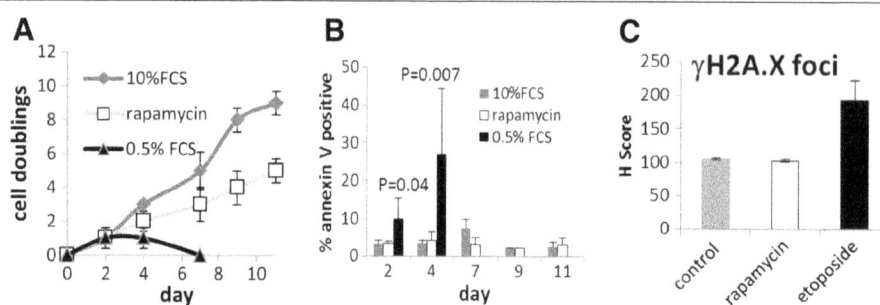

Figure 1 Rapamycin is not toxic to KG1a cells. (A, B) KG1a cells were suspended/re-suspended at 2×10^5/ml on days 0,2,4,7 and 9 of an 11 day culture in medium with 0.5% foetal calf serum, 10% foetal calf serum or 10% foetal calf serum + 100 nM rapamycin. **(A)** Cell growth was measured by haemocytometer; **(B)** apoptosis was measured by Annexin V labelling. Annexin V was measured only at 2 and 4 days on cells grown in 0.5% FCS as there were insufficient cells remaining by 7 days. **(C)** Following 48 hours' culture in RPMI with 10% foetal calf serum with or without 100 nM rapamycin, cells were harvested, and processed for immunohistochemical analysis of γH2A.X foci. Cells treated for 2 hrs with 100 μg/ml etoposide were used as positive control in each assay. (For interpretation, an H score (reference 22) is a staining intensity score of 1–5 per cell for 100 cells, such that a score of 100 represents no staining and a score of 500 represents 100 completely damaged cells.). In each experiment datapoints indicate mean and standard deviation of 3 independent assays.

the parameter we used was cell reduction at $2 \times IC_{50}$. Thus, using an example from Figure 3B, roscovitine reduces unmanipulated cell number by 94% at $2 \times IC_{50}$, i.e. by doubling the IC_{50} concentration roscovitine managed to deplete a futher 44% of cells, whereas araC manages to deplete only a further 9% of cells when the IC_{50} concentration is doubled (Figure 3B). We established that the RP2 inhibitor group of drugs were significantly more effective at reducing cell number at $2 \times IC_{50}$ than the topoisomerase targeting agents or the nucleoside analogues ($P = 0.001$ for topoisomerase targeting agents and $P < 0.001$ for nucleoside analogues compared with RP2 inhibitors in unmanipulated cells, $P = 0.003$ for both comparisons in dormancy-enriched cells, Figure 3B.) (DRB was used as a positive control for RP2 targeting and is not a chemotherapeutic agent: its effects were therefore not included in the statistical analysis).

Targeting of RNA polymerase II and RNA sythesis by RP2 inhibitors

Serine 2 of the elongation factor RNA Polymerase II (RP2S2) is a molecular target of CDK9 [33]. Flavopiridol, roscovitine and TG02 have multiple and diverse targets in addition to RP2. We therefore measured whether RP2S2 and RNA synthesis were being targeted at each drug's IC_{50}. The existing literature, including our own previous work with TG02 [10,13-15] indicated that investigation of these parameters after 6 hours of treatment would show optimal effects. At this timepoint, RP2S2 was significantly downregulated in dormancy-enriched KG1a cells treated with RP2 inhibitors (Figure 4A). RNA synthesis was greatly reduced at the same timepoint (Figure 4B). A number of molecules with short message and protein half-lives are depleted by RNA polymerase II inhibitors [8], including several survival and cycle-related proteins [11-13,15]. Moreover

TG02, flavopiridol and roscovitine are all documented to induce cell cycle arrest in G0/G1 [14,34,35], which we confirmed in the KG1a model (data not shown), so it was important to establish whether the decreases in cell numbers relative to untreated controls were solely due to growth inhibition or whether, as would be necessary for dormant cell targeting, they also undergo apoptosis. We observed apoptosis in all cases at the IC_{50} for DRB, flavopiridol and TG02 (Figure 4C). Roscovitine had notably little ability to induce apoptosis in the dormancy-enriched cells (discussed below).

Sensitivity to RP2 inhibition in dormant CD34+ primary leukaemic cells

We and others have previously documented the *in vitro* toxicity of TG02 to bulk CD34 + CD38- primary AML cells and demonstrated effective cell reduction at 100 nM [14,15]. The CD34 + CD38- subset is enriched for dormant cells, but to address directly the question of whether RP2 inhibitors target dormant primary cells, we sought a flow cytometric assay that would combine a dormancy marker with an apoptotic marker. Annexin V is the standard, extremely sensitive, marker for apoptosis in non-adherent cells, but its use in permeabilised cells is problematic. Ki-67 is the standard marker for excluding, and thus identifying, dormant cells, but detects an intracellular antigen and thus requires cells to be fixed and permeabilised, which compromises Annexin V staining. We looked for a cell surface marker which would discriminate between dormant and cycling cells and could be used in conjunction with Annexin V to investigate apoptosis in dormant cells. The absence of CD71, the transferrin receptor, has been reported in dormant lymphocytes and in cancer stem cells [36,37]. In preliminary experiments, we established that cells which were negative for CD71 (i.e. found in the lower two quadrants

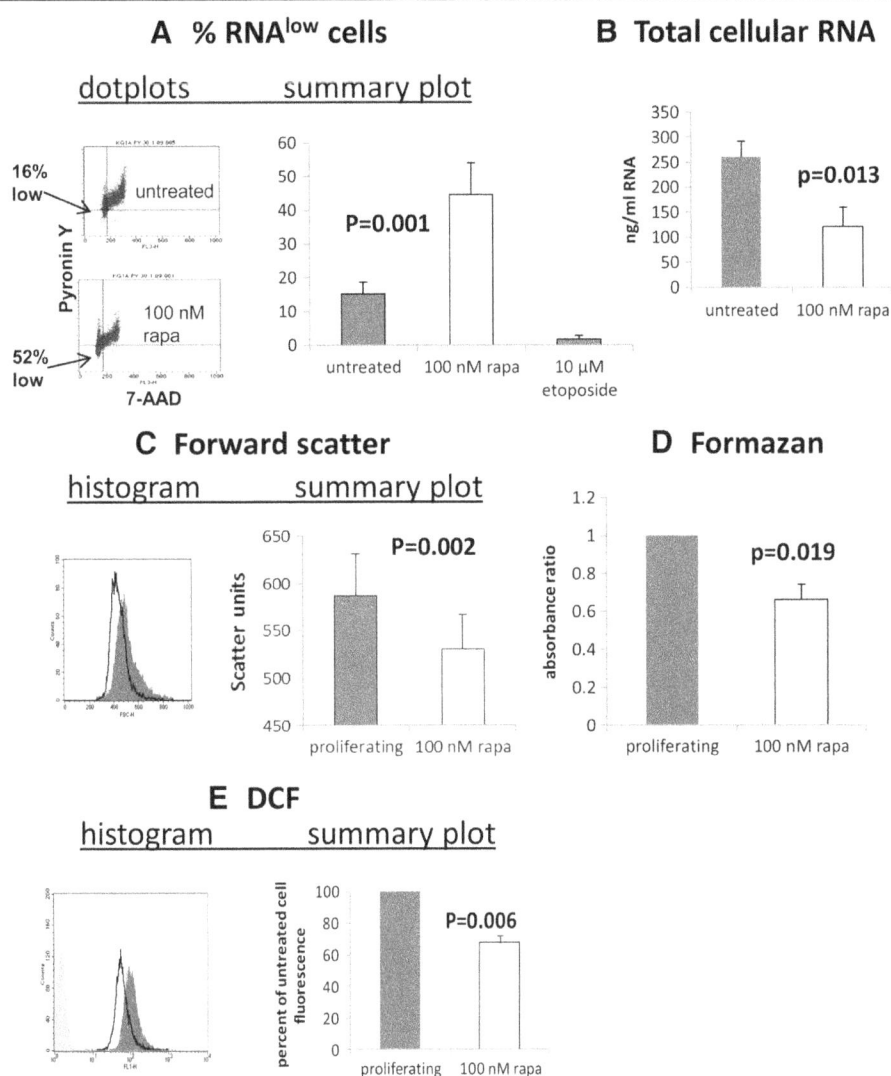

Figure 2 Rapamycin induces key features of dormancy. Evaluation of cellular properties after treatment of KG1a cells with 100 nM rapamycin for 48 hours. (**A**) RNA content: Flow cytometric dotplots indicate the percentage of cells which are low in RNA (Pyronin Y) as well as low in DNA (7-AAD) and summary chart. In the summary chart, the RNA content of KG1a cells treated for 48 hours with etoposide, which induces predominant G2/M arrest, are used as negative control. (**B**) The total RNA content of lysed cells, measured by spectrophotometry. (**C**) Flow cytometric analysis of forward scatter as an indicator of cell size: representative histogram: dark-filled histogram = untreated cells, unfilled histogram = rapamycin-treated cells and summary graph (instrument and voltage-dependent units). (**D**) Reduction of 2,3-bis(2-methoxy-4-nitro5-sulfophenyl)-5-{(phenylamino)carbonyl}-2H-tetrazolium hydroxide to formazan: absorbance ratio (adjusted for cell count) after 48 hours as a measure of mitochondrial metabolism. (**E**) Flow cytometric dichlorofluorescein diacetate as a measure of reactive oxygen species: example, dark-filled histogram = untreated cells, unfilled histogram = rapamycin-treated cells, pale grey histogram = baseline; summary graph. In each experiment datapoints illustrate mean and standard deviation of at least 3 independent assays. All P values are for comparisons between untreated and rapamycin-treated cells.

of the dot plots in Figure 5A) were also almost all Ki-67-negative (i.e. there were very few cells in the lower right quadrants). CD71 negative cells can therefore be classified as dormant. To determine whether RP2 inhibition induces apoptosis in dormant primary AML blasts, we labelled in vitro-treated blasts for Annexin V and CD71. Figure 5B shows our gating strategy. Using eight primary samples, we found clear evidence of CD71[neg] cells in the

Annexin V [lowpos] subset of CD34+ AML blasts treated with DRB, TG02 or flavopiridol (Figure 5C). When compared with etoposide (which had not been effective in targeting dormancy-enriched KG1a cells as shown in Figure 3) a significantly higher proportion of apoptosing cells was found in the CD71[neg] compartment after treatment with all three RP2 inhibitors (P < 0.001 for DRB and TG02, P = 0.007 for flavopiridol). It is important to

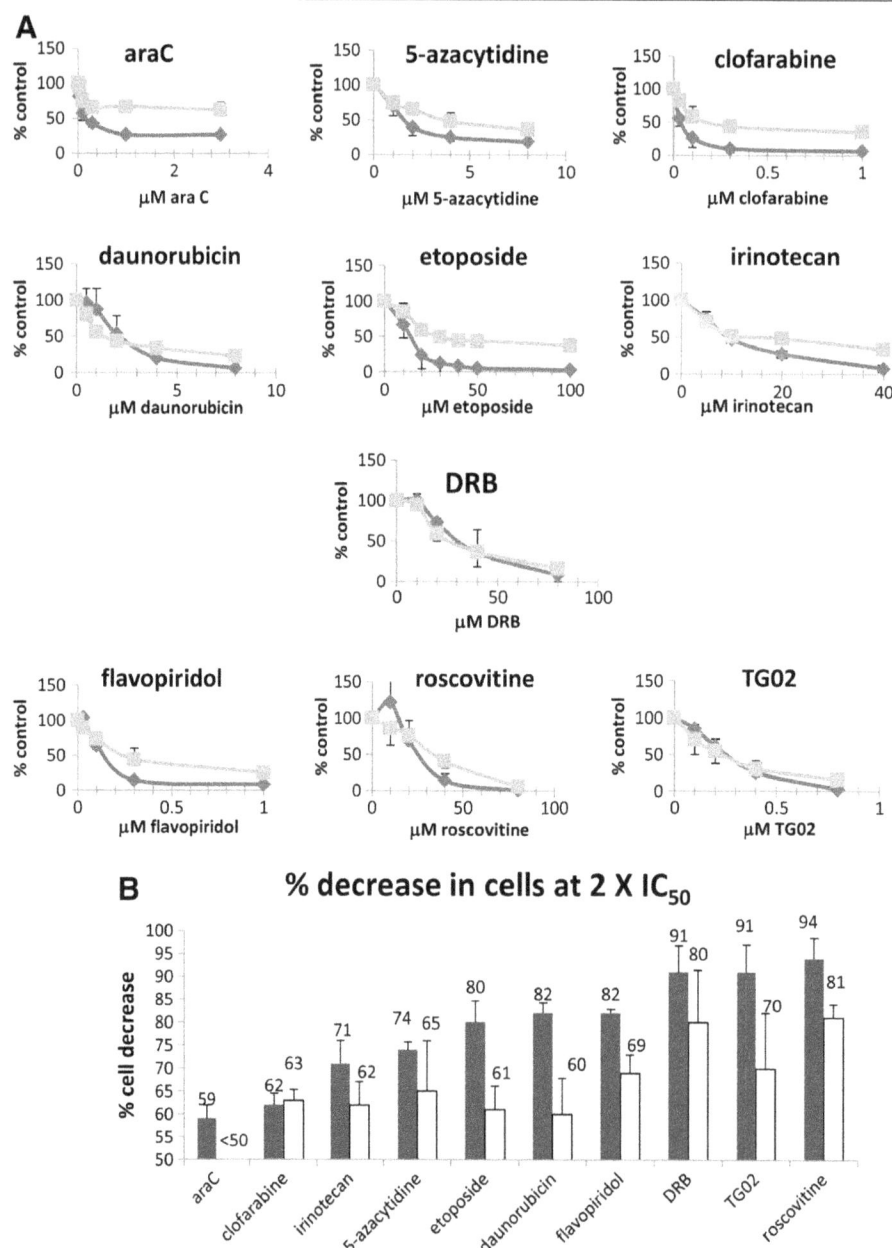

Figure 3 KG1a responses to chemotherapeutic agents. Un-manipulated KG1a cells and cells enriched for dormancy by rapamycin pre-treatment were cultured in the presence of drugs for 48 hours whereupon net cell growth and survival was estimated using the 2,3-bis(2-methoxy-4-nitro5-sulfophenyl)-5-{(phenylamino)carbonyl}-2H-tetrazolium hydroxide (XTT) assay. (**A**) Dose response curves in proliferating and dormancy-enriched cells. Dark lines represent un-manipulated cells and light grey lines represent dormancy-enriched cells. (**B**) Percentage decrease in viable cells at $2 \times IC_{50}$. Dark bars represent unmanipulated cells and unfilled bars represent dormancy-enriched treated cells. Note that for araC no IC_{50} for dormancy-enriched cells was reached, even at 20 times the IC_{50} of proliferating cells. In each experiment datapoints indicate mean and standard deviation of at least 3 independent assays.

understand here that we are not comparing the toxicity of different agents but are selecting cells in which apoptosis is occuring to determine in which compartment (dormant or non-dormant) it is occuring. We also took advantage of the fact that primary AML cells *in vitro* show some spontaneous apoptosis, compared to which all three RP2 inhibitors again were associated with a significantly greater proportion of apoptotic cells in the CD71[neg] compartment (P < 0.001 for DRB, P = 0.003 for TG02 and P = 0.01 for flavopiridol). Roscovitine at doses up to 2 µM only reduced viable cell concentration in a minority of primary samples studied and we therefore have not documented results with this agent.

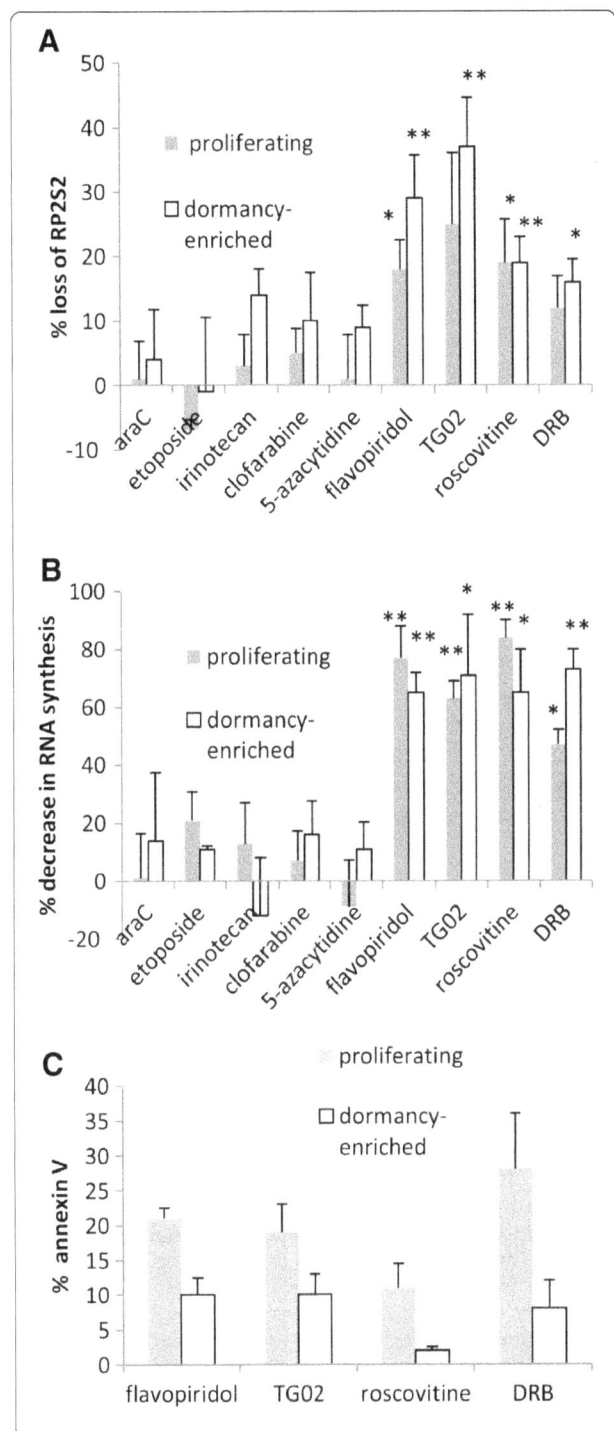

Figure 4 Decreased RNA Polymerase II activity and RNA synthesis in transcriptional RP2i-treated KG1a cells. Unmanipulated KG1a cells and cells enriched for dormancy by rapamycin pre-treatment were cultured with chemotherapy drugs, each drug at its 48 hour IC_{50} concentration. (Daunorubicin was not included in this set of experiments, due to interference from its fluorescent properties). (**A**) Loss of serine 2-phosphorylated RNA Polymerase II (RP2S2) was measured after 6 hours' incubation of proliferating and dormancy-enriched cells with chemotherapeutic agents. For comparisons against untreated controls ** signifies $P < 0.01$; * signifies $P < 0.05$. (**B**) RNA synthesis was measured by 20 μM 5-ethynyl uridine incorporation for the final hour of a six hour treatment with chemotherapeutic agents. For comparisons against untreated controls ** signifies $P < 0.01$; * signifies $P < 0.05$. (**C**) Apoptosis was measured using Annexin V after 18 hours. In each experiment datapoints indicate mean and SEM of at least 3 independent assays.

Discussion

There is a paradox at the centre of chemoresistance research, in that most anti-neoplastic drugs have been designed to target proliferating cells as a surrogate for tumour cells, and therefore the highly chemoresistant dormant tumour cell does not fit into the mainstream chemotherapeutic paradigm. In the AML field, a vanguard of researchers has been investigating possible solutions to this problem for the last twenty years and more. From *in vitro* and animal model work, it is clear that non-proliferating AML cells are resistant to ara-C, and that chemosensitivity increases when cells are induced into cycle by growth factor exposure [38-40]. However over a dozen clinical trials reflecting a great deal of effort in applying this knowledge have yielded equivocal results ([41] and references therein) and fresh approaches are needed.

We reasoned that it would be useful to have *in vitro* models to contribute to the search for ways of targeting dormant leukaemia cells. Whilst there is a need for the creation of suitable *in vivo* models to test longer- term chemosensitivity in dormant leukaemia cells in an appropriate microenvironment, we suggest that the value of *in vitro* work is that it allows the comparison of a broad range of drugs and allows for investigations of their mechanisms of action, as is illustrated in the current work.

The overwhelming evidence that activation of the mTOR pathway pushes haematopoietic and leukaemic cells out of dormancy [25-28] led us to investigate this pathway. Moreover an elegant study published after the current work was completed showed that AML cells with an undifferentiated phenotype have prolonged *in vivo* survival when mTOR activity is knocked out, and that subsequent mTOR re-activation restores the leukaemogenic potential of these cells [42]. In our study, rapamycin slowed, but did not completely arrest growth in KG1a cells (Figure 1A). However, in contrast to serum

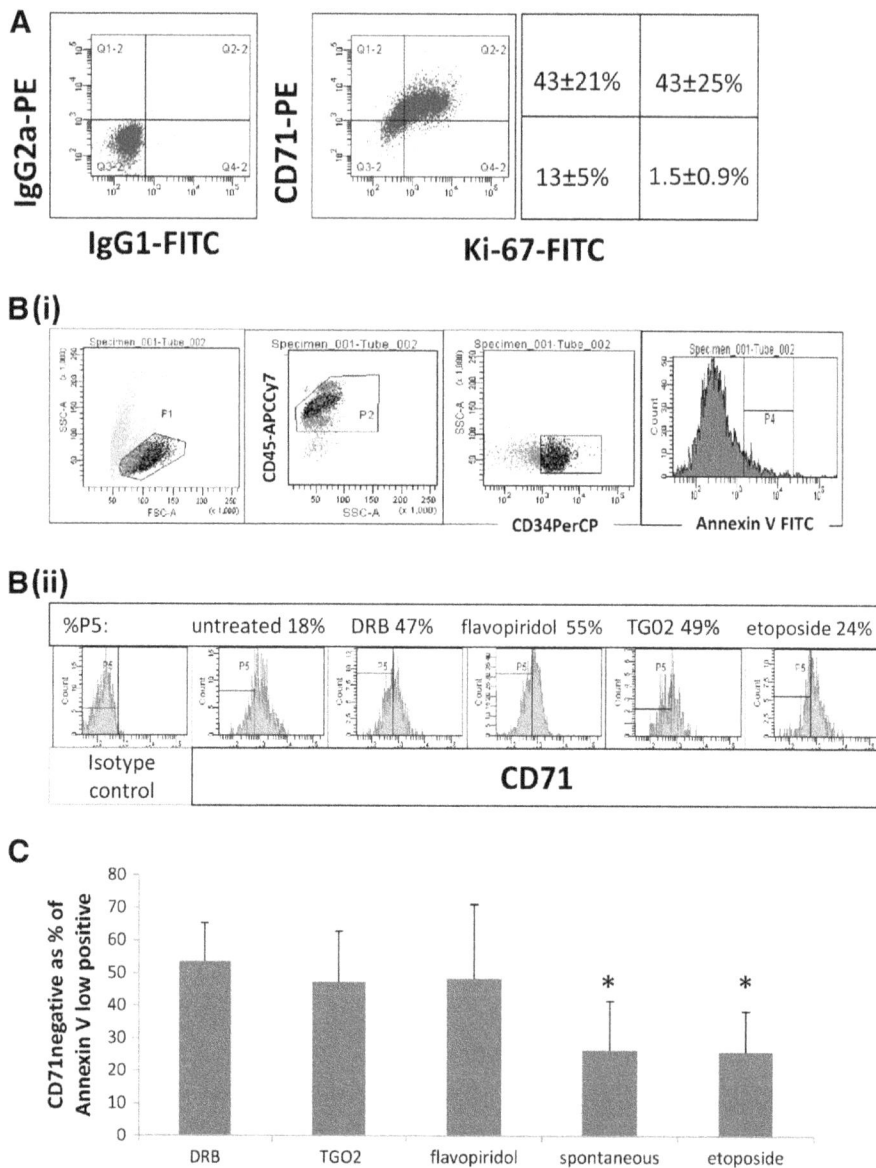

Figure 5 Apoptosis in CD34+ dormant patient cells treated with RP2 inhibitors. (**A**) Ki-67/CD71 co-expression in CD34-gated primary AML cells before culture. For Ki-67 and CD71 quadrant delineation, gating was carried out strictly such that 1% of isotype control fluorescence fell into the positive quadrants. Flow cytometric dotplots of one sample and a diagram summarising mean ± standard deviation of target cell percentage in each quadrant for the seven primary samples studied are shown. (**B**) An example of CD71 expression in CD34+ annexin V + AML blasts. Patient cells were cultured for 16–18 hours with DRB, TG02, flavopiridol or etoposide. They were then labelled with CD71, CD45 and CD34, rinsed and additionally labelled with Annexin V. CD71 expression was determined in CD34+ early apoptotic cells using the four part gating strategy detailed in the Methods section. (i) Illustration of gating strategy showing how gates P1-P4 are applied; note especially that gates P1 and P4 are narrowed to exclude late stages of apoptosis or necrosis in order to alleviate concern that CD71 might be shed. (ii) Flow cytometric histograms showing CD71 expression in the cell subset gated on P1-P4 (MFI = mean fluorescence intensity). (**C**) CD71 negative cells shown as a percentage of total early apoptotic cells from the P1-P4 subset of primary samples (n = 8 for TG02 and etoposide, n = 6 for DRB and flavopiridol). As primary samples are heterogeneous, apoptosis-inducing drug concentrations were sample-specific (30-100 nM for TG02 and flavopiridol, 0.2-2 μM for etoposide, 20 μM for DRB). * The low proportions of CD71neg cells in untreated and etoposide-treated samples compared to RP2 inhibitor-treated samples were statistically significant, as detailed in the text.

withdrawal, which is the most commonly used model for dormancy, rapamycin did not cause apoptosis or DNA damage (Figure 1) - an essential consideration for a model in which the chemosensitivity of previously undamaged cells is to be assessed. We suggest that rapamycin provides a useful model for dormancy because key features, i.e. low RNA, low metabolism and low ROS, are enriched in the rapamycin-treated compared with the untreated cells (Figure 2). Low RNA is of paramount importance, since cells characterised by low RNA content retain the capacity to re-enter the cell cycle and act as progenitors *in vivo* [30,31]. The RNA^{low} characteristic of dormant cells is consistent with their lack of proliferation and low metabolism [3], but for dormant cancer cells this might be difficult to reconcile with addiction to survival gene expression, leading us to suggest that these cells may be sensitive to transcriptional RP2 inhibitors. A publication several years ago showed that flavopiridol targets non-cycling A549 cells [43]. Flavopiridol and roscovitine were initially designed to target cyclin dependent kinases that drive cell proliferation, and it was only subsequently that the effects were noted for both of these agents on down-regulating survival molecules and inhibition of transcription through inactivation of CDK9 [9,10,13,44]. TG02 has been characterised more recently and, like the two other agents, has multiple targets including cycling and transcriptional CDKs [14]. In cell-free assays, TG02 has a 3nM IC$_{50}$ for CDK9 [14]. As all three agents have multiple targets, we also used the RP2-specific inhibitor DRB in our assays [4,32].

We have shown that transcriptional RP2 inhibitors are better able than conventional agents to target dormancy-enriched AML cells. We hypothesised that a therapeutic window might exist for dormant cancer cells because of the addiction of malignant cells to survival gene expression [4,5]. Results from clinical trials with roscovitine and flavopiridol [45] including a trial incorporating flavopiridol in combination chemotherapy of AML [46] have shown some efficacy at sub-toxic doses. TG02 at tolerated doses induced lasting complete remissions in an AML xenograft model [14] and at the time of writing, is in Phase 1 trials for refractory and relapsed leukaemias. We show that the specific transcriptional RP2 inhibitor DRB as well as TG02, roscovitine and flavopiridol down-regulate RNA Polymerase II activation and RNA synthesis in both unmanipulated and dormancy-enriched cells. We have not attempted to pick out specific targets of RP2 down-regulation, as these are multitudinous [8]. Functionally they tend to be genes involved in rapid cellular responses, such as apoptosis regulators, mitosis regulators and genes involved in signalling pathways such as several NFκB target genes [8]. We have shown that apoptosis is induced by the specific RP2 inhibitor DRB and by flavopiridol and TG02 (Figures 4 and 5). Roscovitine appears to work mainly by growth inhibition or a non-apoptotic mechanism of death. It is noteworthy in this respect that gene expression profiling of agents inhibiting transcriptional CDKs found that DRB and flavopiridol had similar broad activity, whereas roscovitine had a narrower range of activity [8]. Moreover, in our hands, micromolar concentrations

of roscovitine were found to reduce viable cell concentration in only 5/12 leukaemia samples studied *in vitro* (data not shown) in contrast to a robust response to TG02 at 100 nM [15].

To further validate our results indicating that RP2 inhibitors target dormancy-enriched KG1a cells, we sought agreement for our findings in primary material. In contrast to cell lines, primary AML samples are enriched for cells in G$_0$ of the cell cycle [39]. We examined the extent of apoptosis induced by RP2 inhibitors in dormant and proliferative compartments of primary cells. As Annexin V is a highly sensitive marker for early apoptosis in primary AML cells, we looked for a cell surface dormancy marker that could be used in conjunction with Annexin V to measure apoptosis in dormant compared to proliferating cells. CD71 (the transferrin receptor) is absent in un-stimulated peripheral blood lymphocytes, in some cancer stem cells and in long term culture-initiating cells from normal bone marrow [36,37,47]. Analysis of patient samples co-labelled with CD71 and Ki-67 indicated that CD71 is not expressed in dormant AML blasts (Figure 5). Co-labelling of cells with CD71 and Annexin V clearly indicated the contrast between the high proportion of CD71^{neg} apoptotic cells following treatment with DRB, flavopiridol or TG02 and the high CD71 expression in etoposide-treated apoptotic cells. Even compensating for the plasma protein binding of the drug, the concentration of TG02 used in this experiment is readily achievable *in vivo* in both animals [14] and humans (as measured following oral administration in ongoing clinical studies - FB, unpublished).

Conclusion

In conclusion, we have shown that RP2 inhibitors effectively target both KG1a cells enriched for dormancy by mTOR inhibition and CD71^{neg} primary leukaemia patient samples thus providing grounds for suggesting that transcriptional RP2 inhibitors may be a useful class of agent for targeting dormant cells thought to contribute to relapses in leukaemia.

Abbreviations
7-AAD: 7-amino actinomycin D; AML: Acute myeloid leukaemia; araC: Cytarabine; CDK: Cyclin dependent kinase; DRB: 5,6-dicholoro-1-β-D-ribofuranoslybenzimidazole; EU: 5-ethynyl uridine; DCF: Dichlorofluorescein; DCFDA: 2′,7′-Dichlorofluorescin diacetate; FCS: Foetal calf serum; FSC: Forward scatter; HSC: Haematopoietic stem cell; mTOR: Mammalian target of rapamycin; rapa: Rapamycin; ROS: Reactive oxygen species; RP2: RNA Polymerase II; RP2S2: RNA Polymerase II serine 2; XTT: 2,3-bis(2-methoxy-4-nitro5-sulfophenyl)-5-{(phenylamino)carbonyl}-2H-tetrazolium hydroxide.

Competing interests
Francis Burrows is an employee of Tragara Pharmaeuticals.
No financial interest/relationships with financial interest relating to the topic of this article have been declared by the remaining authors.

Authors' contributions
MP designed the study, participated in all experiments and drafted the manuscript. FB participated in the design of the study and contributed TG02. AW helped to develop the mTOR inhibition model. NB set up and participated in experiments to determine the effects of transcriptional CDK inhibitors on cell survival and RP2S2 phosphorylation. CS participated in the design of the study, oversaw the RNA experiments and participated in drafting the manuscript. NR participated in the design and co ordination of the study and contributed primary AML samples. All authors read and approved the final manuscript.

Acknowledgments
Financial support was obtained from the Nottinghamshire Leukaemia Appeal.

Author details
[1]Nottingham University Hospitals, Nottingham, UK. [2]Tragara Pharmaceuticals, San Diego, USA. [3]University of Nottingham, Nottingham, UK. [4]Academic Haematology, Clinical Sciences Building, Nottingham University Hospitals City Campus, Nottingham NG5 1PB, UK.

References
1. Aguirre-Ghiso JA: **Models, mechanisms and clinical evidence for cancer dormancy.** *Nat Rev Cancer* 2007, **7**(11):834–846.
2. Goss PE, Chambers AF: **Does tumour dormancy offer a therapeutic target?** *Nat Rev Cancer* 2010, **10**(12):871–877.
3. Blagosklonny MV: **Cell senescence: hypertrophic arrest beyond the restriction point.** *J Cell Physiol* 2006, **209**(3):592–597.
4. Koumenis C, Giaccia A: **Transformed cells require continuous activity of RNA polymerase II to resist oncogene-induced apoptosis.** *Mol Cell Biol* 1997, **17**(12):7306–7316.
5. Certo M, Del Gaizo MV, Nishino M, Wei G, Korsmeyer S, Armstrong SA, Letai A: **Mitochondria primed by death signals determine cellular addiction to antiapoptotic BCL-2 family members.** *Cancer Cell* 2006, **9**(5):351–365.
6. Llambi F, Green DR: **Apoptosis and oncogenesis: give and take in the BCL-2 family.** *Curr Opin Genet Dev* 2011, **21**(1):12–20.
7. Komarnitsky P, Cho EJ, Buratowski S: **Different phosphorylated forms of RNA polymerase II and associated mRNA processing factors during transcription.** *Genes Dev* 2000, **14**(19):2452–2460.
8. Lam LT, Pickeral OK, Peng AC, Rosenwald A, Hurt EM, Giltnane JM, Averett LM, Zhao H, Davis RE, Sathyamoorthy M, *et al*: **Genomic-scale measurement of mRNA turnover and the mechanisms of action of the anti-cancer drug flavopiridol.** *Genome Biol* 2001, **2**(10):RESEARCH0041.
9. Chen R, Keating MJ, Gandhi V, Plunkett W: **Transcription inhibition by flavopiridol: mechanism of chronic lymphocytic leukemia cell death.** *Blood* 2005, **106**(7):2513–2519.
10. Kitada S, Zapata JM, Andreeff M, Reed JC: **Protein kinase inhibitors flavopiridol and 7-hydroxy-staurosporine down-regulate antiapoptosis proteins in B-cell chronic lymphocytic leukemia.** *Blood* 2000, **96**(2):393–397.
11. Rosato RR, Almanara JA, Kolla SS, Maggio SC, Coe S, Gimenez MS, Dent P, Grant S: **Mechanism and functional role of XIAP and Mcl-1 down-regulation in flavopiridol/vorinostat antileukemic interactions.** *Mol Cancer Ther* 2007, **6**(2):692–702.
12. MacCallum DE, Melville J, Frame S, Watt K, Anderson S, Gianella-Borradori A, Lane DP, Green SR: **Seliciclib (CYC202, R-Roscovitine) induces cell death in multiple myeloma cells by inhibition of RNA polymerase II-dependent transcription and down-regulation of Mcl-1.** *Cancer Res* 2005, **65**(12):5399–5407.
13. Alvi AJ, Austen B, Weston VJ, Fegan C, MacCallum D, Gianella-Borradori A, Lane DP, Hubank M, Powell JE, Wei W, *et al*: **A novel CDK inhibitor, CYC202 (R-roscovitine), overcomes the defect in p53-dependent apoptosis in B-CLL by down-regulation of genes involved in transcription regulation and survival.** *Blood* 2005, **105**(11):4484–4491.
14. Goh KC, Novotny-Diermayr V, Hart S, Ong LC, Loh YK, Cheong A, Tan YC, Hu C, Jayaraman R, William AD, *et al*: **TG02, a novel oral multi-kinase inhibitor of CDKs, JAK2 and FLT3 with potent anti-leukemic properties.** *Leukemia* 2012, **26**(2):236–243.

15. Pallis M, Abdul-Aziz A, Burrows F, Seedhouse C, Grundy M, Russell N: **The multi-kinase inhibitor TG02 overcomes signalling activation by survival factors to deplete MCL1 and XIAP and induce cell death in primary acute myeloid leukaemia cells.** *Br J Haematol* 2012, **159**(2):191–203.
16. Fingar DC, Blenis J: **Target of rapamycin (TOR): an integrator of nutrient and growth factor signals and coordinator of cell growth and cell cycle progression.** *Oncogene* 2004, **23**(18):3151–3171.
17. Yang X, Yang C, Farberman A, Rideout TC, de Lange CF, France J, Fan MZ: **The mammalian target of rapamycin-signaling pathway in regulating metabolism and growth.** *J Anim Sci* 2008, **86**(14 Suppl):E36–50.
18. Bailly JD, Muller C, Jaffrezou JP, Demur C, Gassar G, Bordier C, Laurent G: **Lack of correlation between expression and function of P-glycoprotein in acute myeloid leukemia cell lines.** *Leukemia* 1995, **9**(5):799–807.
19. Schmid I, Cole SW, Korin YD, Zack JA, Giorgi JV: **Detection of cell cycle subcompartments by flow cytometric estimation of DNA-RNA content in combination with dual-color immunofluorescence.** *Cytometry* 2000, **39**(2):108–116.
20. Jao CY, Salic A: **Exploring RNA transcription and turnover in vivo by using click chemistry.** *Proc Natl Acad Sci U S A* 2008, **105**(41):15779–15784.
21. Scudiero DA, Shoemaker RH, Paull KD, Monks A, Tierney S, Nofziger TH, Currens MJ, Seniff D, Boyd MR: **Evaluation of a soluble tetrazolium/formazan assay for cell growth and drug sensitivity in culture using human and other tumor cell lines.** *Cancer Res* 1988, **48**(17):4827–4833.
22. Seedhouse C, Grundy M, Shang S, Ronan J, Pimblett H, Russell N, Pallis M: **Impaired S-phase arrest in acute myeloid leukemia cells with a FLT3 internal tandem duplication treated with clofarabine.** *Clin Cancer Res* 2009, **15**(23):7291–7298.
23. Jawad M, Seedhouse C, Mony U, Grundy M, Russell NH, Pallis M: **Analysis of factors that affect in vitro chemosensitivity of leukaemic stem and progenitor cells to gemtuzumab ozogamicin (Mylotarg) in acute myeloid leukaemia.** *Leukemia* 2010, **24**:74–80.
24. Mony U, Jawad M, Seedhouse C, Russell N, Pallis M: **Resistance to FLT3 inhibition in an in vitro model of primary AML cells with a stem cell phenotype in a defined microenvironment.** *Leukemia* 2008, **22**(7):1395–1401.
25. Yilmaz OH, Valdez R, Theisen BK, Guo W, Ferguson DO, Wu H, Morrison SJ: **Pten dependence distinguishes haematopoietic stem cells from leukaemia-initiating cells.** *Nature* 2006, **441**(7092):475–482.
26. Chen C, Liu Y, Liu R, Ikenoue T, Guan KL, Zheng P: **TSC-mTOR maintains quiescence and function of hematopoietic stem cells by repressing mitochondrial biogenesis and reactive oxygen species.** *J Exp Med* 2008, **205**(10):2397–2408.
27. Campbell TB, Basu S, Hangoc G, Tao W, Broxmeyer HE: **Overexpression of Rheb2 enhances mouse hematopoietic progenitor cell growth while impairing stem cell repopulation.** *Blood* 2009, **114**(16):3392–3401.
28. Ito K, Bernardi R, Morotti A, Matsuoka S, Saglio G, Ikeda Y, Rosenblatt J, Avigan DE, Teruya-Feldstein J, Pandolfi PP: **PML targeting eradicates quiescent leukaemia-initiating cells.** *Nature* 2008, **453**(7198):1072–1078.
29. Shang S, Seedhouse C, Russell N, Pallis M: **Low dose rapamycin does not modulate p-glycoprotein function in acute myeloid leukaemia.** *Leuk Res* 2008, **32**(5):836–837.
30. Gothot A, Pyatt R, McMahel J, Rice S, Srour EF: **Functional heterogeneity of human CD34(+) cells isolated in subcompartments of the G0/G1 phase of the cell cycle.** *Blood* 1997, **90**(11):4384–4393.
31. Guan Y, Gerhard B, Hogge DE: **Detection, Isolation and Stimulation of Quiescent Primitive Leukemic Progenitor Cells from Patients with Acute Myeloid Leukemia (AML).** *Blood* 2003, **101**:3142–3149.
32. Zandomeni R, Mittleman B, Bunick D, Ackerman S, Weinmann R: **Mechanism of action of dichloro-beta-D-ribofuranosylbenzimidazole: effect on in vitro transcription.** *Proc Natl Acad Sci U S A* 1982, **79**(10):3167–3170.
33. Cho EJ, Kobor MS, Kim M, Greenblatt J, Buratowski S: **Opposing effects of Ctk1 kinase and Fcp1 phosphatase at Ser 2 of the RNA polymerase II C-terminal domain.** *Genes Dev* 2001, **15**(24):3319–3329.
34. Carlson BA, Dubay MM, Sausville EA, Brizuela L, Worland PJ: **Flavopiridol induces G1 arrest with inhibition of cyclin-dependent kinase (CDK) 2 and CDK4 in human breast carcinoma cells.** *Cancer Res* 1996, **56**(13):2973–2978.
35. Meijer L, Borgne A, Mulner O, Chong JP, Blow JJ, Inagaki N, Inagaki M, Delcros JG, Moulinoux JP: **Biochemical and cellular effects of roscovitine, a potent and selective inhibitor of the cyclin-dependent kinases cdc2, cdk2 and cdk5.** *Eur J Biochem* 1997, **243**(1–2):527–536.

36. Neckers LM, Cossman J: Transferrin receptor induction in mitogen-stimulated human T lymphocytes is required for DNA synthesis and cell division and is regulated by interleukin 2. *Proc Natl Acad Sci U S A* 1983, **80**(11):3494–3498.

37. Ohkuma M, Haraguchi N, Ishii H, Mimori K, Tanaka F, Kim HM, Shimomura M, Hirose H, Yanaga K, Mori M: Absence of CD71 transferrin receptor characterizes human gastric adenosquamous carcinoma stem cells. *Ann Surg Oncol* 2012, **19**(4):1357–1364.

38. Cannistra SA, Groshek P, Griffin JD: Granulocyte-macrophage colony-stimulating factor enhances the cytotoxic effects of cytosine arabinoside in acute myeloblastic leukemia and in the myeloid blast crisis phase of chronic myeloid leukemia. *Leukemia* 1989, **3**(5):328–334.

39. Tafuri A, Andreeff M: Kinetic rationale for cytokine-induced recruitment of myeloblastic leukemia followed by cycle-specific chemotherapy *in vitro*. *Leukemia* 1990, **4**(12):826–834.

40. Saito Y, Uchida N, Tanaka S, Suzuki N, Tomizawa-Murasawa M, Sone A, Najima Y, Takagi S, Aoki Y, Wake A, *et al*: Induction of cell cycle entry eliminates human leukemia stem cells in a mouse model of AML. *Nat Biotechnol* 2010, **28**(3):275–280.

41. Pabst T, Vellenga E, van Putten W, Schouten HC, Graux C, Vekemans MC, Biemond B, Sonneveld P, Passweg J, Verdonck L, *et al*: Favorable effect of priming with granulocyte colony-stimulating factor in remission induction of acute myeloid leukemia restricted to dose-escalation of cytarabine. *Blood* 2012, **119**:5367–5373.

42. Hoshii T, Tadokoro Y, Naka K, Ooshio T, Muraguchi T, Sugiyama N, Soga T, Araki K, Yamamura K, Hirao A: mTORC1 is essential for leukemia propagation but not stem cell self-renewal. *J Clin Invest* 2012, **122**(6): 2114–2129.

43. Bible KC, Kaufmann SH: Flavopiridol: a cytotoxic flavone that induces cell death in noncycling A549 human lung carcinoma cells. *Cancer Res* 1996, **56**(21):4856–4861.

44. Chao SH, Price DH: Flavopiridol inactivates P-TEFb and blocks most RNA polymerase II transcription *in vivo*. *J Biol Chem* 2001, **276**(34):31793–31799.

45. Rizzolio F, Tuccinardi T, Caligiuri I, Lucchetti C, Giordano A: CDK inhibitors: from the bench to clinical trials. *Curr Drug Targets* 2010, **11**(3):279–290.

46. Karp JE, Garrett-Mayer E, Estey EH, Rudek MA, Smith BD, Greer JM, Drye DM, Mackey K, Dorcy KS, Gore SD, *et al*: Randomized phase II study of two schedules of flavopiridol given as timed sequential therapy with cytosine arabinoside and mitoxantrone for adults with newly diagnosed, poor-risk acute myelogenous leukemia. *Haematologica* 2012, **97**(11):1736–1742.

47. Lansdorp PM, Dragowska W: Long-term erythropoiesis from constant numbers of CD34+ cells in serum-free cultures initiated with highly purified progenitor cells from human bone marrow. *J Exp Med* 1992, **175**(6):1501–1509.

23

Raltegravir does not revert efflux activity of MDR1-P-glycoprotein in human MDR cells

Maria Luisa Dupuis, Alessandro Ascione, Lucia Palmisano, Stefano Vella and Maurizio Cianfriglia[*]

Abstract

Background: Raltegravir (Isentress®)(RALT) has demonstrated excellent efficacy in both treatment-experienced and naïve patients with HIV-1 infection, and is the first strand transfer integrase inhibitor to be approved for use in HIV infected adults worldwide. Since the *in vivo* efficacy of this class of antiviral drugs depends on their access to intracellular sites where HIV-1 replicates, we analyzed the biological effects induced by RALT on human MDR cell systems expressing multidrug transporter MDR1-P-glycoprotein (MDR1-Pgp).

Methods: Our study about RALT was performed by using a set of consolidated methodologies suitable for evaluating the MDR1-Pgp substrate nature of chemical and biological agents, namely: i) assay of drug efflux function; ii) analysis of MDR reversing capability by using cell proliferation assays; iii) monoclonal antibody UIC2 (mAb) shift test, as a sensitive assay to analyze conformational transition associated with MDR1-Pgp function; and iv) induction of MDR1-Pgp expression in MDR cell variant subjected to RALT exposure.

Results: Functional assays demonstrated that the presence of RALT does not remarkably interfere with the efflux mechanism of CEM-VBL100 and HL60 MDR cells. Accordingly, cell proliferation assays clearly indicated that RALT does not revert MDR phenotype in human MDR1-Pgp expressing cells. Furthermore, exposure of CEM-VBL10 cells to RALT does not induce MDR1-Pgp functional conformation intercepted by monoclonal antibody (mAb) UIC2 binding; nor does exposure to RALT increase the expression of this drug transporter in MDR1-Pgp expressing cells.

Conclusions: No evidence of RALT interaction with human MDR1-Pgp was observed in the *in vitro* MDR cell systems used in the present investigation, this incorporating all sets of studies recommended by the FDA guidelines. Taken in aggregate, these data suggest that RALT may express its curative potential in all sites were HIV-1 penetrates, including the MDR1-Pgp protected blood/tissue barrier. Moreover RALT, evading MDR1-Pgp drug efflux function, would not interfere with pharmacokinetic profiles of co-administered MDR1-Pgp substrate antiretroviral drugs.

Keywords: Raltegravir, MDR1-Pgp, Drug substrate, MDR1-Pgp induction, Antiretroviral treatment

Background

The suboptimal penetration of antiretroviral agents into sanctuary sites such as the central nervous system or into target CD4 cells may contribute to viral persistency. Drug transporters are viewed as one of the major mechanisms which account for suboptimal tissue concentrations of antiretroviral agents. MDR1-P-glycoprotein (MDR1-Pgp, ABCB1), as well as other ABC family members of structurally and functionally related proteins, is a plasma membrane transporter which participates in the transport of a wide variety of drugs, including anti-cancer chemotherapeutics [1] and antiretroviral compounds [2]. The antiviral agent Raltegravir (Isentress®)(RALT) is the first integrase inhibitor (IIN) to be approved for treatment of HIV infection in adults [3,4]. However, the involvement of human drug transporters in RALT absorption, disposition, metabolism and excretion (ADME) has not been fully investigated. RALT has been described as being an MDR1-Pgp substrate [5,6], but there are still few data in the public domain, which are not even definitive.

As for all known anti-retrovirals, the emergence of viral mutations conferring resistance to antiretroviral agents has been documented for this compound [7]. However,

* Correspondence: Maurizio.Cianfriglia@iss.it
Department of Therapeutic Research and Medicines Evaluation, Istituto Superiore di Sanità, Viale Regina Elena 299, Rome, Italy

drug resistance may also be caused by the biological activity of MDR1-Pgp and/or other members of the ABC transporter family which, through intercepting drugs by means of the binding transport sites within the MDR1-Pgp binding pocket, delivers them out of the cells *via* an ATP dependent mechanism [8,9]. MDR1-Pgp was initially studied in the setting of anticancer treatment; it was identified as the biological entity conferring the multidrug resistance (MDR) in tumor cells, this by reducing the level of cytotoxic drug under sub-lethal concentration [10]. *In vitro* and *in vivo* studies have shown that all protease inhibitors display a high affinity for MDR1-Pgp [11-13], as well the CCR5 inhibitor maraviroc [6,14] and quinolonyl diketoacid derivatives (DKA) with anti-integrase activity [15]. These latter compounds, although different in chemical structure from RALT, exert a similar inhibition on strand transfer activity of HIV-1 integrase. Since *in vivo* efficacy of this class of drugs depends on their access to intracellular sites where HIV-1 replicates, and given that limited information exists on RALT interaction with human MDR1-Pgp expressing cells, we performed a set of well-established *in vitro* studies on the human CD4 positive lymphoblastoid CCRF-CEM cell line and its derivative MDR variants, in line with FDA concept paper on drug interactions [16]. In order to strengthen the data about the interaction between RALT and human MDR1-Pgp, we incorporated an additional human MDR cell system in this investigation. In line with FDA recommendations, we evaluated RALT as substrate, inhibitor and inducer of MDR1-Pgp by performing the following studies: i) inhibition of drug transport function by using the classical efflux assay [17]; ii) down-modulation of multidrug resistance (MDR) phenotype in cell proliferation assay [18]; iii) up-modulation of the monoclonal antibody (mAb) UIC2 epitope in MDR cells during MDR1-Pgp-mediated drug transport [19]; and iv) induction of MDR1-Pgp expression by exposing MDR CEM-VBL10 cells to MDR1-Pgp substrates [20].

Results and discussion

Assessment of MDR1-Pgp expression level in human MDR cell lines

The studies for evaluating the functional and biological interaction of RALT with human MDR1-Pgp were conducted by using two different human cell systems consisting of: a) the lymphoblastoid CD4 positive cell line CCRF-CEM and its derivative MDR variants CEM-VBL10 and CEM-VBL100 expressing increased level of MDR1-Pgp binding sites and relative resistance; b) the drug sensitive/resistant HL60 and HL60-DNR cell pairs of acute myeloid leukemia (AML) origin. The MDR phenotype of such cells was tested and monitored by the highly specific mAb MM4.17 to the external MDR1-Pgp domain [21]. The binding profiles shown in Figure 1 confirm the

MDR nature of CEM-VBL10, CEM VBL100 and HL60-DNR cells, while the parental drug sensitive cell lines CCRF-CEM and HL60 were not recognized by the mAb, thereby indicating the absence of detectable MDR1-Pgp molecules.

Drug efflux

Rhodamine 123 (Rh123) is a fluorescent marker substrate for MDR1-Pgp; incubation of MDR1-Pgp-positive cells with this drug, followed by washing and further incubation at 37°C, results in a diminished fluorescence profile due to the active drug transport exerted by the MDR1-Pgp efflux system expressed in MDR cells. The presence of a MDR1-Pgp inhibitor such as Verapamil (Vrp) during incubation and/or drug extrusion, restores Rh123 fluorescence [17]. As shown in Figure 2, differently from the potent MDR1-Pgp drug transporter inhibitor Vrp, RALT is not capable at the indicated concentrations to inhibit drug efflux and does not produce Rh123 accumulation in both CEM-VBL100 and HL60-DNR MDR cells. In order to verify the absence of inhibitory effect of RALT on MDR1-Pgp function, additional drug efflux assays were performed with VBL-bodipy and Calcein-AM: these studies showed that the drug does not affect the efflux of the fluorescent dye substrate VBL-bodipy while a little shift involving 5-10% of the Calcein-AM treated cells was observed (Additional file 1: Figure S1). Therefore, these data confirm the absence of a remarkable inhibitory activity of RALT on MDR1-Pgp expressing cells.

Proliferation assay

To evaluate RALT's potential ability to down modulate the MDR phenotype, standard proliferation assays were used. The experiments were performed by using increasing concentrations of the potent cytotoxic drug vinblastine (VBL) in presence and absence of RALT and the MDR reversing agent Vrp. The concentration of RALT equal to 12.5 µg/mL used in proliferation assays, is twice that observed in plasma of patients treated with conventional RALT dosage [22]. The study was conducted both on drug sensitive parental cells and their derivative variants CEM-VBL100 and HL60-DNR. The growth curves shown in the Figure 3 demonstrate that RALT does not induce any modulation of MDR phenotype on CEM-VBL100 and HL60-DNR cell lines; this suggests that this antiviral drug does not interfere with MDR1-Pgp drug transport function. The cell growth patterns of CEM-VBL100 cells (Figure 3, Panel A) obtained in the presence of VBL and VBL plus RALT are similar as evidenced by their IC50 values (0.226 ± 0.053 µg/mL and 0.201 ± 0.047 µg/mL, respectively) (Figure 3, Panel B). Likewise, the cell growth profiles obtained with HL60-DNR in VBL and VBL plus RALT (Figure 3, Panel A) containing cell culture conditions may be considered comparable in terms of IC50 values

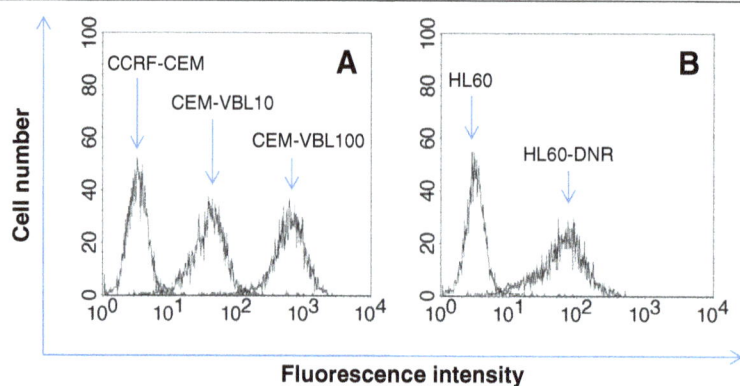

Figure 1 MDR cell lines. MDR1-Pgp expression was determined by the highly specific mAb MM4.17. In **Panel A**, the binding profiles obtained by staining the parental drug sensitive cell line CCRF-CEM and its derivative MDR variants (CEM-VBL10 and CEM-VBL100) are shown. In **Panel B**, there are the binding profiles of the AML drug sensitive/resistant cell pairs HL60 and HL60-DNR.

$(0.062 \pm 0.011$ μg/mL and 0.067 ± 0.010 μg/mL, respectively) (Figure 3, Panel B). In contrast, the growth curve profiles of both CEM-VBL100 and HL60-DNR MDR cells cultured in the presence of VBL and the MDR reversing agent Vrp, show a dramatic inhibition of cell proliferation caused by down modulation of MDR1-Pgp activity. The IC50 values calculated for the CEM-VBL100 and HL60-DNR in the presence of Vrp were 0.0052 ± 0.0010 μg/mL and 0.0050 ± 0.0010 μg/mL, respectively (Figure 3, Panels A and B). The cell growth curve patterns of the parental drug sensitive CCRF-CEM and HL60 cell lines show, as expected, a higher susceptibility to VBL, while no further biological effect was observed in the presence of the various combinations of drugs (Figure 3, Panels A and B). In order to better elucidate the potential interaction of RALT with MDR1-Pgp, we exposed the panel of cell lines to different amounts of RALT ranging from 0.1 to 100 μg/mL. In this case, the parental drug sensitive cells seem to be more susceptible to RALT in respect to their MDR variants (Figure 4). Considering the small magnitude of growth inhibition, this phenomenon may simply reflect a different drug susceptibility among the cell types observed in *in vitro* conditions. However, it cannot be ruled out that RALT may behave as a weak substrate, and that the MDR1-Pgp molecules expressed on MDR cells act as a drug transporter lowering the drug concentration and its related cytotoxic effect. This result might justify the observation of the small fraction of MDR cell population retaining the dye substrate Calcein-AM in the drug efflux studies (Additional file 1: Figure S1). Furthermore, this hypothesis may be in partial in agreement with previous published findings showing that a reduction of RALT efflux of only 32% was observed when the potent reversing agent Tariquidar was used to inhibit ABCB1 in CEM VBL100 cells [5]. To this regard, it should here mentioned as FDA guidelines recommend that a drug should achieve an efflux ratio

greater than a 50% reduction when an ABCB1 inhibitor is used in order for ABCB1 transport to be considered relevant *in vivo* [16]. To further investigate the RALT modulating effect on MDR1-Pgp, the mAb UIC2 shift assay was used. This test is a useful tool for detecting conformational changes associated with the function of MDR1-Pgp and provides a potentially useful diagnostic test for both the expression and the function of MDR1-Pgp [19].

UIC2 shift assay

The UIC2 mAb (IgG2a) reacts with the extracellular moiety of MDR1-Pgp and inhibits MDR1-Pgp-mediated efflux of all tested MDR chemotherapeutic drugs. It has been shown that the reactivity of UIC2 mAb on MDR cells is enhanced in the presence of a large array of compounds recognized as MDR1-Pgp substrates which include cytotoxic agents together with certain classes of MDR reversing agents (Verapamil, Quinidine, Cyclosporine-A) [19]. This phenomenon has been used to develop a highly specific and sensitive method to confirm the MDR1-Pgp substrate and MDR reversal agent nature of several chemical agents [23,24]. Therefore, to elucidate the RALT/MDR1-Pgp interaction, we took advantage of the mAb UIC2 ability to bind with increased affinity to its target in the presence of MDR1-Pgp modulators due to conformational changes in functioning MDR1-Pgp. In order to highlight this phenomenon, we used the cell line CEM-VBL10 as MDR1-Pgp expressing cells instead of CEM-VBL100 cells, because of the former's relatively lower number of MDR1-Pgp binding sites/cell (10,000 binding sites/cell) [M. Cianfriglia, unpublished]. In general, cell lines with a higher level of MDR1-Pgp molecules require higher concentrations of MDR1-Pgp substrates for maximal stimulation [25]. The results of this study show a significant induction of mAb UIC2 binding on CEM-VBL10 cells incubated with VBL (Figure 5, Panel C), while no

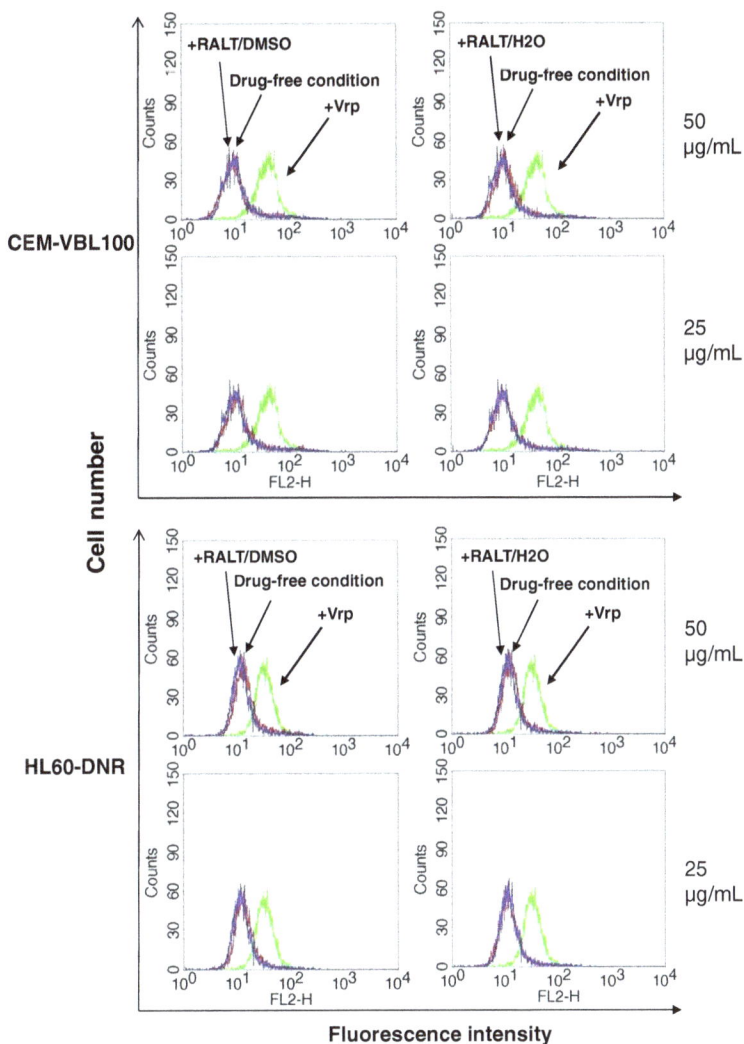

Figure 2 Evaluation of Rh123 transport inhibition mediated by RALT. The efflux of the dye MDR1-Pgp substrate Rh123 in CEM-VBL100 and HL60-DNR MDR cells was monitored in drug-free conditions (blue histogram), in the presence of the potent MDR1-Pgp blocker Vrp (2.5 μg/mL) (green histogram), and following incubation with RALT (red histogram) dissolved in DMSO or H2O at the concentrations shown on the right side of the panels.

UIC2 mAb binding shift was observed in presence of 25 and 50 μg/mL of RALT (Figure 5, Panel A and B).

Induction of MDR1-Pgp expression in MDR cells

Since the discovery of the simultaneous resistance of tumor cells to a large array of anti-cancer compounds in the late 1970s, the inhibition of MDR1-Pgp conferring the MDR has become an attractive therapeutic strategy in order to *de novo* sensitize tumor cells to anticancer drugs in cancer patients [26]. However, drug/drug interactions are critical factors in all therapeutic regimens, the co-administration of MDR modulators with drugs that are MDR1-Pgp substrates needing to be balanced with lower drug concentrations to avoid unpredictable side effects [27]. In this regard, the FDA concept paper on drug interactions recommends that new drug candidates should be evaluated as substrates, inhibitors, and also as inducers of MDR1-Pgp [16]. We therefore decided to study the induction of MDR1-Pgp after a prolonged exposure to various concentrations of RALT of CEM-VBL10 cells, which are very prone to modulate MDR1-Pgp expression in the presence of cytotoxic drugs and/or MDR1-Pgp substrates. In parallel experiments, the cells were cultured with increasing amounts of the potent MDR1-Pgp inducer and substrate VBL. The relationship of RALT and VLB concentrations are absolutely empirical, but congruous to demonstrate different induction phenomena exerted by these drugs. In the presence of VBL, CEM-VBL10 cells "respond" by increasing the percentage of MDR cells in relationship with drug concentration, as evidenced by the

A

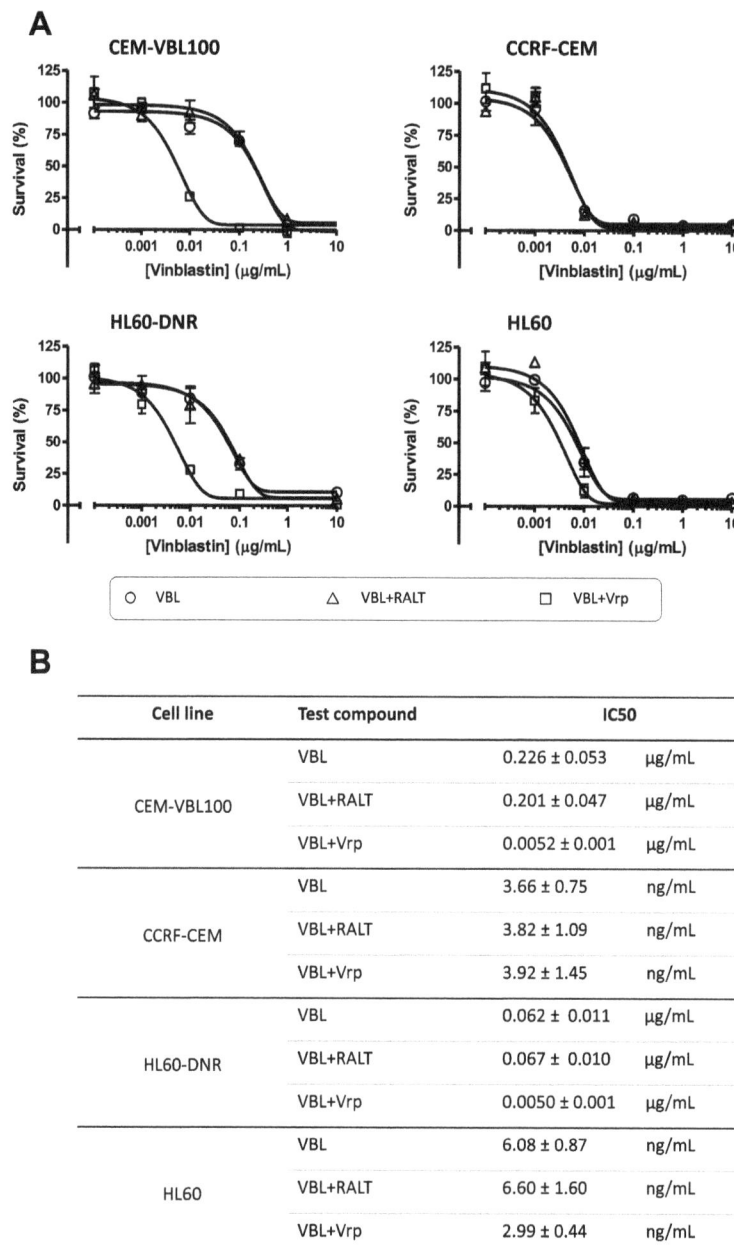

B

Cell line	Test compound	IC50	
CEM-VBL100	VBL	0.226 ± 0.053	µg/mL
	VBL+RALT	0.201 ± 0.047	µg/mL
	VBL+Vrp	0.0052 ± 0.001	µg/mL
CCRF-CEM	VBL	3.66 ± 0.75	ng/mL
	VBL+RALT	3.82 ± 1.09	ng/mL
	VBL+Vrp	3.92 ± 1.45	ng/mL
HL60-DNR	VBL	0.062 ± 0.011	µg/mL
	VBL+RALT	0.067 ± 0.010	µg/mL
	VBL+Vrp	0.0050 ± 0.001	µg/mL
HL60	VBL	6.08 ± 0.87	ng/mL
	VBL+RALT	6.60 ± 1.60	ng/mL
	VBL+Vrp	2.99 ± 0.44	ng/mL

Figure 3 MDR chemosensitization. In the upper part of the figure the dose-response growth curves of drug sensitive parental cell lines (CCRF-CEM and HL60) and their derivative MDR variants (CEM-VBL100 and HL60/DNR) are shown **(Panel A)**. The cells were cultured for 72 h in medium containing increasing concentrations of VBL alone (open circles), VBL plus 12.5 µg/mL of the IIN RALT (open triangles), and VBL plus 2.5 µg/mL of the MDR1-Pgp blocker Vrp (open squares). In the lower part of the figure **(Panel B)**, the IC50 values (concentrations of the compound that inhibits cell growth by 50%) for each cell culture condition are reported. Values are means of three independent experiments, each done in triplicate.

progressive shift of the fluorescence profiles obtained with the MDR1-Pgp specific antibody MM4.17 (left part of Figure 6). In contrast, RALT is totally ineffective in inducing MDR1-Pgp expression up to the maximum tested concentration of 50 µg/mL (right part of Figure 6). By exposing CEM-VBL10 to an additional increase of drug concentrations (100 ng/mL of VBL and 100 µg/mL of

RALT), a large phenomenon of cell death in the VBL containing cultures was observed, but no particular biological effect with regard to the RALT (data not shown).

Several clinical trials have shown a sustained antiretroviral effect and a good tolerability of RALT in naive and treatment-experienced HIV-1 infected patients [28]. Previous investigations have already reported that RALT has a

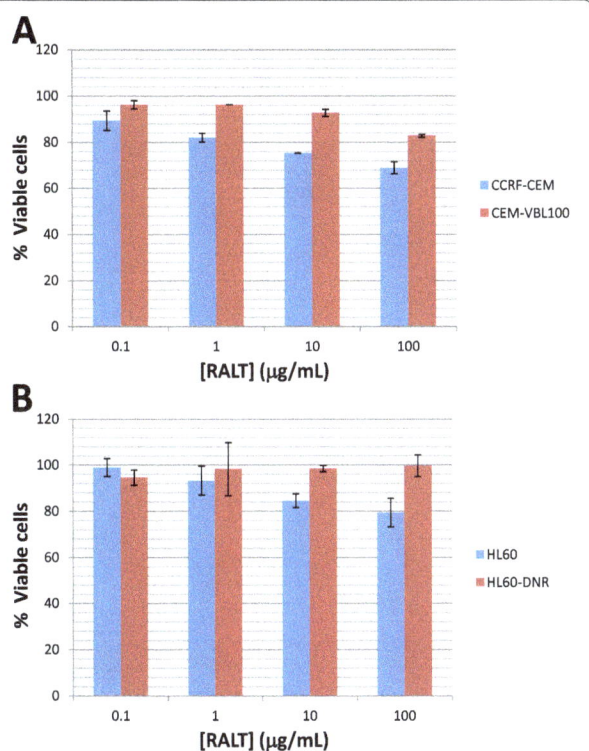

Figure 4 Growth inhibition assay. Concentration-dependent effect of the RALT on proliferation rate of drug sensitive/resistant cell pairs CCRF-CEM and HL60 (**Panels A** and **B**, respectively) after 72 h of culture. The figure depicts one representative experiment, and data are expressed as % of untreated control cells with each concentration tested in triplicate.

or CYP3A4-dependent testosterone 6 beta-hydroxylase activity [14]. In previous studies conducted by our group, a series of diketoacid-containing derivatives (DKA) functioning as inhibitors of HIV-1 integrase have been described as being MDR1-Pgp ABCB1 substrates [15] with strong MDR1-Pgp inhibitory activity. Elvitegravir [4,6], which has a biochemical formulation similar to DKA, shows marked drug interaction with MDR1-Pgp multi-drug transporter and acts as a strong MDR reversing agent [15]. Our study performed with human MDR cell lines clearly shows that the RALT compound does not inhibit MDR1-Pgp mediated drug transport function. The different level of cytotoxic effect exerted by RALT on drug sensitive/resistant cell pairs (Figure 4) and the low shift of a small fraction of MDR cell population incubated in presence of Calcein-AM may be cell type and dye-substrate related, and not sufficient to establish the existence of an authentic interaction with MDR1-Pgp. In this context, Zambruski et al. [6], include elvitegravir, vicriviroc and to a lesser extent RALT in the list of MDR1-Pgp substrates. However, our own findings concerning RALT seem to suggest otherwise, a possible explanation being in the different cell system used and in the interpretation of data. Again in this regard, Moss et al. showed that RALT has minimal interactions with known drug transporters, and that the rate of MDR1-Pgp-mediated transport *in vitro* is so low that the potential for interactions of this entity is expected to be small [5]. The very low rate of RALT transport by MDR1-Pgp expressing cells may explain the absence of major drug interactions with known potent MDR1-Pgp inhibitors. Furthermore, very recently, Tempestilli et al., [30] showed that darunavir, unlike RALT, may modify the expression and functionality of MDR1-Pgp on human lymphocytes. Taken in aggregate, the above mentioned studies are consistent with a previous report where the co-administration of low-dose ritonavir had no major effect on RALT pharmacokinetics, and no dose adjustment was required for patients [31].

low propensity for involvement in drug–drug interactions [6]. Update studies on pharmacology profile of RALT are described in the recently published review article by Brainard et al. [29], which reports that RALT is not an inhibitor of the major CYP isozymes, including CYP3A4, UGTs, and MDR1-Pgp. Additionally, it has been reported that RALT is not an inducer of CYP3A4 RNA expression

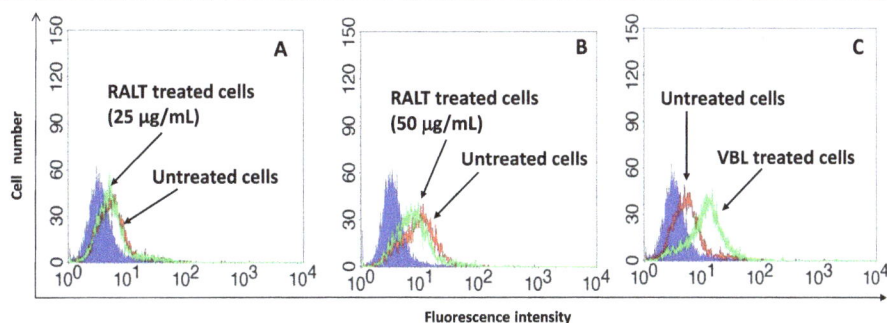

Figure 5 Modulation of the UIC2 epitope. In the **Panel A** and **B** the binding profiles of the mAb UIC2 on CEM-VBL10 MDR cells are shown (red histogram); incubation of the cells with RALT (25 and 50 μg/mL) does not interfere with mAb UIC2 binding (green histogram). Conversely, a marked shift of mAb binding UIC2 is observed incubating CEM-VBL10 cells with VBL (10 μg/mL) (**Panel C**, green histogram). The filled profile represents cells stained with secondary antibody alone.

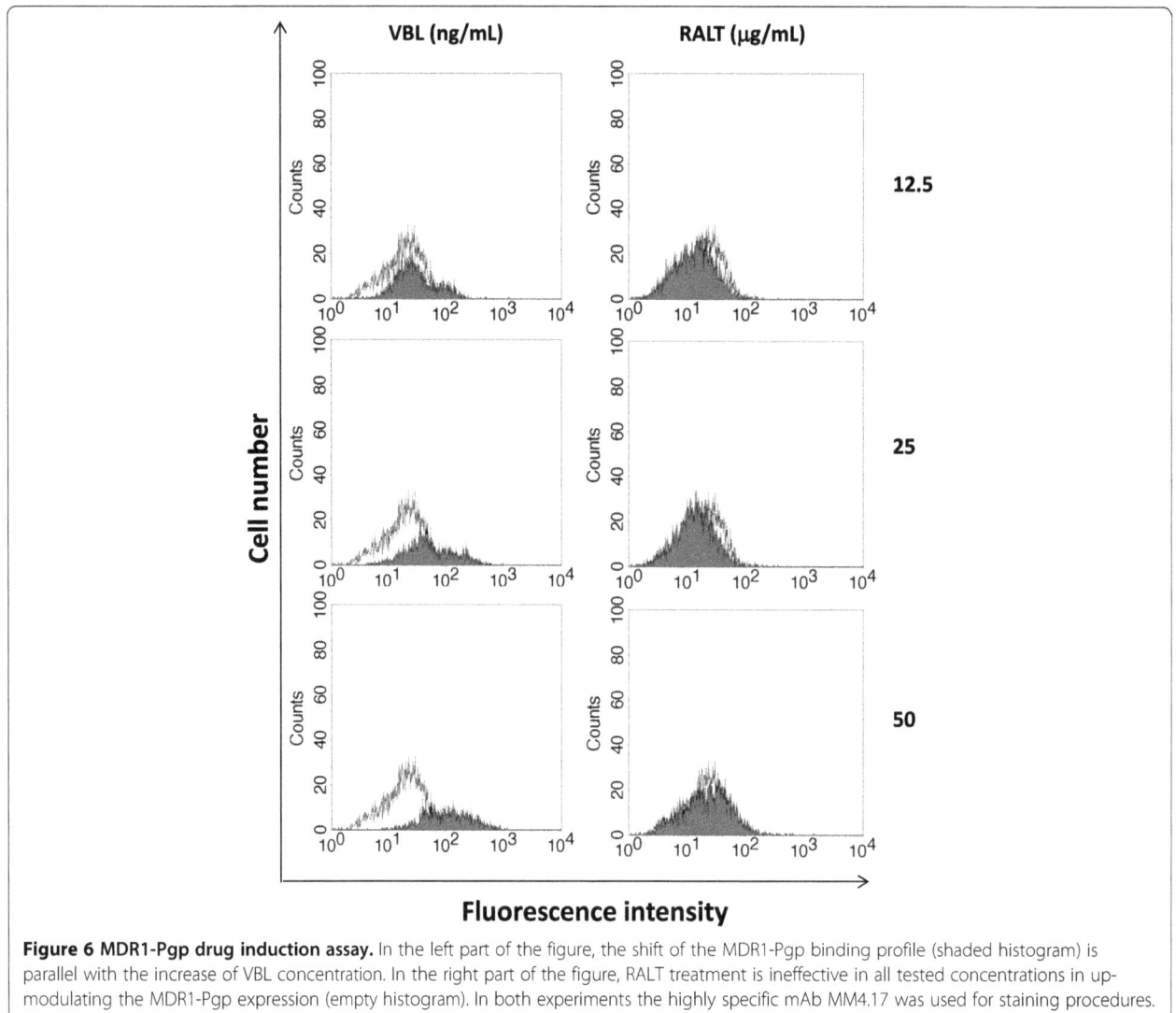

Figure 6 MDR1-Pgp drug induction assay. In the left part of the figure, the shift of the MDR1-Pgp binding profile (shaded histogram) is parallel with the increase of VBL concentration. In the right part of the figure, RALT treatment is ineffective in all tested concentrations in up-modulating the MDR1-Pgp expression (empty histogram). In both experiments the highly specific mAb MM4.17 was used for staining procedures.

Overall, these findings suggest that, in addition to its well known efficacy and safety, RALT may present an advantage in respect to other anti-retrovirals that are MDR1-Pgp substrate. Indeed, RALT's biological properties may endow it with a higher therapeutic potential against HIV-1 residing in sanctuaries sites pharmacologically protected by MDR1-Pgp expressed on blood tissue barriers. However, in this context, it is important to remember that, despite MDR1-Pgp is the first discovered and probably the most widely studied ABC transporter protein, there are other ABC transporters involved in clinical MDR and in drug absorption and distribution; these include multidrug resistance proteins (MRPs, ABCCs) and breast cancer resistant protein (BCRP, ABCG2) [32,33]. In particular, MRP1, MRP2, MRP4 and BCRP/ABCG2, together with MDR1-Pgp, are present on many barrier sites such as the blood-brain barrier and on many circulating cells such as lymphocytes, and consequently they could contribute

to reduce antiretroviral agents in sanctuary or HIV-1 target sites [34].

Conclusions

Our investigations demonstrate that RALT is ineffective in inhibiting drug efflux and in down-modulating the MDR phenotype of human CEM and HL60 MDR cells to an extent considered relevant *in vivo* by FDA guidelines [16]. In addition, exposure of CEM-VBL10 to RALT does not induce the functional conformation of MDR1-Pgp intercepted by the shift of UIC2 mAb binding. Furthermore, in contrast to other licensed anti-HIV-1 drugs such as the protease inhibitors, RALT has proved to be ineffective in inducing an increase of MDR1-Pgp expression level in MDR cells in culture conditions. The absence of remarkable RALT/MDR1-Pgp interaction may represent a medically relevant property, although at present its impact in the clinical setting is not totally clear. Further studies are warranted to better define i) the mechanisms underlying the profound functional differences of RALT in comparison with other IINs which behave as MDR-Pgp substrates and MDR reversing agents and, ii) the potential involvement of other ABC drug transporters in RALT absorption and disposition.

Methods

Chemicals

The RALT was a kind gift of the Merck company (Pomezia, Rome, Italy); Verapamil (Isoptin) was purchased by Abbott (Latina, Italy); Vinblastine (Velbe) by Eli Lilly (Paris, France); Rhodamine-123 was purchased from Sigma (St. Louis, MO). Vinblastine-bodipy (VBL-bodipy) and Calcein acetoxymethlyl ester (Calcein-AM) were purchased from Molecular Probes (Eugene, OH).

Cell lines

The multidrug resistant (MDR) variants CEM-VBL10 and CEM-VBL100 cells were isolated by stepwise selection of the parental drug sensitive CCRF-CEM (CEM) in the presence of increasing concentrations of VBL [up to the final concentration of 10 and 100 ng/mL, respectively]. Cells were grown under standard conditions for mammalian cells cultured in suspension. The basic medium (BM) for cell culturing consisted of RPMI-1640 supplemented with 10% foetal calf serum (FCS), L-glutamine (2 mM) penicillin (100 U/mL) and streptomycin (100 U/mL). All these components were purchased from Hyclone (Logan, Utah, USA). Identical culture conditions were adopted for the multidrug resistant (MDR) variants HL60-DNR, kindly provided by Dr. Ruoping Tang (Hopitaux de Paris, Paris, France).

MDR efflux assay

CEM-VBL100 and HL60-DNR cell lines (1×10^6) were loaded with Rh123 (5 µg/mL)(or with VBL-bodipy, 50 ng/mL, or Calcein-AM, 50 ng/mL) in 1 mL of BM in the presence of RALT (concentrations: 50 and 25 µg/mL) or Vrp (2.5 µg/mL) for 1 h at 37°C. The cells were incubated with Rh123 at the indicated concentrations or with drug diluents (DMSO: 0.5%; H2O). At the end of incubation, the cells were washed in serum-free medium and re-suspended in BM in the presence of RALT or Vrp (drug diluents was added in control samples) for a further 1 h at 37°C. Finally, cells were washed twice with ice cold phosphate-buffered saline (PBS)/FACS, and analyzed in a flow cytometer (FACScan, Becton Dickinson, San Josè, CA).

Cell proliferation assay

The parental drug sensitive and their MDR derivative cell lines in exponential phase of growth were collected, extensively washed with warm RPMI-1640 and seeded in (in triplicate) in 96-well microtiter Costar plates (Costar, Rochester, NY) at a density of 5×10^3 cells/mL.

For MDR chemosensitization studies, the cells were cultured in BM containing increasing concentrations of VBL ranging from 0 to 10 µg/mL; in parallel, MDR cell cultures containing the different concentrations of VBL were grown in the presence of RALT (12.5 µg/mL) dissolved in water. As a control the MDR reversing agent Vrp was used at the concentration of 2.5 µg/mL in an additionally parallel culture. In growth inhibition assays RALT was tested alone at 4 concentrations spread over a range between 0 and 100 µg/mL. For all above described experiments cell survival was determined by WST-1 assay (PreMix WST-1 cell proliferation kit, Vinci Biochem, Firenze, Italy) after 72 h treatment at 37°C in 5% CO2. The values describing the concentration-response profiles are calculated as % of appropriated control and represent the mean of three independent experiments, each done in triplicate. The GraphPad Prism statistical analysis program was used.

Monoclonal antibodies and UIC-2 Shift assay

The mAb UIC2 [19] was kindly provided by Dr. E. Mechetner (Chemicon Inc, Temecula, CA). For determination of MDR1-Pgp expression, the mAb MM4.17 recognizing an extracellular MDR1-P-gp epitope on intact/living human MDR cells [21] was used (data not shown). Both UIC2 and MM4.17 mAbs were used in a highly purified form. The UIC2 shift assay was performed under physiological conditions as previously described [19]. CEM-VBL10 cells (1×10^6) were resuspended in 1 mL of PBS containing 2% FCS and allowed to equilibrate at 37°C in a water bath for 10 min. The RALT was added to samples (final concentration 25 and 50 µg/mL) and incubated for additional 15 min at 37°C with purified UIC2 mAb (final concentration 12.5 µg/mL). VBL (10 µg/mL), a well known UIC2 shifting agent, was used as positive control do detect the conformation of MDR1-Pgp during drug efflux function. Cells were then washed twice in ice-cold PBS containing 2% FCS with 0.01% sodium azide (Shift Stop Buffer, SSB), stained on ice in SSB for additional 15 min with 5 µg/mL of fluorescein-conjugated goat-antimouse antibody (FITC-GAM, Cappel, West Chester, Pa, USA), washed twice with ice cold PBS/FACS and maintained in ice until flow cytometry analysis.

Induction of MDR1-Pgp expression in MDR cells

For the evaluation of the induction of MDR phenotype, CEM-VBL10 cells in exponential phase of growth were collected, extensively washed with warm RPMI-1640 and resuspended at the concentration of 5×10^4 cells/mL in BM alone, or in the presence of different VBL concentrations (from 100 ng/mL to 12.5 ng /mL) or RALT (from 100 µg/mL to 12.5 µg/mL) and were seeded in

24-wells Costar plates (Costar, Rochester, NY) for 96 h. At the end of the incubation, the cells were harvested, washed with BM alone, and incubated with 12.5 µg/mL of mAb MM4.17. After 30 min of incubation at 4°C, the cells were washed, pelleted, resuspended and incubated for an additional 30 min at 4°C in the presence of fluorescein-conjugated goat antimouse antibody (FITC-GAM, Cappel). After incubation, the cells were washed, resuspended in PBS and processed for flow cytometry analysis.

Data presentation
All the experiments were repeated at least thrice. The significance was assessed by Student's t-test and the criterion for statistical significance was set at P < 0.05.

Additional file

Additional file 1: Figure S1. Evaluation of VBL-bodipy and Calcein-AM transport inhibition mediated by RALT. The efflux of the fluorescent dyes MDR1-Pgp substrate VBL-bodipy (upper part of the Figure) and Calcein-AM (lower part of the Figure) on CEM-VBL100 MDR cells was monitored in drug-free conditions (red histogram), in the presence of the potent MDR1-Pgp blocker Vrp (2.5 µg/mL) (green histogram), and following incubation with 50 µg/mL RALT (blue histogram) dissolved in DMSO or H2O.

Abbreviations
RALT: Raltegravir; IIN: Integrase inhibitor; MDR1-Pgp and ABCB1: MDR1-P-glycoprotein; MDR: Multidrug resistance; DKA: Quinolonyl diketoacid derivatives; mAb: Monoclonal antibody; Rh123: Rhodamine-123; Vrp: Verapamil; VBL: Vinblastine.

Competing interests
The authors declare that they have no competing interests.

Authors' contributions
CM and LP: conceived and planned the biological approach of this study, participated in the design and coordination of the research and drafted the manuscript. DML and AA: conceived and conducted all the cell biological experiments to demonstrate the biological function of the integrase inhibitor. SV: coordinated and supervised the study. All authors read and approved the final manuscript.

Acknowledgements
This work has been possible thanks to funding received from EC in the Project: The European AIDS Treatment Network, (NEAT) with contract number LSHP-CT-2006-037570, which is a FP 6 Network of Excellence within the "Integrating and Strengthening the European Research Area". This work was supported by AIDS grants of Istituto Superiore di Sanità and Italian Ministry of Health, and partly by an ISS-NIH research grant. It was also supported by a research grant from the Investigator Initiated Studies Program of Merck Sharp & Dohme Corp. The opinions expressed in this paper are those of the authors and do not necessarily represent those of Merck Sharp & Dohme Corp. We thank Mrs Stefania Donnini for secretarial support and Martin Bennett for his help in revising the manuscript for grammar and style.

References
1. Gottesman MM, Fojo T, Bates SE: Multidrug resistance in cancer: role of ATP-dependent transporters. Nat Rev Cancer 2002, 2:248–258.
2. Sakaeda T, Nakamura T, Okumura K: Pharmacogenetics of MDR1 and its impact on the pharmacokinetics and pharmacodynamics of drugs. Pharmacogenomics 2003, 4:397–410.
3. Summa V, Petrocchi A, Bonelli F, Crescenzi B, Donghi M, Ferrara M, Fiore F, Gardelli C, Gonzalez Paz O, Hazuda DJ, Jones P, Kinzel O, Laufer R, Monteagudo E, Muraglia E, Nizi E, Orvieto F, Pace P, Pescatore G, Scarpelli R, Stillmock K, Witmer MV, Rowley M: Discovery of raltegravir, a potent, selective orally bioavailable HIV-integrase inhibitor for the treatment of HIV-AIDS infection. J Med Chem 2008, 51:584–237.
4. Pandey KK: Raltegravir in HIV-1 infection: safety and efficacy in treatment-naïve patients. Clin Med Rev Ther 2012, 2011:13–30.
5. Moss DM, Kwan WS, Liptrott NJ, Smith DL, Siccardi M, Khoo SH, Back DJ, Owen A: Raltegravir Is a Substrate for SLC22A6: a Putative Mechanism for the Interaction between Raltegravir and Tenofovir. Antimicrob Agents Chemother 2011, 55:879–887.
6. Zembruski NC, Büchel G, Jödicke L, Herzog M, Haefeli WE, Weiss J: Potential of novel antiretrovirals to modulate expression and function of drug transporters in vitro. J Antimicrob Chemother 2011, 66:802–812.
7. Malet I, Delelis O, Valantin MA, Montes B, Soulie C, Wirden M, Tchertanov L, Peytavin G, Reynes J, Mouscadet JF, Katlama C, Calvez V, Marcelin AG: Mutations associated with failure of raltegravir treatment affect integrase sensitivity to the inhibitor in vitro. Antimicrob Agents Chemother 2008, 52:1351–1358.
8. Evans WE, McLeod HL: Pharmacogenomics – drug disposition, drug targets, and side effects. N Engl J Med 2003, 348:538–549.
9. Kartner N, Riordan JR, Ling V: Cell surface P-glycoprotein associated with multidrug resistance in mammalian cell lines. Science 1983, 221:1285–1288.
10. Germann UA, Pastan I, Gottesman MM: P-glycoproteins: mediators of multidrug resistance. Semin Cell Biol 1993, 4:63–76.
11. Huisman MT, Smit JW, Schinkel AH: Significance of P-glycoprotein for the pharmacology and clinical use of HIV protease inhibitors. AIDS 2000, 14:237–242.
12. Lee CG, Gottesman MM, Cardarelli CO, Ramachandra M, Jeang KT, Ambudkar SV, Pastan I, Dey S: HIV-1 protease inhibitors are substrates for the MDR1 multidrug transporter. Biochemistry 1998, 37:3594–3601.
13. Kim RB, Fromm MF, Wandel C, Leake B, Wood AJ, Roden DM, Wilkinson GR: The drug transporter P-glycoprotein limits oral absorption and brain entry of HIV-1 protease inhibitors. J Clin Invest 1998, 101:289–294.
14. Walker DK, Bowers SJ, Mitchell RJ, Potchoiba MJ, Schroeder CM, Small HF: Preclinical assessment of the distribution of maraviroc to potential human immunodeficiency virus (HIV) sanctuary sites in the central nervous system (CNS) and gut-associated lymphoid tissue (GALT). Xenobiotica 2008, 38:1330–1339.
15. Di Santo R, Costi R, Roux A, Artico M, Lavecchia A, Marinelli L, Novellino E, Palmisano L, Andreotti M, Amici R, Galluzzo CM, Nencioni L, Palamara AT, Pommier Y, Marchand C: Novel bifunctional quinolonyl diketo acid derivatives as HIV-1 integrase inhibitors: design, synthesis, biological activities, and mechanism of action. J Med Chem 2006, 49:1939–1945.
16. Huang SM, Strong JM, Zhang L, Reynolds KS, Nallani S, Temple R, Abraham S, Habet SA, Baweja RK, Burckart GJ, Chung S, Colangelo P, Frucht D, Green MD, Hepp P, Karnaukhova E, Ko HS, Lee JI, Marroum PJ, Norden JM, Qiu W, Rahman A, Sobel S, Stifano T, Thummel K, Wei XX, Yasuda S, Zheng JH, Zhao H, Lesko LJ: New era in drug interaction evaluation: US Food and Drug Administration update on CYP enzymes, transporters, and the guidance process. J Clin Pharmacol 2008, 48:662–670.
17. Chaudhary PM, Mechetner EB, Roninson IB: Expression and activity of the multidrug resistance P-glycoprotein in human peripheral blood lymphocytes. Blood 1992, 80:2735–2739.
18. Cianfriglia M, Dupuis ML, Molinari A, Verdoliva A, Costi R, Galluzzo CM, Andreotti M, Cara A, Di Santo R, Palmisano L: HIV-1 integrase inhibitors are substrates for the multidrug transporter MDR1-P-glycoprotein. Retrovirology 2007, 7:4–17.
19. Mechetner EB, Schott B, Morse BS, Stein WD, Druley T, Davis KA, Tsuruo T, Roninson IB: P-Glycoprotein function involves conformational transitions detectable by differential immunoreactivity. Proc Natl Acad Sci USA 1997, 94:12908–12913.
20. Dupuis ML, Flego M, Molinari A, Cianfriglia M: Saquinavir induces stable and functional expression of the multidrug transporter P-glycoprotein in human CD4 T-lymphoblastoid CEMrev cells. HIV Med 2003, 4:338–345.

21. Cianfriglia M, Willingham MC, Tombesi M, Scagliotti GV, Frasca G, Chersi A: P-glycoprotein epitope mapping. I: Identification of a linear human-specific epitope in the fourth loop of the Pglycoprotein extracellular domain by MM4.17 murine monoclonal antibody to human multi-drug-resistant cells. *Int J Cancer* 1994, **56:**153–160.

22. Yilmaz A, Gissle´n M, Spudich S, Lee E, Jayewardene A, Aweeka F, Price RW: **Raltegravir Cerebrospinal Fluid Concentrations in HIV-1 Infection.** *Plos One* 2009, **4:**e6877.

23. Meschini S, Marra M, Condello M, Calcabrini A, Federici E, Dupuis ML, Cianfriglia M, Arancia G: **Voacamine, an alkaloid extracted from Peschiera fuchsiaefolia, inhibits P-glycoprotein action in multidrug-resistant tumor cells.** *Int J Oncol* 2005, **27:**1597–1603.

24. Nagy H, Goda K, Fenyvesi F, Bacsó Z, Szilasi M, Kappelmayer J, Lustyik G, Cianfriglia M, Szabó G Jr: **Distinct groups of multidrug resistance modulating agents are distinguished by competition of P-glycoprotein-specific antibodies.** *Biochem Biophys Res Commun* 2004, **315:**942–949.

25. Dupuis ML, Tombesi M, Sabatini M, Cianfriglia M: **Differential effect of HIV-1 protease inhibitors on P-glycoprotein function in multidrug-resistant variants of the human CD4+ T lymphoblastoid CEM cell line.** *Chemotherapy* 2003, **49:**8–16.

26. Wu CP, Calcagno AM, Ambudkar SV: **Reversal of ABC drug transporter-mediated multidrug resistance in cancer cells: Evaluation of current strategies.** *Curr Mol Pharmacol* 2008, **1:**93–105.

27. Ramanathan S, Abel S, Tweedy S, *et al*: **Pharmacokinetic interaction of ritonavir-boosted elvitegravir and maraviroc.** *J Acquir Immune Defic Syndr* 2010, **53:**209–214.

28. Markowitz M, Morales-Ramirez JO, Nguyen B-Y, Kovacs CM, Steigbigel RT, Cooper DA, Liporace R, Schwartz R, isaacs R, Gilde LR, Wenning L, Zhao J, Teppler H: **Antiretroviral activity, pharmacokinetics, and tolerability of MK-0518 a novel inhibitor of HIV-1 integrase, dosed as monotherapy for 10 days in treatment- naive HIV-1-infected individuals.** *J Acquir Immune Defic Syndr* 2006, **43:**509–515.

29. Brainard DM, Wenning LA, Stone JA, Wagner JA, Iwamoto M: **Clinical pharmacology profile of raltegravir, an HIV-1 integrase strand transfer inhibitor.** *J Clin Pharmacol* 2011, **51:**1376–1402.

30. Tempestilli M, Gentilotti E, Tommasi C, Nicastri E, Martini F, De Nardo P, Narciso P, Pucillo LP: **Determination of P-glycoprotein surface expression and functional ability after in vitro treatment with darunavir or raltegravir in lymphocytes of healthy donors.** *Int Immunopharmacol* 2013, **16:**492–497.

31. Iwamoto M, Wenning LA, Petry AS, Laethem M, De Smet M, Kost JT, Breidinger SA, Mangin EC, Azrolan N, Greenberg HE, Haazen W, Stone JA, Gottesdiener KM, Wagner JA: **Minimal effects of ritonavir and efavirenz on the pharmacokinetics of raltegravir.** *Antimicrob Agents Chemother* 2008, **52:**4338–4343.

32. Dean M, Allikmets R: **Complete characterization of the human ABC gene family.** *J Bioenerg Biomembr* 2001, **33:**475–479.

33. Leslie EM, Deeley RG, Cole SP: **Multidrug resistance proteins: role of P-glycoprotein, MRP1, MRP2, and BCRP (ABCG2) in tissue defense.** *Toxicol Appl Pharmacol* 2005, **204:**216–237.

34. Glavinas H, Krajcsi P, Cserepes J, Sarkadi B: **The role of ABC transporters in drug resistance, metabolism and toxicity.** *Curr Drug Deliv* 2004, **1:**27–42.

Permissions

All chapters in this book were first published in BMCPT, by BioMed Central; hereby published with permission under the Creative Commons Attribution License or equivalent. Every chapter published in this book has been scrutinized by our experts. Their significance has been extensively debated. The topics covered herein carry significant findings which will fuel the growth of the discipline. They may even be implemented as practical applications or may be referred to as a beginning point for another development.

The contributors of this book come from diverse backgrounds, making this book a truly international effort. This book will bring forth new frontiers with its revolutionizing research information and detailed analysis of the nascent developments around the world.

We would like to thank all the contributing authors for lending their expertise to make the book truly unique. They have played a crucial role in the development of this book. Without their invaluable contributions this book wouldn't have been possible. They have made vital efforts to compile up to date information on the varied aspects of this subject to make this book a valuable addition to the collection of many professionals and students.

This book was conceptualized with the vision of imparting up-to-date information and advanced data in this field. To ensure the same, a matchless editorial board was set up. Every individual on the board went through rigorous rounds of assessment to prove their worth. After which they invested a large part of their time researching and compiling the most relevant data for our readers.

The editorial board has been involved in producing this book since its inception. They have spent rigorous hours researching and exploring the diverse topics which have resulted in the successful publishing of this book. They have passed on their knowledge of decades through this book. To expedite this challenging task, the publisher supported the team at every step. A small team of assistant editors was also appointed to further simplify the editing procedure and attain best results for the readers.

Apart from the editorial board, the designing team has also invested a significant amount of their time in understanding the subject and creating the most relevant covers. They scrutinized every image to scout for the most suitable representation of the subject and create an appropriate cover for the book.

The publishing team has been an ardent support to the editorial, designing and production team. Their endless efforts to recruit the best for this project, has resulted in the accomplishment of this book. They are a veteran in the field of academics and their pool of knowledge is as vast as their experience in printing. Their expertise and guidance has proved useful at every step. Their uncompromising quality standards have made this book an exceptional effort. Their encouragement from time to time has been an inspiration for everyone.

The publisher and the editorial board hope that this book will prove to be a valuable piece of knowledge for researchers, students, practitioners and scholars across the globe.

List of Contributors

Jean Lachaine
Faculty of Pharmacy, University of Montreal, Montreal, Quebec, Canada

Catherine Beauchemin
Faculty of Pharmacy, University of Montreal, Montreal, Quebec, Canada

Elodie Ramos
Health Economics and Outcomes Research, Pfizer Canada Inc., Kirkland, Quebec, Canada

Arkadiusz Gertych
Translational Cytomics Group, Department of Surgery, Cedars-Sinai Medical Center, Los Angeles, CA 90048, USA
Bioinformatics Laboratory, Department of Surgery, Cedars-Sinai Medical Center, Los Angeles, CA 90048, USA

Jin Ho Oh
Translational Cytomics Group, Department of Surgery, Cedars-Sinai Medical Center, Los Angeles, CA 90048, USA
Chromatin Biology Laboratory, Department of Surgery, Cedars-Sinai Medical Center, Los Angeles, CA 90048, USA

Kolja A Wawrowsky
Translational Cytomics Group, Department of Surgery, Cedars-Sinai Medical Center, Los Angeles, CA 90048, USA
Department of Biomedical Sciences, Cedars-Sinai Medical Center, Los Angeles, CA 90048, USA

Daniel J Weisenberger
USC Epigenome Center, Keck School of Medicine, University of Southern California, Los Angeles, CA 90089, USA

Jian Tajbakhsh
Translational Cytomics Group, Department of Surgery, Cedars-Sinai Medical Center, Los Angeles, CA 90048, USA
Chromatin Biology Laboratory, Department of Surgery, Cedars-Sinai Medical Center, Los Angeles, CA 90048, USA

Min-Wei Huang
Institute of Biomedical Engineering, National Cheng Kung University, Tainan 70403, Taiwan
Department of Psychiatry, Chiayi Branch, Taichung Veterans General Hospital, Chia-Yi 60090, Taiwan

Tsung-Tsair Yang
Department of Psychiatry, Cardinal Tien Ken-Sin Hospital, Taipei 23148, Taiwan

Po-Ren Ten
Department of Psychiatry, Show Chwan Memorial Hospital, Changhua 50008, Taiwan

Po-Wen Su
Department of Psychiatry, Chu-Tung Branch, National Taiwan University Hospital, Hsinchu 31064, Taiwan

Bo-Jian Wu
Department of Psychiatry, Yuli Hospital, Hualien 98147, Taiwan

Chin-Hong Chan
Department of Psychiatry, Taichung Veterans General Hospital, Taichung 40705, Taiwan

Tsuo-Hung Lan
Department of Psychiatry, Taichung Veterans General Hospital, Taichung 40705, Taiwan

I-Chao Liu
Department of Psychiatry, Cardinal Tien Ken-Sin Hospital, Taipei 23148, Taiwan

Wei-Cheh Chiu
Department of Psychiatry, Cathay General Hospital, Taipei 10630, Taiwan

Chun-Ying Li
Institute of Biomedical Engineering, National Cheng Kung University, Tainan 70403, Taiwan

Kuo-Sheng Cheng
Institute of Biomedical Engineering, National Cheng Kung University, Tainan 70403, Taiwan
Medical Devices Innovation Center, National Cheng Kung University, Tainan 70403, Taiwan

Yu-Chi Yeh
Department of Psychiatry, Cathay General Hospital, Taipei 10630, Taiwan

Timothy E Richardson
Institute for Aging and Alzheimer's Disease Research, Department of Pharmacology & Neuroscience, University of North Texas Health Science Center, Fort Worth, TX 76107, USA
Texas College of Osteopathic Medicine, University of North Texas Health Science Center, Fort Worth, TX 76107, USA

James W Simpkins
Institute for Aging and Alzheimer's Disease Research, Department of Pharmacology & Neuroscience, University of North Texas Health Science Center, Fort Worth, TX 76107, USA

Mohamed A Ibrahim
Wilmer Eye Institute, Johns Hopkins University School of Medicine, 600 North Wolfe Street, Maumenee 745, Baltimore, MD 21287, USA

Diana V Do
Wilmer Eye Institute, Johns Hopkins University School of Medicine, 600 North Wolfe Street, Maumenee 745, Baltimore, MD 21287, USA
Stanley M. Truhlsen Eye Institute, University of Nebraska Medical Center, Omaha, NE, USA

Yasir J Sepah
Wilmer Eye Institute, Johns Hopkins University School of Medicine, 600 North Wolfe Street, Maumenee 745, Baltimore, MD 21287, USA

Syed M Shah
Wilmer Eye Institute, Johns Hopkins University School of Medicine, 600 North Wolfe Street, Maumenee 745, Baltimore, MD 21287, USA

Elizabeth Van Anden
Wilmer Eye Institute, Johns Hopkins University School of Medicine, 600 North Wolfe Street, Maumenee 745, Baltimore, MD 21287, USA

Gulnar Hafiz
Wilmer Eye Institute, Johns Hopkins University School of Medicine, 600 North Wolfe Street, Maumenee 745, Baltimore, MD 21287, USA

J Kevin Donahue
Division of Cardiology, Department of Medicine, Johns Hopkins University School of Medicine, Baltimore, MD, USA
Department of Medicine, Case Western Reserve University School of Medicine, Cleveland, OH, USA

Richard Rivers
Department of Anesthesia, Johns Hopkins University School of Medicine, Baltimore, MD, USA

Jai Balkissoon
OxiGene, Inc., South San Francisco, California, CA, USA

James T Handa
Wilmer Eye Institute, Johns Hopkins University School of Medicine, 600 North Wolfe Street, Maumenee 745, Baltimore, MD 21287, USA

Peter A Campochiaro
Wilmer Eye Institute, Johns Hopkins University School of Medicine, 600 North Wolfe Street, Maumenee 745, Baltimore, MD 21287, USA

Quan Dong Nguyen
Wilmer Eye Institute, Johns Hopkins University School of Medicine, 600 North Wolfe Street, Maumenee 745, Baltimore, MD 21287, USA
Stanley M. Truhlsen Eye Institute, University of Nebraska Medical Center, Omaha, NE, USA

Dohan Weeraratne
Amgen Inc., One Amgen Center Drive, Thousand Oaks, CA 91320, USA

Alin Chen
Amgen Inc., One Amgen Center Drive, Thousand Oaks, CA 91320, USA

Jason J Pennucci
Amgen Inc., One Amgen Center Drive, Thousand Oaks, CA 91320, USA

Chi-Yuan Wu
Amgen Inc., One Amgen Center Drive, Thousand Oaks, CA 91320, USA

Kathy Zhang
Amgen Inc., One Amgen Center Drive, Thousand Oaks, CA 91320, USA

Jacqueline Wright
Amgen Inc., One Amgen Center Drive, Thousand Oaks, CA 91320, USA

Juan José Pérez-Ruixo
Amgen Inc., One Amgen Center Drive, Thousand Oaks, CA 91320, USA

Bing-Bing Yang
Amgen Inc., One Amgen Center Drive, Thousand Oaks, CA 91320, USA

Arunan Kaliyaperumal
Amgen Inc., One Amgen Center Drive, Thousand Oaks, CA 91320, USA

Shalini Gupta
Amgen Inc., One Amgen Center Drive, Thousand Oaks, CA 91320, USA

Steven J Swanson
Amgen Inc., One Amgen Center Drive, Thousand Oaks, CA 91320, USA

Narendra Chirmule
Amgen Inc., One Amgen Center Drive, Thousand Oaks, CA 91320, USA

Marta Starcevic
Amgen Inc., One Amgen Center Drive, Thousand Oaks, CA 91320, USA

Panagiotis Apostolou
Research Genetic Cancer Centre Ltd (R.G.C.C. Ltd), Filotas, Florina, Greece

Maria Toloudi
Research Genetic Cancer Centre Ltd (R.G.C.C. Ltd), Filotas, Florina, Greece

Marina Chatziioannou
Research Genetic Cancer Centre Ltd (R.G.C.C. Ltd), Filotas, Florina, Greece

Eleni Ioannou
Research Genetic Cancer Centre Ltd (R.G.C.C. Ltd), Filotas, Florina, Greece

Dennis R Knocke
Nerium Biotechnology, Inc. San Antonio, Texas, USA

Joe Nester
Nerium Biotechnology, Inc. San Antonio, Texas, USA

Dimitrios Komiotis
Department of Biochemistry & Biotechnology, University of Thessaly, Larisa, Greece

Ioannis Papasotiriou
Research Genetic Cancer Centre Ltd (R.G.C.C. Ltd), Filotas, Florina, Greece

Mariel Núñez
Radioisotopes Laboratory, School of Pharmacy and Biochemistry, University of Buenos Aires, Buenos Aires, Argentina

Vanina Medina
Radioisotopes Laboratory, School of Pharmacy and Biochemistry, University of Buenos Aires, Buenos Aires, Argentina

Graciela Cricco
Radioisotopes Laboratory, School of Pharmacy and Biochemistry, University of Buenos Aires, Buenos Aires, Argentina

Máximo Croci
Institute of Immunooncology Dr. EJV Crescenti, Buenos Aires, Argentina

Claudia Cocca
Radioisotopes Laboratory, School of Pharmacy and Biochemistry, University of Buenos Aires, Buenos Aires, Argentina

Elena Rivera
Radioisotopes Laboratory, School of Pharmacy and Biochemistry, University of Buenos Aires, Buenos Aires, Argentina

Rosa Bergoc
Radioisotopes Laboratory, School of Pharmacy and Biochemistry, University of Buenos Aires, Buenos Aires, Argentina
Institute of Health Sciences Barceló, Buenos Aires, Argentina

Gabriela Martín
Radioisotopes Laboratory, School of Pharmacy and Biochemistry, University of Buenos Aires, Buenos Aires, Argentina

Farshad Kajbaf
Service d'Endocrinologie-Nutrition, Hôpital Sud, Amiens cedex 1 F-80054, France

Jean-Daniel Lalau
Service d'Endocrinologie-Nutrition, Hôpital Sud, Amiens cedex 1 F-80054, France
Université de Picardie Jules Verne, Amiens, France

S M D K Ganga Senarathna
Department of Pharmacology, Faculty of Medicine, University of Colombo, Colombo, Sri Lanka
South Asian Clinical Toxicology Research Collaboration, Kandy, Sri Lanka
Pharmacy Program, Department of Medical Education and Health Sciences, Faculty of Medical Sciences, University of Sri Jayewardenepura, Nugegoda , Sri Lanka

Shalini Sri Ranganathan
Department of Pharmacology, Faculty of Medicine, University of Colombo, Colombo, Sri Lanka

Nick Buckley
South Asian Clinical Toxicology Research Collaboration, Kandy, Sri Lanka
Faculty of Medicine, University of New South Wales, Sydney, Australia

Rohini Fernandopulle
Department of Pharmacology, Faculty of Medicine, University of Colombo, Colombo, Sri Lanka

Alla Kushnir
Division of Neonatology, Department of Pediatrics; Albany Medical Center 43 New Scotland Avenue, Albany, NY 12208 USA
Division of Neonatology, Department of Pediatrics; Cooper Hospital 1 Cooper Plaza, Camden, NJ 08103 USA

Joaquim MB Pinheiro
Division of Neonatology, Department of Pediatrics; Albany Medical Center 43 New Scotland Avenue, Albany, NY 12208 USA

Elizabeth K Hussey
GlaxoSmithKline, 5 Moore Drive, Research Triangle Park, NC 27709, USA

Anita Kapur
GlaxoSmithKline, 5 Moore Drive, Research Triangle Park, NC 27709, USA

Robin O'Connor-Semmes
GlaxoSmithKline, 5 Moore Drive, Research Triangle Park, NC 27709, USA

Wenli Tao
GlaxoSmithKline, 5 Moore Drive, Research Triangle Park, NC 27709, USA

Bryan Rafferty
GlaxoSmithKline, 5 Moore Drive, Research Triangle Park, NC 27709, USA

Joseph W Polli
GlaxoSmithKline, 5 Moore Drive, Research Triangle Park, NC 27709, USA

Charles D James Jr
Tandem Labs, Durham, NC, USA

Robert L Dobbins
GlaxoSmithKline, 5 Moore Drive, Research Triangle Park, NC 27709, USA

Menna Alene
Regulatory Unit, Beker Pharmaceuticals General Business Plc, Lideta Kifle Ketema, Addis Ababa, Ethiopia

Michael D Wiese
Division of Health Sciences, School of Pharmacy and Medical Sciences, University of South Australia, Adelaide, Australia

Mulugeta T Angamo
Clinical Pharmacy Unit, Pharmacy Department, College of Public Health and Medical Science, Jimma University, Jimma, Ethiopia

Beata V Bajorek
School of Pharmacy, Graduate School of Health, The University of technology Sydney (UTS), Sydney, Australia

Elias A Yesuf
Regulatory Unit, Beker Pharmaceuticals General Business Plc, Lideta Kifle Ketema, Addis Ababa, Ethiopia

Nasir Tajure Wabe
Clinical Pharmacy Unit, Pharmacy Department, College of Public Health and Medical Science, Jimma University, Jimma, Ethiopia

Coralith García
Instituto de Medicina Tropical Alexander von Humboldt, Universidad Peruana Cayetano Heredia, Lima, Perú
Hospital Nacional Cayetano Heredia, Lima, Perú

Liz P Llamocca
Instituto de Medicina Tropical Alexander von Humboldt, Universidad Peruana Cayetano Heredia, Lima, Perú

Krystel García
Instituto de Medicina Tropical Alexander von Humboldt, Universidad Peruana Cayetano Heredia, Lima, Perú

Aimee Jiménez
Instituto de Medicina Tropical Alexander von Humboldt, Universidad Peruana Cayetano Heredia, Lima, Perú

Frine Samalvides
Instituto de Medicina Tropical Alexander von Humboldt, Universidad Peruana Cayetano Heredia, Lima, Perú
Hospital Nacional Cayetano Heredia, Lima, Perú

Eduardo Gotuzzo
Instituto de Medicina Tropical Alexander von Humboldt, Universidad Peruana Cayetano Heredia, Lima, Perú
Hospital Nacional Cayetano Heredia, Lima, Perú

Jan Jacobs
Institute of Tropical Medicine Antwerp, Antwerp, Belgium
Department of Medical Microbiology, Faculty of Health, Life Sciences and Medicine, Maastricht University, The Netherlands

Maria Gustafsson
Maria Gustafsson, Department of Pharmacology and Clinical Neuroscience, Umeå University, 901 85, Umeå, Sweden

Stig Karlsson
Stig Karlsson, Department of Nursing, Umeå University, Umeå, Sweden

Hugo Lövheim
Hugo Lövheim, Department of Community Medicine and Rehabilitation, Geriatric Medicine, Umeå University, Umeå, Sweden

Stefano Bianchi
Department of Pharmacy, University Hospital of Ferrara, Corso Giovecca 203, 44123 Ferrara Italy

Erica Bianchini
Department of Pharmacy, University Hospital of Ferrara, Corso Giovecca 203, 44123 Ferrara Italy

Paola Scanavacca
Department of Pharmacy, University Hospital of Ferrara, Corso Giovecca 203, 44123 Ferrara Italy

Anita Kapur
GlaxoSmithKline, 5 Moore Drive, Research Triangle Park, NC 27709, USA

Robin O'Connor-Semmes
GlaxoSmithKline, 5 Moore Drive, Research Triangle Park, NC 27709, USA

Elizabeth K Hussey
GlaxoSmithKline, 5 Moore Drive, Research Triangle Park, NC 27709, USA

Robert L Dobbins
GlaxoSmithKline, 5 Moore Drive, Research Triangle Park, NC 27709, USA

Wenli Tao
GlaxoSmithKline, 5 Moore Drive, Research Triangle Park, NC 27709, USA

Marcus Hompesch
Profil Institute for Clinical Research, Chula Vista, CA, USA

Glenn A Smith
GlaxoSmithKline, 5 Moore Drive, Research Triangle Park, NC 27709, USA

Joseph W Polli
GlaxoSmithKline, 5 Moore Drive, Research Triangle Park, NC 27709, USA

Charles D James Jr
Tandem Labs, Durham, NC, USA

Imao Mikoshiba
Kissei Pharmaceutical Company LTD, Matsumoto City, Japan

Derek J Nunez
GlaxoSmithKline, 5 Moore Drive, Research Triangle Park, NC 27709, USA

Ahmed E Enayetallah
Compound Safety Prediction, Pfizer Inc., Groton, CT, USA
Drug Safety Research & Development, Pfizer Inc., Groton, CT, USA

Dinesh Puppala
Compound Safety Prediction, Pfizer Inc., Groton, CT, USA

Daniel Ziemek
Computational Sciences CoE, Pfizer Inc., Cambridge, MA, USA

James E Fischer
Compound Safety Prediction, Pfizer Inc., Groton, CT, USA

Sheila Kantesaria
Compound Safety Prediction, Pfizer Inc., Groton, CT, USA

Mathew T Pletcher
Compound Safety Prediction, Pfizer Inc., Groton, CT, USA
Rare Disease Research Unit, Pfizer Inc., Cambridge, MA, USA

Shu Liu
Thoracic Oncology Laboratory, Department of Surgery, Helen Diller Family Comprehensive Cancer Center, University of California, 2340 Sutter Street, N-221, San Francisco, CA 94115, USA

David Hsieh
Thoracic Oncology Laboratory, Department of Surgery, Helen Diller Family Comprehensive Cancer Center, University of California, 2340 Sutter Street, N-221, San Francisco, CA 94115, USA

Yi-Lin Yang
Thoracic Oncology Laboratory, Department of Surgery, Helen Diller Family Comprehensive Cancer Center, University of California, 2340 Sutter Street, N-221, San Francisco, CA 94115, USA

Zhidong Xu
Thoracic Oncology Laboratory, Department of Surgery, Helen Diller Family Comprehensive Cancer Center, University of California, 2340 Sutter Street, N-221, San Francisco, CA 94115, USA

Csaba Peto
Thoracic Oncology Laboratory, Department of Surgery, Helen Diller Family Comprehensive Cancer Center, University of California, 2340 Sutter Street, N-221, San Francisco, CA 94115, USA

David M Jablons
Thoracic Oncology Laboratory, Department of Surgery, Helen Diller Family Comprehensive Cancer Center, University of California, 2340 Sutter Street, N-221, San Francisco, CA 94115, USA

Liang You
Thoracic Oncology Laboratory, Department of Surgery, Helen Diller Family Comprehensive Cancer Center, University of California, 2340 Sutter Street, N-221, San Francisco, CA 94115, USA

Saik Urien
CIC-0901 Inserm Necker-Cochin (Assistance Publique-Hopitaux de Paris), Paris EA-3620, France Université Paris Descartes Sorbonne Paris Cité et Institut IMAGINE, Paris, France

Christophe Bardin
Pharmacologie, Hôpital Cochin, Assistance Publique-Hopitaux de Paris, Paris, France

Brigitte Bader-Meunier
Université Paris Descartes Sorbonne Paris Cité et Institut IMAGINE, Paris, France
Unité d'Immuno-Hématologie et Rhumatologie pédiatriques, Hôpital Necker-Enfants Malades, Assistance Publique-Hopitaux de Paris, Paris, France

Richard Mouy
Unité d'Immuno-Hématologie et Rhumatologie pédiatriques, Hôpital Necker-Enfants Malades, Assistance Publique-Hopitaux de Paris, Paris, France

Sandrine Compeyrot-Lacassagne
Unité d'Immuno-Hématologie et Rhumatologie pédiatriques, Hôpital Necker-Enfants Malades, Assistance Publique-Hopitaux de Paris, Paris, France

Franz Foissac
CIC-0901 Inserm Necker-Cochin (Assistance Publique-Hopitaux de Paris), Paris EA-3620, France Université Paris Descartes Sorbonne Paris Cité et Institut IMAGINE, Paris, France

Benoît Florkin
Unité d'Immuno-Hématologie et Rhumatologie pédiatriques, Hôpital Necker-Enfants Malades, Assistance Publique-Hopitaux de Paris, Paris, France

Carine Wouters
Unité d'Immuno-Hématologie et Rhumatologie pédiatriques, Hôpital Necker-Enfants Malades, Assistance Publique-Hopitaux de Paris, Paris, France

Bénédicte Neven
Université Paris Descartes Sorbonne Paris Cité et Institut IMAGINE, Paris, France
Unité d'Immuno-Hématologie et Rhumatologie pédiatriques, Hôpital Necker-Enfants Malades, Assistance Publique-Hopitaux de Paris, Paris, France

Jean-Marc Treluyer
CIC-0901 Inserm Necker-Cochin (Assistance Publique-Hopitaux de Paris), Paris EA-3620, France Université Paris Descartes Sorbonne Paris Cité et Institut IMAGINE, Paris, France
Pharmacologie, Hôpital Cochin, Assistance Publique-Hopitaux de Paris, Paris, France

Pierre Quartier
Université Paris Descartes Sorbonne Paris Cité et Institut IMAGINE, Paris, France
Unité d'Immuno-Hématologie et Rhumatologie pédiatriques, Hôpital Necker-Enfants Malades, Assistance Publique-Hopitaux de Paris, Paris, France

Isis B Yera-Alos
Center for the Development of Pharmacoepidemiology, Havana, Cuba

Liuba Alonso-Carbonell
Center for the Development of Pharmacoepidemiology, Havana, Cuba

Carmen M Valenzuela-Silva
Center for Genetic Engineering and Biotechnology, Havana, Cuba

Angela D Tuero-Iglesias
Center for Genetic Engineering and Biotechnology, Havana, Cuba

Martha Moreira-Martínez
"Abel Santamaría" Hospital, Pinar del Río, Cuba

Ivonne Marrero-Rodríguez
"Gustavo Aldereguía" Hospital, Cienfuegos, Cuba

Ernesto López-Mola
Center for Genetic Engineering and Biotechnology, Havana, Cuba

Pedro A López-Saura
Center for Genetic Engineering and Biotechnology, Havana, Cuba

Monica Pallis
Nottingham University Hospitals, Nottingham, UK
Academic Haematology, Clinical Sciences Building, Nottingham University Hospitals City Campus, Nottingham NG5 1PB, UK

Francis Burrows
Tragara Pharmaceuticals, San Diego, USA

Abigail Whittall
University of Nottingham, Nottingham, UK

Nicholas Boddy
University of Nottingham, Nottingham, UK

Claire Seedhouse
University of Nottingham, Nottingham, UK

Nigel Russell
Nottingham University Hospitals, Nottingham, UK
University of Nottingham, Nottingham, UK

Maria Luisa Dupuis
Department of Therapeutic Research and Medicines Evaluation, Istituto Superiore di Sanità, Viale Regina Elena 299, Rome, Italy

Alessandro Ascione
Department of Therapeutic Research and Medicines Evaluation, Istituto Superiore di Sanità, Viale Regina Elena 299, Rome, Italy

Lucia Palmisano
Department of Therapeutic Research and Medicines Evaluation, Istituto Superiore di Sanità, Viale Regina Elena 299, Rome, Italy

Stefano Vella
Department of Therapeutic Research and Medicines Evaluation, Istituto Superiore di Sanità, Viale Regina Elena 299, Rome, Italy

Maurizio Cianfriglia
Department of Therapeutic Research and Medicines Evaluation, Istituto Superiore di Sanità, Viale Regina Elena 299, Rome, Italy

www.ingramcontent.com/pod-product-compliance
Lightning Source LLC
Chambersburg PA
CBHW080253230326
41458CB00097B/4427